T0229898

CAMBRIDGE PUBLIC H

UNDER THE EDITORSHIP OF

G. S. Graham-Smith, M.D. and    J. E. Purvis, M.A.

University Lecturer in Hygiene and
Secretary to the Sub-Syndicate for
Tropical Medicine

University Lecturer in Chemistry
and Physics in their application
to Hygiene and Preventive Medicine, and Secretary to the State
Medicine Syndicate

# FLIES IN RELATION TO DISEASE

## BLOODSUCKING FLIES

# FLIES IN RELATION TO DISEASE
## BLOODSUCKING FLIES

by

EDWARD HINDLE, B.A., Ph.D.

Assistant to the Quick Professor of Biology, Cambridge

Cambridge:

at the University Press

1914

CAMBRIDGE UNIVERSITY PRESS
Cambridge, New York, Melbourne, Madrid, Cape Town,
Singapore, São Paulo, Delhi, Tokyo, Mexico City

Cambridge University Press
The Edinburgh Building, Cambridge CB2 8RU, UK

Published in the United States of America by Cambridge University Press, New York

www.cambridge.org
Information on this title: www.cambridge.org/9780521235648

First published 1914
First paperback edition 2011

*A catalogue record for this publication is available from the British Library*

ISBN 978-0-521-23564-8 Paperback

TO

# OTTO BEIT

IN RECOGNITION OF
HIS GENEROUS GIFTS TOWARD
THE ADVANCEMENT OF
SCIENTIFIC RESEARCH

# EDITORS' PREFACE

IN view of the increasing importance of the study of public hygiene and the recognition by doctors, teachers, administrators and members of Public Health and Hygiene Committees alike that the *salus populi* must rest, in part at least, upon a scientific basis, the Syndics of the Cambridge University Press have decided to publish a series of volumes dealing with the various subjects connected with Public Health.

The books included in the Series present in a useful and handy form the knowledge now available in many branches of the subject. They are written by experts, and the authors are occupied, or have been occupied, either in investigations connected with the various themes or in their application and administration. They include the latest scientific and practical information offered in a manner which is not too technical. The bibliographies contain references to the literature of each subject which will ensure their utility to the specialist.

It has been the desire of the editors to arrange that the books should appeal to various classes of readers : and it is hoped that they will be useful to the medical profession at home and abroad, to bacteriologists and laboratory students, to municipal engineers and architects, to medical officers of health and sanitary inspectors and to teachers and administrators.

Many of the volumes will contain material which will be suggestive and instructive to members of Public Health and Hygiene Committees ; and it is intended that they shall seek to influence the large body of educated and intelligent public opinion interested in the problems of public health.

# PREFACE

ALTHOUGH it is now generally recognized that flies are very important agencies in the dissemination of infectious diseases, few people are aware of the remarkable advances which have resulted from modern research in this field. To the general public the practical application of these researches appeals with greater force than the detailed accounts of investigations, of absorbing interest though many of them are, in the varied subjects which have to be called to our aid in combating disease. Some of the results hitherto obtained may be illustrated by two examples, both of which have brought this subject into some prominence.

In the first of these, Yellow Fever, owing to the factors involved being relatively simple, it is literally possible within a few months to remove this most deadly disease from the list of human ailments. All that is required is public appreciation of the remedies at our disposal, as demonstrated by the result of the admirable measures adopted by the Americans first in Cuba and afterwards in Panama, which alone rendered possible the completion of the Canal. Similar measures in other regions directed against the mosquito (*Stegomyia fasciata*), which is responsible for the transmission of the infection, would render the reappearance of Yellow Fever in the highest degree improbable in the future.

Sleeping Sickness may be taken as our second example. The difficulties in this case are undoubtedly more formidable, owing to the extreme complexity of the modes of dissemination.

Nevertheless much has already been accomplished, though it is little to what might be done if more adequate funds were at the disposal of our Colonial Medical and Administrative Authorities. The enlightened policy of the Colonial Office contrasts sadly with the lack of interest displayed by the public as a whole, both at home and in the Colonies affected. Public and private funds could not be directed more profitably to the service of humanity than in the fields which the farsighted enterprise of this Department has opened up of recent years.

New and formidable developments in the problem of Sleeping Sickness, to confine ourselves to the second example we have chosen, render it imperative that immediate steps should be taken to combat the spread of a particularly deadly variety of this infection, which, although at present confined to small areas in Nyasaland and the adjoining provinces, threatens to extend over a large part of Africa.

In addition to these two examples, Malaria in all its forms is gradually becoming subject to human control, though some countries are slow to realize that they cannot remain neutral in this war waged by science against their most deadly internal enemies, the mosquitoes. Verily the fly's proboscis is more successful in retarding the progress of civilization and the alleviation of human suffering than all the armaments of our most Christian Powers!

The author's main object in writing this book has been to collocate the more important observations concerning the part taken by biting flies in the transmission of disease. In doing this it seemed advisable to include notes on the classification of the flies concerned and also descriptions of the infections transmitted, but no attempt has been made to give any account of the clinical symptoms of the various diseases,

whether of man or animals. Special attention has been
devoted to the modes of life of the more important insects
mentioned, to the manner in which the infection is transmitted
from one host to another, and also to any preventive measures
directed either against the flies or the infections themselves.

Hitherto those interested in this subject have been obliged
to refer to entomological treatises for a knowledge of the
insects, while information concerning the infections transmitted was only likely to be contained in medical or zoological
publications. Thus there is danger of the interdependence of
the two subjects being overlooked. The entomologist working in this field, without a more or less complete knowledge
of the factors influencing the transmission of any particular
malady, is liable to waste his efforts in unprofitable directions;
whilst the Medical Officer or Administrator who is ignorant
of the main results of entomological research is equally handi-
capped in his attempts to combat the group of diseases under
discussion. It is hoped, therefore, that this book will appeal
to both classes and at the same time that its significance for
the prevention of disease will be apparent to that wider public
already indicated.

The present volume together with that published by
Dr Graham-Smith in the same series[1], covers the whole field
marked out by their general title, *Flies and Disease*.

It may be useful to give the reader some idea of the general
arrangement of the subject matter that we have adopted.
After a short introduction, follow chapters on the structure
and classification of the Diptera, accompanied by a list of
biting flies known to transmit any infection. Each family,
including any such carriers of disease, is then dealt with

---

[1] Graham-Smith. *Flies and Disease—Non-bloodsucking Flies.* Cambridge
Public Health Series.

separately and in most cases some important member of the family is described in greater detail. As far as possible the description of the infections immediately follows that of the family concerned in their transmission. Thus the account of the Psychodidæ and *Phlebotomus* is succeeded by a chapter devoted to Pappataci Fever (Three Day Fever), whilst the account of Malaria follows that of the Anophelinæ. Certain difficulties have arisen in the case of diseases (*e.g.* trypanosomiasis) transmitted by members of more than one family, but such infections have been described in connection with their more important carrier. At the end of each chapter are given a few references to the literature on the subject, but it should be emphasised that the bibliography is not in any way complete, but merely contains the titles of publications that will be of assistance to students requiring detailed information in any particular branch. The present edition does not profess to deal with works published later than the beginning of 1913, although in isolated cases it has been found possible to include references to later work.

The writer has great pleasure in acknowledging the extremely valuable assistance which he has received from Major S. R. Christophers, I.M.S., in the preparation of chapters VIII and IX, devoted respectively to the classification of the Culicidæ, and an account of Malaria. These are almost entirely the work of that distinguished authority and considering their importance in the present work, his name ought to have appeared as a joint author. However, Major Christophers would not consent to this arrangement and therefore the author can only express his great indebtedness for this generous help.

For permission to reproduce illustrations, which had previously appeared in other publications, and also for the loan of the original blocks, I am indebted to the following: the Publisher (G. Fischer) and Editors of the *Archiv für Protistenkunde*, for permission to reproduce Fig. 87; the Editor of the *Bulletin of Entomological Research* for the loan of the blocks of Figs. 18, 19, 59–61, 67, 73 and 74; the President and Fellows of the Cambridge Philosophical Society for the loan of the block of Fig. 57; the Editors of the *Journals of Parasitology* and *Hygiene* for the block of Fig. 41 and permission to reproduce Figs. 4, 8, 25, 26, 27, 29 and 31; the Director of the Tropical Diseases Bureau for the loan of the blocks of Figs. 42–45 and 65; Dr P. H. Bahr and Messrs Witherby and Co. for the loan of the blocks of Figs. 54 and 56; Maclure, Philips and Co. for permission to reproduce Figs. 46, 47 and 49. Dr E. Roubaud for the loan of the blocks of Figs. 62, 64, 66, 68, 70, 76–78; Dr G. S. Graham-Smith for the loan of the blocks of Figs. 1–3 and 82 and 83; Professor G. H. F. Nuttall for permission to reproduce Figs. 30, 32 and 55; Surgeon-General Sir David Bruce for permission to reproduce Figs. 79 and 80; and Miss Muriel Robertson for permission to reproduce the drawings from which Fig. 75 was constructed; Mr Edwin Wilson, F.E.S., kindly prepared the drawing of the stridulating organ of *Anopheles* (Fig. 28).

It is the author's pleasant duty to return thanks for the assistance afforded by these gentlemen.

In conclusion, I should like to express the great debt I owe to Professor G. H. F. Nuttall, who by his friendly criticism and helpful suggestions has lightened the author's labours and also prevented many serious omissions.

E. H.

*September*, 1914.

# CONTENTS

CHAP.                                                      PAGE

I.     Introduction . . . . . . . .   1

II.    Diptera—General description and classification .   12

III.   Biting-Flies as carriers of disease . . . .   25

IV.   Orthorrhapha Nematocera . . . . .   32

V.    Family Psychodidæ (Moth-flies and Sand-flies) . .   35

VI.   Diseases carried by *Phlebotomus*—Pappataci Fever .   44

VII.   Family Culicidæ (Gnats or Mosquitoes) . . .   50

VIII.  Culicidæ (Mosquitoes) continued. Classification .   75

IX.   Anopheline-transmitted diseases . . . .   119

X.    Culicinæ . . . . . . . . .   165

XI.   Diseases transmitted by Culicinæ. Yellow Fever, Dengue, Bird Malaria, etc. . . . . .   177

XII.   Diseases transmitted by Anophelinæ and Culicinæ. Filariasis . . . . . . . .   202

XIII.  Orthorrhapha Brachycera . . . . . .   224

XIV.  Family Tabanidæ (Breeze-flies, Cleggs, Horse-flies, Gad-flies, Seroot-flies) . . . . .   226

XV.   Cyclorrhapha Schizophora . . . . . .   239

XVI.  The Tsetse-flies—Genus *Glossina* Wied., 1830 . .   243

XVII.  *Glossina* and Disease. The Trypanosomes . .   293

XVIII. *Glossina* and Disease (continued) . . . .   300

XIX.  *Stomoxys* . . . . . . . . .   355

XX.   Infections transmitted by *Stomoxys* . . . .   361

XXI.  *Lyperosia* . . . . . . . . .   369

XXII.  Family Hippoboscidæ (Tick-flies) . . . .   372

XXIII. Infections transmitted by Hippoboscidæ . . .   379

INDEX . . . . . . . . .   387

# LIST OF FIGURES

FIG.                                                                    PAGE

1. An Anthomyid fly immediately after emerging from the
   puparium . . . . . . . . . .                                          14
2. Ventral view of head of the same fly . . . .                         14
3. Side view of head of the same fly . . . . .                          14
4. Side view of a female *Anopheles maculipennis* Meigen
   (× about 20) . . . . . . . .                                         16
5. Wing of *Tabanus* sp. shewing the venation . . .                     17
6. Acephalous larva of *Stomoxys calcitrans* (× 7) . . .                20
7. Eucephalous larva of *Phlebotomus papatasii* . . .                   20
8. Obtectate pupa of *Anopheles maculipennis* . . .                     22
9. Coarctate pupa of *Stomoxys calcitrans* . . . .                      22
10. Wing of *Kelloggina*, a blepharocerid . . . .                       34
11. Thorax of *Tipula* . . . . . . . .                                  34
12. Wing of *Ryphus* . . . . . . . .                                    34
13. Wing of *Cecidomyia* . . . . . . . .                                34
14. Antenna of *Orphnephila* . . . . . . .                              34
15. Right hind-leg of *Mycetophilus* . . . . .                          34
16. Head of *Bibio* . . . . . . . . .                                   34
17. Wing of *Chironomus* sp. . . . . . . .                              34
18. Head of *Phlebotomus papatasii* . . . . . .                         36
19. Wing venation of *Phlebotomus papatasii* . . . .                    36
20. *Phlebotomus papatasii*. Male . . . . . .                           37
21. *Phlebotomus papatasii*. Female . . . . .                           38
22. Freshly extruded egg of *Phlebotomus papatasii* . . .               40
23. Adult larva of *P. papatasii* . . . . . .                           40
24. Pupa of *P. papatasii* . . . . . . .                                41
25. *Anopheles maculipennis*. *A*, enlarged view of male ; *B*, head
    of female . . . . . . . . .                                         51
26. Transverse section through proboscis of a female *Anopheles
    maculipennis*, shewing the relative position of the parts
    when at rest . . . . . . . . .                                      52
27. Side view of the head of a female *Anopheles maculipennis*,
    with the various mouth parts separated, but in the
    relative position in which they lie when enclosed in
    the groove of the labium . . . . . .                                53
28. View of under-surface of the base of the wing of *Anopheles
    maculipennis*, shewing stridulating organ . . .                     55
29. Schematic longitudinal section of a female *Anopheles macu-
    lipennis* . . . . . . . . .                                         57

FIG.                                                       PAGE

30. Diagram shewing the corresponding stages in the life-cycle of *Anopheles* and *Culex* . . . . . . . 63

31. *Anopheles maculipennis.* *A*, side view and *B*, dorsal view of egg ; *C*, young larva and *D*, fully-grown larva ; *E* flabellum, or flap overhanging base of certain thoracic hairs ; *F*, a palmate hair ; *G*, ventral view of head of fully-grown larva . . . . . . . . 65

32. *Anopheles maculipennis* ♂, captured in Cambridge, shewing acarine parasites attached to the body . . . 73

33. *Anopheles bifurcatus* . . . . . . . . 80

34. *Anopheles (Patagiamyia) gigas* . . . . . . 82

35. *Anopheles (Myzorhynchus) barbirostris* . . . . 84

36. *Anopheles (Myzomyia) listoni* . . . . . . 86

37. *Anopheles (Pyretophorus) neavei* . . . . . 88

38. *Anopheles (Nyssorhynchus) maculatus* . . . . 91

39. *Anopheles (Cellia) pulcherrimus* . . . . . 93

40. Diagrammatic representation of the life-cycle of the parasite of pernicious malaria . . . . . 130

41. Photomicrograph of sporozoites of malaria from salivary glands of *Anopheles (Pyretophorus) costalis* . . . 135

42. Breeding places of Anophelines. Railway cutting at Kurunegala . . . . . . . . . 137

43. Breeding places of Anophelines. Flooded Paddy Fields in Ceylon . . . . . . . . . . 139

44. Indian fish of utility as mosquito-destroyers. *A* (♂) and *B* (♀), *Lebias dispar* ; *C, Nuria danrica* . . . 150

45. Indian fish of utility as mosquito-destroyers. *A, Haplochilus panchax* ; *B, Ambassis ranga* ; *C, Trichogaster fasciatus* . . . . . . . . . . 152

46. *Stegomyia fasciata*, adult female . . . . . 166

47. *Stegomyia fasciata*, adult male . . . . . 168

48. Distribution of *Stegomyia fasciata* . . . . . 169

49. Larva and pupa of *Stegomyia fasciata* . . . . 174

50. Approximate distribution of Yellow Fever . . . 179

51. Distribution of Dengue . . . . . . . 191

52. Distribution of *Culex fatigans* . . . . . . 193

53. Stomach of *Culex* shewing large numbers of the sporocysts of *Plasmodium præcox* on its walls . . . . 199

54. Microfilariæ of *F. bancrofti* emerging from the uterus of the parent filaria . . . . . . . . 207

55. *Filaria bancrofti.* Stages in development within mosquito 211

56. Head and proboscis of *Stegomyia pseudoscutellaris*, 15 days after feeding, shewing two filariæ lying in the head and three in the proboscis . . . . . . . 213

57. *A*, view of the heart of a dog infested with *Filaria immitis* ; *B*, a female worm removed from the heart to shew its length . . . . . . . . . 220

FIG.                                                        PAGE
58. Part of the Malpighian tubule of an *Anopheles claviger*,
    infected with the embryos of *Filaria immitis*   .   .   221
59. *Tabanus kingi* ♀   .   .   .   .   .   .   .   .   227
60. A rock at Khor Arbat, Anglo-Egyptian Sudan, shewing
    sites selected by *Tabanus kingi* for ovipositing .   .   228
61. Egg-mass and mature larva of *Tabanus kingi* .   .   .   229
62. Comparative morphology of the proboscis of *Glossina* (I),
    *Melophagus* (II) and *Stomoxys* (III) .   .   .   .   244
63. Wing of *Glossina palpalis* to shew the venation   .   .   245
64. Gravid uterus of *G. palpalis*, containing a larva at an ad-
    vanced stage of development   .   .   .   .   .   246
65. *Glossina palpalis*. Photographs shewing the flies in a
    position of rest .   .   .   .   .   .   .   .   257
66. Internal anatomy of *Glossina palpalis*   .   .   .   .   259
67. View on River Gambia to shew a typical haunt of *Glossina
    palpalis* .   .   .   .   .   .   .   .   .   261
68. *Glossina palpalis* in the act of feeding   .   .   .   .   264
69. *Glossina palpalis*. Female in the act of parturition .   .   266
70. Freshly laid larva of *G. palpalis* shewing the changes in
    the body form .   .   .   .   .   .   .   .   267
71. *G. palpalis*. Puparia before and after the escape of the
    imago   .   .   .   .   .   .   .   .   .   268
72. *Glossina morsitans*. Dorsal view of female   .   .   .   276
73. Path through thin deciduous bush, to shew a typical haunt
    of *G. morsitans* .   .   .   .   .   .   .   .   279
74. Base of a tree in Nyasaland shewing one of the positions
    in which the pupæ of *G. morsitans* may be found .   .   284
75. Diagram of the life-cycle of *Trypanosoma gambiense* .   .   312
76. Transverse section (semi-diagrammatic) of the proboscis
    of an infected *Glossina*   .   .   .   .   .   .   314
77. Culture of *Trypanosoma pecaudi*, from the intestine of
    *G. palpalis* .   .   .   .   .   .   .   .   334
78. Culture of *Trypanosoma congolense* from the intestine of
    *G. palpalis* .   .   .   .   .   .   .   .   351
79. *Trypanosoma simiæ*. Successive stages in the division .   354
80. *Trypanosoma simiæ*. Large multinucleate form   .   .   354
81. Wing venation of *Stomoxys calcitrans*   .   .   .   .   356
82. Side view of head of Stable-fly. *A*, proboscis in resting
    position ; *B*, proboscis extended   .   .   .   .   356
83. Stable-fly, *Stomoxys calcitrans* .   .   .   .   .   .   357
84. *Stomoxys calcitrans*. Eggs   .   .   .   .   .   .   359
85. *Lynchia maura* ♀   .   .   .   .   .   .   .   .   376
86. *Hippobosca rufipes* .   .   .   .   .   .   .   .   378
87. Developmental cycle of *Hæmoproteus columbæ*   .   .   381
88. *Trypanosoma theileri*. *A*, small crithidial form ; *B*, large
    individual from blood of cow   .   .   .   .   .   385

# CHAPTER I

## INTRODUCTION

Although biting-flies had long been suspected of being responsible for the spread of various diseases, it was not until 1877 that any direct proof was brought forward in support of this hypothesis. In that year Manson, working in China, discovered that the minute worm, *Filaria bancrofti*, present in the blood of a large percentage of the natives that he examined, underwent a development inside the body of the common grey-legged mosquito, *Culex fatigans*. Although these observations were incomplete and the exact mode of transmission remained undiscovered until more than twenty years later, yet they were of the highest importance, since Manson's work laid the foundation for all subsequent investigations on the part played by biting-flies as carriers of disease.

With the exception of these few observations on the development of *Filaria* in the mosquito, practically the whole of our knowledge of the transmission of disease by insects, has been acquired within the last twenty years. Thus Bruce, in 1895, discovered the cause of Nagana, *Trypanosoma brucei*, and its transmission by the tsetse-fly, whilst two years later Ross, by his brilliant researches on the development of *Proteosoma* and the manner in which it is spread by the mosquito, placed the methods of eradicating malaria on a scientific basis. The rapid progress in this subject may be appreciated by the fact that, with the exception of the specific descriptions of certain insects and the above-mentioned work on *Filaria*, the present volume is entirely concerned with discoveries of the last twenty years. Within this period biting-flies have been shewn to transmit in addition to numerous infections of animals the following human diseases : malaria, sleeping sickness, yellow fever, three-day fever; and evidence has been brought forward also suggesting that dengue and epidemic polyomyelitis are spread by these insects. Before proceeding to a discussion of individual infections, however, and the part played by flies in their transmission, it will be convenient to give a short general account of some of the problems connected with this subject.

It has never been proved that, under natural conditions, biting-flies normally transmit any other than animal parasites from one host to another. In those cases in which the pathogenic agent is unknown, *e.g.* yellow fever, three-day fever, the clinical symptoms seem to indicate that these diseases are also due to animal parasites and not to bacteria. There is no *a priori* reason why biting-flies should not transmit bacterial infections as well as animal, but certainly no bacterial disease is known to be normally transmitted by these insects. Since a biting-fly feeds on blood and can only become infected by ingesting the parasite, it necessarily follows that the latter, at least during some part of its life-cycle, must be present in the blood of the vertebrate host, and the manner in which the infection is conveyed by the insect may be either " direct " or " indirect."

(*a*)   *Direct transmission.*

When the pathogenic agent does not develop in the body of the biting-fly, but is merely carried on the mouth-parts and *directly* inoculated into the next host which the insect feeds upon, the transmission is said to be *direct* or *mechanical*. This kind of transmission somewhat resembles the method of infecting a healthy animal by means of the prick of a needle that has been thrust previously into an infected animal and which is thereby soiled with the infective blood from the latter.

The efficiency of any particular species to act as the direct carrier of a disease agent obviously depends on such mechanical details as the size and shape of the mouth-parts, the number of parasites in the blood, etc. It is possible that bacterial as well as animal infections may be occasionally carried in this manner, especially in those cases where the bacteria are present in the peripheral circulation in considerable numbers, *e.g.* anthrax, Mediterranean fever. Moreover, by feeding sufficient numbers of any species of biting-fly on an animal containing large numbers of some parasite in its blood, and subsequently, without any interval, on a normal susceptible animal, it is possible to obtain experimentally the direct transmission of practically any blood-inhabiting parasite. Employing such methods the transmission of sleeping sickness and relapsing fever may be effected by means of the bites of *Stegomyia*, and Mediterranean fever by the bites of *Culex*; it is almost certain, however, that such transmission rarely, if ever, occurs in nature. Nevertheless, the possibility must not be ignored and all biting-flies should be regarded with suspicion from the point of view of preventive medicine.

Although under experimental conditions it is comparatively easy to demonstrate the direct transmission of certain diseases it is becoming more and more evident that, compared with indirect transmission, this mode of infection plays a relatively unimportant part in the spread of disease. The pathogenic agent of the disease, even under the most favourable conditions, can only survive for a very limited time (at most two to three days) on the mouth-parts of the biting-fly and unless the latter feeds on another host before the expiration of this period no infection is produced. As a rule a fly which has had a full meal of blood rarely desires to feed again for some days and it is only those flies which are interrupted during their feeding that are liable to bite another host within a short space of time. El Debab, a trypanosomiasis of camels occurring in North Africa, is one of the best examples of a disease which seems to be transmitted in this manner. Edmond and Etienne Sergent have shewn that the outbreaks of this disease can be explained on the supposition that it is directly transmitted from infected to healthy animals by various species of tabanids, and they note that in nature these insects frequently bite two or more animals in quick succession, being disturbed whilst feeding, through the efforts of their unwilling victims.

It is, of course, quite possible for a biting-fly to transmit any particular infection both directly and indirectly, as in the case of the transmission of Nagana (*Trypanosoma brucei*) by *Glossina pallidipes*. Bruce shewed that if a tsetse fed on blood containing these trypanosomes, the fly remained infective for about forty-eight hours, during which period, if it bit another animal, the latter became infected. It has since been proved, however, that in addition this trypanosome develops in the alimentary canal of the tsetse-fly and after a certain incubation period, during which the fly is non-infective, it again becomes infective. This infection, therefore, is transmitted both directly and indirectly, but the epidemiology of the disease is strongly against the view that transmission is usually effected by the direct method.

### (b)   *Indirect transmission.*

When the pathogenic agent causing the disease undergoes some developmental cycle in the biting-fly, resulting in the latter becoming more or less permanently infective after this development has taken place, the transmission is said to be *indirect* or *cyclical*. In these cases there is always a definite biological relationship between the biting-fly and the parasite which it conveys, and the latter is only capable of development within the members of certain species or families of insects. The best known example of this indirect method of transmission is that of the malarial parasite by the mosquito. When the parasite, at a suitable stage of its life-history, is taken into the stomach of a susceptible species of mosquito, it undergoes a complicated cycle of development in its new host, finally resulting in the salivary glands of the latter becoming invaded by a stage of the parasite adapted for entry into the blood of the next person that the mosquito bites.

It will be noticed that in this, and all other cases of indirect transmission by biting-flies, the parasite develops in two hosts, vertebrate and invertebrate, respectively. The host in which the parasite undergoes its sexual life-cycle is called the *definitive host*. In the case of the majority, if not all, protozoal parasites, the sexual part of their life-cycle takes place in the invertebrate carrier, and therefore the latter is the definitive host. On the other hand, the sexual cycle of *Filaria bancrofti* takes place in its vertebrate host, man, and in this case man is the definitive host.

The host in which the parasite merely multiplies asexually is called the *intermediate host*, and in the case of protozoal infections is the vertebrate, but in *Filaria* is the invertebrate, host.

The term " intermediate host " has given rise to much confusion, for many writers still persist in considering the expression synonymous with " invertebrate host." As a matter of fact, in the majority of cases the vertebrate is the intermediate host, and it is only obscuring the true relations of parasite and host to persist in the erroneous application of this term.

In all cases the equilibrium between parasite and host is much better established in the definitive than in the intermediate host. As a general rule parasites do not have a very harmful action on their definitive hosts, whether invertebrate or vertebrate, whilst on the other hand there are many examples of parasites seriously affecting the health of their intermediate hosts. Thus the malarial parasite does not seem to affect injuriously the health of its definitive host, the mosquito, whilst in the intermediate host, man, it produces malaria, a serious and often fatal disease. Similarly, the presence of *Filaria bancrofti* in its definitive host, man, does not produce any obvious ill-effects, whilst a large proportion of the infected mosquitoes succumb to the infection.

Although so many parasites have an injurious effect upon their hosts, sometimes causing death, it is obviously a short-sighted policy for a parasite to kill its host, as by so doing it also destroys itself. A parasite which invariably killed its host would eventually die out, owing to the extermination of the latter, and it is not inconceivable that, in this way, excessively fatal infections have disappeared from the world, together with the animals they affected.

At the present time the great majority of blood parasites do not cause the death of their hosts. An equilibrium between the parasite and its host has become established and the former does not increase beyond a certain limit, with the result that the health of the animal from which it is deriving nourishment is not very seriously affected. This is the case with numerous parasites, such as the majority of trypanosomes in vertebrates, *Hæmoproteus* in birds, Hæmogregarines in reptiles, etc. It is only in rare cases that the parasites increase to such an extent that they markedly affect the health of their hosts, but since our attention is only called to diseased animals, the cases in which disease is caused by the parasites are more generally noticed.

A pathogenic blood parasite cannot persist indefinitely unless one or more of the following conditions are fulfilled :

(1) The disease which it produces may be of long duration so that the invertebrate host has numerous opportunities of becoming infected with the parasite and spreading the infection to other hosts. Of course the parasite must be present in the blood in sufficient numbers and at a suitable stage of development to ensure the infection of the biting host which transmits the disease. If these conditions were fulfilled an excessively fatal, though chronic disease, possessed of efficient means of distribution would be able to persist until the extermination of its host had been accomplished, after which it would also cease to exist, unless it became adapted to some other host.

(2) The infection may be hereditarily transmitted in the invertebrate host, so that the offspring of an infected parent also carries the infection. Fortunately, with the doubtful exception of yellow fever in *Stegomyia*, no biting-fly is known to transmit any disease agent to its offspring. One of the best examples of this mode of hereditary infection in other groups is that of *Spirochæta duttoni* in its invertebrate host the tick, *Ornithodorus moubata*.

(3) The parasite may infest more than one species of vertebrate host, in one or more of which the equilibrium between parasite and host has become established. This is by far the most important condition from an epidemiological point of view. If a parasite is able to live in several vertebrate hosts and is non-pathogenic towards any one of them,

the latter serves as a reservoir for the infection and in the presence of an efficient transmitting agent the parasite may persist indefinitely.

It is now known that the parasite of sleeping sickness (*Trypanosoma gambiense*) is maintained in this manner, since in addition to man it infests other vertebrate hosts, *e.g.* antelopes, which are practically unaffected by it.

In the case of the malaria parasite an equilibrium is becoming established between it and its vertebrate host, man, but only in those races that have been exposed to infection for a considerable period. As a result the latter serve as reservoirs of infection for those races that have not become immunized, in whom the parasite produces malaria, a disease which is often fatal unless checked by suitable treatment.

The relations between the parasites and their hosts are very complicated and are not yet thoroughly understood. From a biological point of view, it is probable that all protozoal blood parasites carried by biting-flies are primarily insect parasites and have only secondarily become adapted for living in the blood of vertebrates. Certainly in every case where the life-cycle of the parasite is known the insect is the definitive host, and the equilibrium between the parasite and its insect host seems to be well established, whilst this is not the case with regard to the mutual relations in the vertebrate host.

The extreme pathogenicity of certain protozoal infections in vertebrates, *e.g.* yellow fever in man, the various trypanosomiases of man and animals, etc., strongly suggests that these diseases are of comparatively recent origin and there has not yet been time for any balance to become established between the parasites and their respective hosts.

The trypanosomes constitute an excellent example of a group of flagellates which primitively inhabited the alimentary tracts of various invertebrates, and have recently become adapted to a parasitic mode of life in the blood of vertebrates.

A large variety of insects, both biting and non-biting, contain parasitic flagellates, *Crithidia*, *Leptomonas*, etc., in their digestive tracts, and there are all stages between flagellates which are just capable of living in the blood of vertebrates, but are usually insect parasites (*e.g. Trypanosoma boylei* Lafont), and such forms as *Trypanosoma gambiense*, which have become well-adapted to a parasitic mode of life in many of the larger vertebrates. In the latter case the tsetse-fly, the insect host of *T. gambiense*, has apparently developed an immunity against infection with this flagellate, for only a comparatively small proportion of the flies becomes infected after ingesting blood containing the parasites.

When once a biting-fly becomes infected with the particular species of blood parasite of which it is the definitive host, it generally remains infective for a very considerable period, often for the remainder of its life. It is obvious, therefore, that when a parasite is transmitted by a true definitive host, it is much more difficult to eradicate than when it is spread mechanically. In the latter case it is only necessary to protect all infected vertebrates from the bites of flies for a period of not more than three days and the insects cease to be infective. In the former case, however, the eradication of the parasite can only be accomplished effectively by the destruction of the insect host. In fact the prevention of protozoal infections, which include many of the more important tropical diseases, is mainly an entomological problem, as it depends on the destruction of insects and to do this a knowledge of their habits and life-cycles is essential.

In the case of yellow fever the destruction of the invertebrate host, *Stegomyia fasciata*, is comparatively simple, and as a result this disease is rapidly disappearing from the more civilized parts of the world. On the other hand, no effective means have yet been discovered of destroying *Glossina morsitans*, one of the most important disease carriers in Africa. Yet there is little doubt that when we have acquired a complete knowledge of the bionomics of this redoubtable insect, it will be possible to devise some means of considerably reducing its numbers.

An infected invertebrate host may spread infection from one vertebrate to another in a variety of ways, but in the case of biting-flies, the infected insect whilst feeding generally inoculates the parasite directly into the body of the host.

The possibility of other modes of infection, however, should not be ignored, for they are known to occur in closely related groups, and therefore it is considered advisable to include a short account of some of the ways in which the infective agent may be spread by its invertebrate host.

The simplest case is that in which the parasite, without undergoing any morphological or biological changes, merely multiplies in the alimentary canal of its invertebrate host. The parasite may then enter a vertebrate either by regurgitation of the contents of the alimentary canal when the invertebrate host is feeding, or else by the fæces of the latter, containing the parasites, entering the open wound caused by its bite. The plague bacillus, which multiplies in the gut of the flea, is probably transmitted in this way.

Usually, however, the parasite undergoes a cyclical development, passing through various stages that are generally incapable of living in the blood of vertebrates, and therefore during this developmental period the host is non-infective. This negative interval is known as the *incubation period* and may vary from two or three days up to as long as 12 or 13 weeks, its duration depending mainly on the temperature, as development is accelerated by increased warmth and retarded, or even completely arrested, by cold.

The development of various species of trypanosomes in the alimentary canal of the tsetse-fly includes some of the simplest examples of cyclical evolution. In the case of *Trypanosoma cazalboui*, when ingested by the tsetse some of the parasites remain in the fly's proboscis. In this region they develop, also undergoing certain biological changes, and for a period of about seven days they are incapable of living in the blood of vertebrates. At the expiration of this short incubation period, however, the trypanosomes recover their infectivity for vertebrates, and after this the tsetse is infective for a considerable period. In other trypanosomes, *e.g. T. gambiense* and *T. brucei*, the evolution in the tsetse-fly is more complicated, the parasites developing in the digestive tract and passing through a crithidial stage before finally becoming infective, but in every case during this development they are restricted to the lumen of the alimentary canal and its ducts. It is probable that the evolution of *Hæmoproteus columbæ* is also restricted to the alimentary canal of its invertebrate host, *Lynchia*, but in this case the development is rather more complicated than that of the trypanosomes, as it includes a sexual phenomenon.

The most complex type of evolution is that of the malaria parasite (*Plasmodium*) in its definitive host, the mosquito. In this case the development commences with the production of sexual forms which only become mature in the stomach of the mosquito, and the result of conjugation is a motile body which bores its way through the gut-wall and comes to rest in or near the outer lining of the gut. It then grows at the expense of the tissues of the mosquito and forms a large spherical cyst in which are developed minute sickle-shaped bodies, the sporozoites. Eventually the latter are set free into the body-cavity of the insect and make their way to the salivary glands, where they come to rest in the salivary ducts. These forms are capable of developing in the blood of the vertebrate host and are inoculated, together with the salivary fluid, when the mosquito feeds. The development of the Hæmogregarines and Piroplasmidæ in their respective invertebrate hosts seems to resemble that of *Plasmodium*. Between the simple evolution of *T. cazalboui* and the highly complicated development of *Plasmodium* there are numerous gradations, but the majority of protozoal parasites probably pass through a life-cycle comparable with that of *Plasmodium*.

The development of the ultra-microscopic virus of yellow fever is peculiar from the fact that it is possible to transmit the infection from one mosquito to another without the mediation of the vertebrate host. The incubation period of the virus in the mosquito is about 12 days, but after the insect has become infective, if it is crushed up and fed to another *Stegomyia* the latter becomes infective.

The evolution of *Filaria* in the invertebrate host is very different from that of the Protozoa, as the sexual part of the life-cycle takes place in the vertebrate, in this case the definitive host, and the embryonic filariæ, contained in the blood, merely require to complete part of their larval development in the tissues of the mosquito.

The manner in which the infective agent re-enters the vertebrate host is of considerable interest and varies in different cases.

As a rule the infective agent is directly inoculated into the body when the infected invertebrate feeds on some vertebrate host. The parasites may be present in the proboscis of the infected arthropod or leech, or contained in the salivary fluid, but in either case the result is the same and the infection is passed directly into the blood.

In the case of *Filaria*, the parasite is contained in the proboscis of the infected insect and when it feeds escapes on to the surface of the skin. The parasite subsequently bores its way through the skin and thus reaches the general circulation of its vertebrate host.

Sometimes the infective agent is merely deposited on the surface of the skin in the fæces of the invertebrate host. From this site the parasite may reach the blood circulation by means of the open wound caused by the bite of the invertebrate host (as in the case of *Spirochæta duttoni*), or through an excoriated part of the skin.

Sometimes the same result is obtained by the host licking up the parasite from the surface of its body. This is one of the modes of infection of *Trypanosoma lewisi*, in which the infection reaches the circulation through the mucous membrane of the alimentary canal of the rat.

The transmission of *Spirochæta recurrentis* by the louse is comparable with that of *S. duttoni* by the human tick, for in the former case the parasites, set free only by crushing the insect, pass through the excoriations produced by scratching with the finger-nails. As lice are frequently crushed between the nails, it is easy to see how the infective agent can reach the circulation.

Occasionally it is necessary for the vertebrate to swallow the parasite, which subsequently bores its way through the alimentary canal. The best known example of this method is that of *Filaria medinensis*, which develops in the body of

*Cyclops.* When an infected specimen of the latter is taken into the stomach, the filariæ are set free and penetrate into the tissues of the vertebrate host. The transmission of the *Leucocytozoon* of the rat by *Lælaps* is of the same nature, for the rats can only become infected by swallowing *Lælaps* containing the parasites. As mentioned above the transmission of *Trypanosoma lewisi* by the rat-flea is also of this nature, and Strickland has shewn that the surest way of infecting rats with this trypanosome is to feed them with fleas containing the parasite.

REFERENCES.

Brumpt, E. (1910). *Précis de Parasitologie.* Paris : Masson et Cie.
Castellani and Chalmers (1912). *Manual of Tropical Medicine,* 2nd edition. London : Baillière, Tindall and Cox.
Hindle, E. (1911). The Transmission of *Spirochæta duttoni. Parasitology,* vol. IV. pp. 133–149.
Manson, P. (1908). *Tropical Diseases,* 5th edition. London : Cassell and Co. Ltd.
Mesnil, F. (1912). Modes de propagation des Trypanosomiases. Les Trypanosomes chez l'hôte invertébré. *Bull. Inst. Pasteur,* vol. X. pp. 1–17 and 49–63.
Minchin, E. A. (1912). *An Introduction to the Study of the Protozoa.* London : Edward Arnold.
Strickland, C. (1911). Mechanism of Transmission of *T. lewisi* by the Rat-flea. *Brit. Med. Journ.* 1911, p. 1049.

# CHAPTER II

DIPTERA.—GENERAL DESCRIPTION AND CLASSIFICATION

*Definition.* The large Order of Diptera includes all those insects provided with two well-developed wings and, in addition, a hinder pair of rudimentary wings known as halteres, or balancers. The mouth-parts are usually adapted for piercing and sucking, and are more or less modified according to the habits of the insect. The various stages of development, larva, pupa, and adult, or imago, are quite distinct, metamorphosis being complete. In addition, all the members of the Order possess a distinctly segmented abdomen with the exception of the Pupipara, a very aberrant group which has become modified for an exclusively parasitic mode of existence.

### General Morphology.

The **head** is connected with the thorax by an extremely slender neck and in consequence is very mobile, being capable of undergoing semi-rotation. The majority of the exposed surface is occupied by the large faceted eyes, which are usually much larger in the male than in the female, probably owing to the fact that the former has to seek out its mate. The eyes may actually meet in the middle line, in which case they are termed *holoptic*, in contradistinction to when they are separate, or *dichoptic*. The holoptic condition is especially characteristic of the male but occasionally is found in both sexes.

In certain families, *e.g.* Muscidæ, the head shews anteriorly a small depression, the *lunula*, which is bounded by an arched suture passing over the bases of the antennæ. This structure is the remnant of a peculiar organ, the *ptilinum*, which, in the fly emerging from the pupal case, appears as a bladder-like expansion of the front of the head. The ptilinum can be expanded and retracted and consequently it is of great use in helping the fly to break through the pupal case, and also to force its way through any material in which the latter may be buried. It is only present during the first few hours after the fly has emerged and subsequently it becomes completely introverted, forming the inconspicuous lunula of the mature fly (Figs. 1–3).

The **antennæ** are of great use to the systematist as they offer a simple means of classification, the number of segments being of considerable importance.

In the more primitive families of the Order, *e.g.* Culicidæ, there are a series of segments of approximately equal size, the number of which varies from eight to sixteen. In some cases the antennæ of the male are larger and composed of more segments than those of the female. The majority of flies, however, possess antennæ of a totally distinct form, peculiar to the order, consisting of three segments, the outer one of which, at its distal extremity, bears a fine process known as the *arista*, which is occasionally segmented and often covered with hairs. It probably represents the remaining segments of the more primitive type of antennæ.

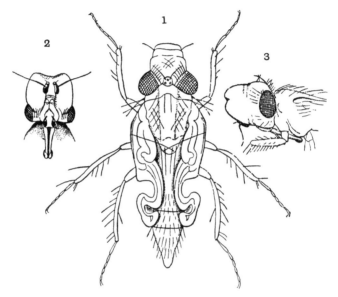

Fig. 1. An Anthomyid fly immediately after emerging from the puparium, shewing the greatly distended ptilinum and unexpanded wings.

Figs. 2 and 3. Ventral and side views of the head of the same fly. After Graham-Smith.

The **mouth-parts** are composed typically of the following structures : labrum, epipharynx, maxillæ, mandibles, hypopharynx and labium. These are liable to great variation, even within the same family, but all blood-sucking Diptera agree in the possession of a mouth that is adapted for piercing and cutting. The *labrum*, or upper lip, together with the *epipharynx*, is usually elongated ; the *hypopharynx*, or tongue, is also much prolonged and, together with the labrum, may form a tube for the ingestion of blood or other liquids ; the *labium*, or lower lip, is more or less membranous or fleshy, and usually functions as a sheath for the protection of the other mouth-parts. The *mandibles* and *maxillæ* are each represented by a pair of long pointed processes adapted for piercing. In addition, a pair of well-developed *maxillary palps* is always present, situated one on each side of the base of the labium. The palps are extraordinarily well developed in the Culicidæ (Fig. 4), in the genus *Megarhinus* being nearly as long as the whole body of the insect.

The **thorax** is composed almost entirely of mesothorax, the prothorax and metathorax being very small and fused with it. A small part of the metathorax projects backwards over the base of the abdomen and is known as the *scutellum*.

The **abdomen** is composed of a variable number of segments, more or less closely fused together. The number of segments externally visible may vary from nine to five, or rarely four. In certain cases the first two segments are fused together and the first one is often very much shortened. In the male the terminal segments are curled under the body, forming what is termed the *hypopygium*, which serves to protect the copulatory appendages.

The three pairs of **legs** are attached to the prothorax, mesothorax and metathorax, respectively. The legs are in-variably composed of five parts known as the coxa, trochanter, femur, tibia and tarsus. The *tarsus* is generally five-jointed ; its terminal joint bears a well-developed pair of claws, and underneath each of these is often a free pad or membrane, the *pulvillus*. This structure is often absent amongst the Orthorrhapha and is usually better developed in the male than in the female. Between each pair of claws is situated a median structure known as the *empodium*, which may have the form of a pad, or a bristle. Occasionally the pulvilli are absent and the empodium takes on their function.

The **wings** are of very great importance from a classificatory point of view. As in all insects they consist of simple folds supported by veins or nervures, the arrangement of which is known as the *venation*. The wings are membranous but may be covered with hairs or scales, and the shape and disposition

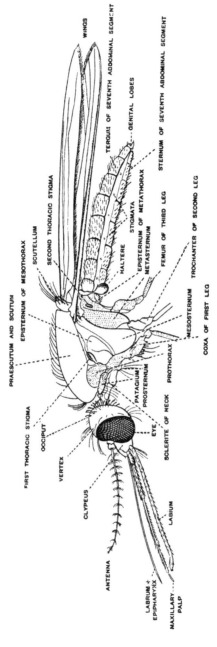

Fig. 4. Side view of a female *Anopheles maculipennis* Meigen (× about 20), to shew the various parts of the body. The prothorax and metathorax with their respective legs are dotted. After Nuttall and Shipley.

of the latter is of great use in the identification of various species of mosquitoes. The venation, although comparatively simple, has been greatly complicated by the fact that entomologists are not agreed as to the terminology of the various parts and in consequence different writers use different names for the same structures.

In the following description of the wing of *Tabanus*, which is taken as an example because the venation is rather complicated, we have adopted the system of nomenclature most generally used by descriptive entomologists.

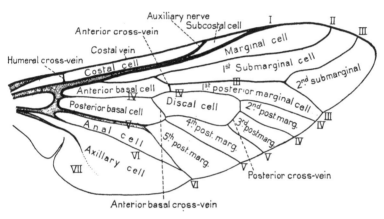

Fig. 5. Wing of *Tabanus* sp. shewing the venation. The numbers I, II, III, etc. indicate respectively the first, second and third longitudinal veins, etc.

The most easy way of recognizing the veins is to commence with the *discal* cell, which is a large cell situated about the middle of the wing. It is present in the great majority of flies, but is absent in the Culicidæ. Anteriorly, the discal cell is bounded by the *fourth longitudinal* vein, and somewhere along its length will be seen a short connecting vein, the *anterior cross-vein*. The latter is constantly present in all flies. In front it is connected with the *third longitudinal*, and behind with that part of the fourth longitudinal that bounds the discal cell.

Counting forwards from the third longitudinal, which is forked, occur the *second* and *first longitudinals*, these three veins arising from a common stem and radiating to the *costal* vein, which runs round the edge of the wing. Between the costal vein and first longitudinal, is present an *auxiliary*, or *subcostal* vein, which runs parallel with the costal for a short distance and then curves into it. Near the base of the wing the two latter veins are connected by the short *humeral cross-vein*, which is very constant. The subcostal, and the first three longitudinals support the anterior half of the wing. The *fourth* and *fifth longitudinals* arise together and diverge towards the margin ; each of them forks before reaching the edge of the wing. The *sixth longitudinal* arises more or less independently, and runs towards the hind margin of the wing. The three latter veins together support the posterior half of the wing. The fourth and fifth longitudinals are connected by two cross-veins, the *anterior basal* near the axil and the *posterior cross-vein* in the outer half of the wing. Between the fifth and sixth longitudinals is a *posterior basal cross-vein*. It will be seen that the wing is divided by its longitudinal nervures into two fields separated by an interval which is traversed only by the anterior cross-vein.

The various spaces or cells included between the veins are distinguished by special names ; their arrangement may be understood by referring to the figure (Fig. 5).

In addition to this system of nomenclature, that proposed by Schiner is used by a certain number of writers. One great source of confusion between this and the older system is the different meaning of the subcostal ; Schiner employs the term *mediastinal* for the subcostal, and *subcostal* for the first longitudinal ; moreover, the corresponding cells are similarly named.

The **surface of the body** in flies differs considerably in the nature of its vestiture. Sometimes the integument is almost naked, but generally it is covered with hairs, or bristles, or sometimes scales. Those flies which are provided with an armature of bristles, or *macrochætæ*, may be termed *chæto-phorous* ; and where there is no definite arrangement of bristles, the fly is said to be *eremochætous*. Osten Sacken has drawn up an elaborate system of nomenclature for the arrangement of the bristles, which is of considerable value for purposes of classification.

### Internal Anatomy.

The **alimentary canal** is provided with a muscular pharynx. The œosphagus usually gives off a large diverticulum known as the crop or sucking stomach, but in some insects, *e.g.* Culicidæ, its place is taken by two or three long thin-walled sacs, the œsophageal diverticula. The stomach is large and consists of an anterior portion, the proventriculus, and a true stomach behind it ; the latter usually gives off cæca. The intestine is coiled and ends in a rectum ; at its junction with the stomach open the long Malpighian tubules, generally four in number. The salivary glands are large and their common duct opens at the top of the hypopharynx.

The **heart** consists of a thin-walled tube running along beneath the dorsal surface of the insect. Usually it is divided into several chambers but in the more specialized families there are only two.

The **respiratory system** consists of two main tracheæ running longitudinally one on each side of the body and opening to the exterior by means of the spiracles. The latter are arranged on each side of the body, two large pairs in the thorax and one pair to each abdominal segment. The two main tracheal trunks expand at the base of the abdomen into conspicuous air-sacs, which are probably of use when the insect is flying.

The **nervous system** is very variable. In the elongate Nematocera there are five or six abdominal ganglia and three distinct thoracic ganglia, but in the more specialized forms, such as the Muscidæ, all the thoracic and abdominal ganglia are fused into a single mass. Various gradations may be found between these two extremes and it is interesting to trace the gradual concentration of the nervous system side by side with the higher specialization of the insects.

The **reproductive organs** present some interesting peculiarities. The ovaries consist of a very large number of egg-tubes.    The female, in addition, has three spermathecæ, paired accessory organs, and no true bursa copulatrix.    The male has two oval testes with short ducts, communicating with a well-developed penis, surrounded by accessory copulatory appendages.

### Reproduction.

The great majority of flies lay **eggs**, which are generally deposited in such a position that the young larva will be in easy reach of its food-supply.    A number of families, however, are more or less viviparous, the eggs hatching within the body of the parent and the resulting larvæ nourished for varying periods before being liberated.    In the majority of such cases the larvæ are deposited whilst quite young, but in the Pupipara and *Glossina* the larvæ are nourished within the oviduct of the mother until quite full-grown and when set free at once proceed to pupate.

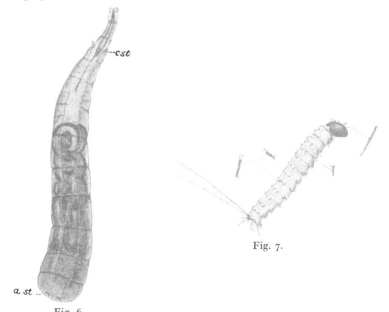

Fig. 7.

Fig. 6.

Fig. 6.    Acephalous larva of *Stomoxys calcitrans* (×7).    After Newstead.
    *cst*, compound thoracic stigmen ; *ast*, posterior stigmen.

Fig. 7.    Fucephalous larva of *Phlebotomus papatasii*.    After Newstead.

The larvæ are generally of the form known as maggots. They are without exception destitute of true thoracic legs, although in some groups stumpy pseudopods, resembling those of the caterpillar, may be present. These pseudopods vary greatly in their arrangement ; sometimes they are provided with recurved hairs.

The larvæ may be divided into two groups according to the size of the head. In the *eruciform* maggots the head is so small as to be almost invisible and these are termed *acephalous* larvæ (*e.g. Glossina*). In the *eucephalous* larvæ there is a well-marked head provided with mandibles, and usually there is a distinct thorax and abdomen (*e.g. Anopheles*).

The tracheal system exhibits great variety and the larvæ may be classified according to the arrangement of their spiracles. In the *peripneustic* forms, the spiracles are arranged along the sides of the body, one pair to each segment ; in the *amphipneustic* forms there are two pairs of spiracles, one at each end of the body ; whilst in the *metapneustic* forms there is only one pair of spiracles placed at the posterior extremity of the body. The great majority of aquatic larvæ belong to the latter type and there are often very elaborate devices for keeping the tip of the body in communication with the atmosphere so that air can enter the spiracles.

The habitat of the larvæ is much more variable than their structure, and they display great diversity in their mode of life. The majority of the maggot-like forms live in decaying organic matter, whilst nearly all the eucephalous larvæ are aquatic, occurring in both fresh- and salt-water and feeding either on vegetable matter, or preying on other small animals. A certain number of them are parasites, occurring in both plants and animals, and there is one form, the Congo floor-maggot, which sucks the blood of human beings and in its method of feeding somewhat resembles the bed-bug.

The pupa may be either *obtectate* or *coarctate*. In the former case the pupa is merely protected by a thin chitinous pellicle and the outlines of the various appendages of the future insect can be clearly distinguished through this covering—as, for example, in the mosquito. In these obtectate forms the larva casts off its skin before pupating. This type of pupa is found, with few exceptions, throughout the members of the Brachycera and Nematocera. In the coarctate forms there are no external protuberances, with the possible exception of a pair of projections at one end of the body, but the whole pupa looks like a tiny barrel, with rounded ends. In this case the pupating larva does not escape from its skin at the last moult but merely shrinks within it, and the larval skin

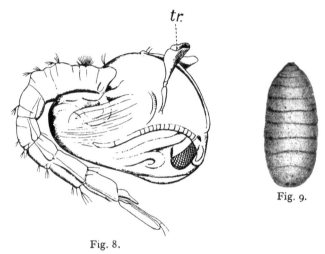

Fig. 8.

Fig. 8.   Obtectate pupa of *Anopheles maculipennis*.   *tr*, respiratory trumpet. After Nuttall and Shipley.

Fig. 9.   Coarctate pupa of *Stomoxys calcitrans*.   After Newstead.

is strengthened by the secretion of chitin so that it forms an adequate protection for the pupa. The external case is frequently known as the *puparium*. This type of pupa is found in the Cyclorrhapha, which includes the house-fly, *Stomoxys*, *Glossina*, etc.

The adult fly escapes from the pupal case in one of two ways. In the obtectate forms the dorsal surface of the pupal sheath splits longitudinally or in a T-shaped fashion, and the insect draws itself out through the opening. In the coarctate pupæ the anterior end of the pupal case is pushed off by means of the expanded ptilinum of the emerging fly (*vide supra*, p. 14).

The obtectate pupæ, as for example in the mosquito, are often actively motile, progressing almost as freely as the larvæ. The coarctate. pupæ, however, are devoid of all movement and are usually to be found buried in the earth, in crannies, or in similar localities. The mature fly, after breaking out of the pupal case, is aided in forcing its way through any covering of earth, or similar material, by the alternate expansions and contractions of the ptilinum, which becomes completely retracted soon after the fly has emerged.

*Classification.*

The most generally adopted classification is that of Brauer who divides the Diptera into two suborders, the *Orthorrhapha* and *Cyclorrhapha*, according to the manner in which the adult fly emerges from the pupal case, either by a T-shaped opening along the back (Orthorrhapha) or by a circular opening at the anterior extremity (Cyclorrhapha). Although this distinction is of great importance it is rather difficult of practical application when the immature stages are unknown, and the only method of distinguishing the adult fly is the presence or absence of a suture over the insertion of the antennæ. The position of the Pupipara is somewhat doubtful, but from Roubaud's researches it seems probable that the Hippoboscidæ, at any rate, are merely a highly specialized group of the Muscidæ. For the present, however, they will be regarded as a separate division and accordingly, following Sharp's arrangement, the Diptera may be divided into five sections:

Series 1. *Orthorrhapha Nematocera.* Flies in which the antennæ are composed of more than six segments of which all except the first two are equal in size. An arista is not present. The palpi are long and flexible, and usually four- or five-jointed. The second longitudinal vein is often forked and with the exception of the Tipulidæ and Rhyphidæ a discal cell is not present. This section includes the mosquitoes, sand-flies, *Chironomus*, etc., all of which are what may be termed gnat-like flies.

Series 2. *Orthorrhapha Brachycera.* Flies in which the antennæ are composed of three dissimilar segments, the last of which often carries an arista, usually terminal in position. When an arista is not present the flagellum ends in an appendage consisting of a number of indistinctly separated segments. The maxillary palps are composed of one or two segments and are not flexible. There is no definite arched suture above the insertion of the antennæ. The second longitudinal vein is not forked, but frequently the third is forked ; the venation is often very complex. This section includes the important family of Tabanidæ, in addition to a few other less well-known forms.

These first two divisions together constitute Brauer's suborder Orthorrhapha, which includes all those Diptera in which the imago escapes from its pupal case by means of a dorsal T-shaped opening or longitudinal slit ; accordingly ptilinum and lunula are absent in the adult insect. The larva possesses a distinct head and the pupa is usually obtectate.

Series 3. *Cyclorrhapha Aschiza*. Flies without a frontal suture and with a somewhat indefinite lunula. The antennæ are composed of not more than three segments of which the end one bears an arista, which is not terminal, but usually superior, in position. This group includes a large number of very minute flies and also the great family Syrphidæ, but none of the members are known to suck blood and are therefore of no interest in the present connection.

Series 4. *Cyclorrhapha Schizophora* or Eumyiid flies. Flies in which the antennæ are composed of three segments and an arista. None of the veins of the wing are forked. In the Calyptratæ the frontal suture is well-marked leaving a distinct lunula over the insertion of the antennæ. In the Acalyptratæ, the form of the head is less characteristic, but the members of this section can generally be distinguished from the Brachycera by their less complex wing venation. This group includes the important family Muscidæ, of which the common house-fly, also *Stomoxys*, and *Glossina* are well-known examples.

The latter two series together constitute the suborder Cyclorrhapha, which may be defined as Diptera in which the imago escapes from the pupal case by means of a circular aperture at the anterior extremity produced by the pressure of the expanded ptilinum. In consequence a frontal lunula is generally present. The larva is without a distinct head (maggot-like) and the pupa is coarctate. The antenna is composed of three segments, the terminal one of which bears an arista, usually dorsal in position. The maxillary palps are each composed of a single segment, the maxillæ are rudimentary and the mandibles absent. The third longitudinal vein is not forked and there are not more than three complete posterior cells. The number of abdominal segments never exceeds seven and is usually less.

Series 5. *Pupipara*. Abnormal Diptera of parasitic habit in which the wings are often rudimentary or absent. The head fits into a hollow of the thorax and the abdomen is not distinctly segmented. The larva, until it is mature, develops within the body of the female and when deposited at once pupates.

This group consists of an assembly of diverse forms, probably of varied affinities but all agreeing in their habit of depositing fully-grown larvæ. The best-known family is the Hippoboscidæ, including *Hippobosca*, and *Melophagus*, the sheep-ked.

REFERENCES.

Alcock, A. (1911). *Entomology for Medical Officers*. London : Gurney and Jackson.
Brauer, F. (1880). *Denk. Kais. Akad. Wissensch. Math.-Naturwissensch. Klasse*, vol. 42, p. 105.
Sharp, D. (1899). *Insects*, Part II in the *Cambridge Natural History*. London : Macmillan and Co.
Williston, S. W. (1908). *Manual of North American Diptera*. New Haven, U.S.A. : G. T. Hathaway.

# CHAPTER III

## BITING-FLIES AS CARRIERS OF DISEASE

The term " Biting-Flies " has been selected in order to include all those members of the Order of Diptera that either habitually, or occasionally, feed by sucking the blood of vertebrates. As a result of their feeding habits they are mainly

**TABLE I.** *Giving a list of the families of the Diptera containing any blood-sucking members; in addition, those species known to transmit any infective agents are mentioned.*

| | Disease transmitted | Locality | Authority |
|---|---|---|---|
| **Orthorrhapha Nematocera.** | | | |
| **Family Psychodidæ.** | | | |
| *Phlebotomus papatasii* .. :: .. | Pappataci Fever. (Three-Day Fever.) | Mediterranean Region, India, etc. | Doerr, Franz and Taussig |
| | Verruga Peruviana (?). | Peru. | Townsend. |
| **Family "Chironomidæ.** | | | |
| *Ceratopogon,* the female of which is a notorious blood-sucker .. .. .. | — | — | — |
| **Family Simuliidæ.** | | | |
| *Simulium* .. .. .. .. | Pellagra (?). (Some causal connection suggested.) | Italy, etc. | Sambon. |
| **Family Culicidæ.** | | | |
| **Sub-family Anophelinæ.** | | | |
| *Anopheles maculipennis,* Meigen | Malaria. | Europe and North America. | Grassi, Bignami, Bastianelli, Schaudinn, etc. |
| | *Filaria immitis.* | Europe. | Noé, Fülleborn. |
| ,, *pursati,* Laveran | Malaria. | Camboge. | Laveran. |
| ,, *bifurcatus,* L. | ,, | Europe and North America. | Grassi. |
| ,, *pseudopunctipennis,* Theob. | Malaria (?). | North America. | Darling. |
| ,, *aikeni,* James | Malaria. | India and Malay. | Daniels, Christophers. |
| ,, *algeriensis,* Theob. | ,, | North Africa. | Ed. and Et. Sergent. |
| ,, *arabiensis,* Patton | *Filaria bancrofti.* | Aden. | Patton. |
| ,, *(Myzomyia) rossii,* Giles | Malaria. | India. | James. |
| ,, *funesta,* Giles | ,, | ,, | Stephens and Christophers. |
| ,, *listoni,* Liston | ,, | Africa. | Ross, Annett and Austen, Stephens and Christophers. |
| ,, *formosaensis* I and II, Tsuzuki | ,, | Southern Asia. | Kinoshita, Stephens and Christophers. |
| ,, *culicifacies,* Giles | ,, | Formosa. | Tsuzuki. |
| ,, *albirostris,* Theob. | ,, | Southern Asia. | Stephens and Christophers. |
| | ,, | Malay. | Staunton, James. |

| Species | Disease / development | Locality | Observer(s) |
|---|---|---|---|
| Anopheles (Myzomyia) d' thali, Patton .. | Malaria (?). | Aden. | Patton. |
| ,, ,, turkhudi, Liston .. | Malaria. | India. | Stephens and Christophers. |
| ,, ,, lutzi, Theob. .. | ,, | Tropical America. | Lutz. |
| ,, ,, hispaniola, Theob. .. | ,, | North Africa, Spain. | Ed. and Et. Sergent. |
| ,, (Pseudomyzomyia) ludlowi, Theob. .. | ,, | Malay | Christophers. |
| ,, (Pyretophorus) costalis, Loew. .. | ,, | Tropical Africa. | Ross, Stephens and Christophers. |
| ,, ,, chaudoyei, Theob. .. | Filaria bancrofti. | West Africa. | Annett, Dutton and Elliott. |
| ,, ,, superpictus, Grassi .. | Malaria. | Algeria, etc. | Billet. |
| ,, ,, myzomyfacies, Theob. .. | ,, | Europe. | Grassi. |
| ,, (Myzorhynchus) pseudopictus, Grassi .. | ,, | Algeria. | Ed. Sergent. |
| ,, ,, barbirostris, van der Wulp. | Malaria (?). | Italy. | Grassi. |
| | F. bancrofti. | Asia. | Christophers. |
| ,, ,, ,, | ,, | Malay. | Leicester. |
| ,, ,, sinensis, Wiedemann .. | (Incomplete development.) Malaria. | Asia. | Tsuzuki and Kinoshita. |
| | F. bancrofti. | Malay. | Leicester. |
| ,, ,, mauritianus, Grandpré .. | (Incomplete development.) Malaria (?). | Mauritius. | Ross. |
| ,, ,, umbrosus, Theob. .. | Malaria. | Malay. | Staunton. |
| ,, ,, nigerrimus, Giles .. | F. bancrofti (?). | India. | Alcock. |
| ,, ,, minutus, Theob. .. | F. bancrofti. | Malay States. | ,, Leicester. |
| ,, ,, peditaeniatus, Leicester .. | (Incomplete development.) Malaria (?). | South America. | Darling. |
| ,, (Cellia) argyrotarsis, Rob.-Desv. .. | F. bancrofti. | West Indies. | Low and Vincent. |
| ,, ,, alhipes, Theob. ,, .. | Malaria. | Egypt. | Newstead, Dutton and Todd. |
| ,, ,, pharoensis, Theob. .. | ,, | ,, | Darling. |
| ,, ,, tarsimaculatus, Goeldi .. | ,, | South America. | Stephens and Christophers. |
| ,, (Neocellia) stephensi, Liston .. | ,, | India, Philippines. | Liston, Bentley. |
| ,, ,, willmori, James .. | ,, | Oriental Region. | — |
| ,, (Nyssorhynchus) fuliginosus, Giles .. | Malaria (?). | India. | Stephens and Christophers. |
| ,, ,, maculatus, Theob. .. | Malaria. | ,, | Staunton. |
| ,, ,, willmori, James .. | ,, | ,, | Mrs Adie. |
| ,, ,, maculipalpis var. indiensis, Theob. | ,, | ,, | Stephens and Christophers, Bentley, Robertson, Liston. |
| ,, ,, theobaldi, Giles .. | ,, | ,, | Stephens and Christophers. |

TABLE I (continued).

| | Disease transmitted | Locality | Authority |
|---|---|---|---|
| Anopheles (Cycloleppteron) mediopunctatus, Theob. .. .. | Malaria. | Brazil. | Cruz. |
| ,, (Arribalzagia) pseudomaculipes, Chagas .. .. | ,, | | ,, |
| ,, (Patagiamyia) punctipennis, Say... .. .. | ,, | North America. | Hirschberg. |
| **Sub-family Culicinæ.** | | | |
| Culex pipiens, L. .. | Filaria bancrofti. | China. | Manson. |
| ,, ,, .. | Plasmodium præcox. | Europe. | Ruge. |
| ,, ,, .. | Hæmoproteus noctua. | Austria. | Schaudinn. |
| ,, ,, .. | Leucocytozoon ziemanni (?). | — | ,, |
| ,, ,, .. | Mediterranean Fever. (Direct transmission in laboratory.) | — | Kennedy. |
| ,, fatigans .. .. | F. bancrofti. | St Lucia, West Indies. | Low. |
| ,, ,, .. .. | Plasmodium præcox. | India. | Ross. |
| ,, (Culicada) nemorosus .. | Dengue. | Philippines. | Ashburn and Craig. |
| ,, (Leucomyia) gelidus, Theob. .. | Plasmodium præcox. | Europe. | Neumann. |
| ,, ,, sitiens, Wied. .. | F. bancrofti. (Incomplete development.) | Malay. | Leicester. |
| Stegomyia fasciata, Fab. .. .. | Yellow Fever. | Tropical America and West Africa. | Finlay, Reed, Carroll, Agramonte and Lazear, etc. |
| ,, ,, .. .. | Plasmodium præcox. | India, Europe and North Africa. | Ross, Ed. Sergent, Neumann. |
| ,, ,, .. .. | F. bancrofti (?). (Non-efficient host.) | West Indies. | Low. |
| ,, ,, .. .. | Trypanosoma gambiense. (Direct transmission in laboratory.) | — | — |
| ,, scutellaris, Walker .. | F. bancrofti. (Incomplete development.) | — | Fülleborn and Mayer. |
| ,, pseudoscutellaris, Theob. .. | F. bancrofti. (Complete development.) | Fiji. | Bahr. |

| Species | Parasite / Development | Locality | Observer |
|---|---|---|---|
| *Stegomyia gracilis*, Leicester | *F. bancrofti.* | Malay. | Leicester. |
| ,, *perplexa*, Leicester | *F. bancrofti.* (Incomplete development.) | Malay. | Leicester. |
| *Mansonia uniformis*, Theob. | *F. bancrofti.* (Incomplete development.) | Central Africa, Malay. | Daniels, Leicester. |
| ,, ,, | *Trypanosoma brucei.* (Direct transmission in laboratory.) | — | Martin, Lebeuf and Roubaud. |
| ,, *annulipes*, Theob. | *F. bancrofti.* (Incomplete development.) | Malay. | Leicester |
| *Tæniorhynchus domesticus*, Leicester | *F. bancrofti.* (Incomplete development.) | ,, | |
| *Scutomyia albolineata*, Theob. | *F. bancrofti.* (Incomplete development.) | , | |

## Orthorrhapha Brachycera.
### Family Leptidæ. (Includes a few blood-sucking species.)
### Family Tabanidæ.

| Species | Parasite / Development | Locality | Observer |
|---|---|---|---|
| *Tabanus striatus* | *Trypanosoma evansi.* | Philippines. | Mitzmain. |
| ,, *nemoralis*, Meig. <br> ,, *tomentosus*, Macq. } | { *T. soudanense,* <br> *T. brucei, T. equiperdum,* <br> and "Mal de la Zousfana." | Algeria. | Ed. and Et. Sergent. |
| ,, *fumifer* <br> ,, *partitus* <br> ,, *vagus* <br> ,, *minimus* } | *T. evansi* (?). | Malay. | Rogers, Fraser and Symonds. |
| ,, *atratus*.. <br> ,, *ditæniatus*, Macq. <br> ,, *biguttatus*, Wied. } | { *T. evansi* (?). <br> { *T. evansi* var. *mbori,* <br> *T. cazalboui.* | New York. <br> Timbuctoo and Ségou. | Mohler and Thompson. <br> Cazalbou. |
| ,, *secedens*, Walk. | *T. pecorum* (?). | Uganda. | |
| ,, sp. | *T. evansi.* | Malay, India. <br> East Africa. | Bruce, Hamerton, Bateman and Mackey. <br> Rogers, Leese, Baldrey. <br> Jowett. |
| *Hæmatopola* sp. (mixed with *Stomoxys*) | Dimorphic cattle trypanosome. | Eastern Rhodesia. | Hart. |
| *Pangonia* sp. (together with *Stomoxys nigra*) | ,, (?) | West Africa. | Leiper. |
| *Chrysops* sp. | *Filaria loa.* | | |

TABLE I (continued).

### Cyclorrhapha Schizophora.

Family Muscidæ.

| | Disease transmitted | Locality | Authority |
|---|---|---|---|
| Glossina palpalis, Rob.-Des. .. | Trypanosoma gambiense. | Uganda. | Bruce. |
| ,, ,, .. | T. brucei. | East Africa. | Kleine. |
| ,, ,, .. | T. cazalboui. | West Africa, | Bouffard, Bruce and others. |
| ,, ,, .. | T. dimorphon. | Uganda. | Bouet and Roubaud. |
| ,, ,, .. | T. pecaudi. | West Africa. | ,, |
| ,, ,, .. | T. nanum. | Dahomey. | Duke. |
| ,, ,, .. | T. pecorum (?). | Uganda. | Fraser and Duke. |
| ,, tachinoides Westw. .. | { T. cazalboui. / T. dimorphon. | West Africa. | Bouet and Roubaud. |
| ,, pallidipes, Austen .. | T. brucei. | Zululand. | Bruce. |
| ,, longipalpis, Wied. .. | Dimorphic cattle trypanosome. | East Africa. | P. H. Ross. |
| ,, ,, ,, .. | T. dimorphon. | Dahomey. | Bouet and Roubaud. |
| ,, morsitans, Westw. .. | { T. pecaudi. / T. cazalboui. | West Africa. | ,, |
| ,, ,, .. | T. rhodesiense. | Rhodesia, Nyasaland. | Kinghorn and Yorke. |
| ,, ,, .. | T. gambiense. | Tanganyika. | Fischer. |
| ,, ,, .. | T. brucei. | East Africa. | Kleine. |
| ,, ,, .. | T. pecaudi. | Sudan. | Bouet and Roubaud. |
| ,, ,, .. | T. cazalboui. | { West Africa. / Katanga. | Belgian S.S. Commission. Bouet and Roubaud. |
| ,, ,, .. | T. dimorphon. | West Africa. | Kinghorn and Yorke. |
| ,, ,, .. | T. pecorum. | Rhodesia. | Rodhain, van der Branden, Pons and Bequaert. |
| ,, ,, .. | T. congolense. | Katanga. | Kinghorn and Yorke. |
| ,, ,, .. | T. simiæ. | Rhodesia. Nyasaland. | Bruce, Harvey, Hamilton, Davey and Lady Bruce. |

| Organism | Trypanosome / Disease | Locality | Authority |
|---|---|---|---|
| *Glossina brevipalpis*, Newstead | { *T. gambiense.* (Direct transmission.) } | East Africa. | P. H. Ross. |
| | *T. brucei* (?). | ,, | Koch and Stuhlmann. |
| ,, ,, *longipennis*, Corti | Dimorphic trypanosome. | ,, | P. H. Ross. |
| | Aïno (? = *T. brucei*)? | Somaliland. | Brumpt. |
| *Stomoxys calcitrans*, L. | *Trypanosoma evansi.* | Malay. | Fraser and Symonds. |
| ,, ,, | *Filaria labiato-papillosa.* | Italy. | Noë. |
| ,, ,, | Epidemic polyomyelitis (?). | United States. | Rosenau, Anderson and Frost. |
| ,, ,, | Anthrax (?). (Direct transmission in laboratory.) | — | Schuberg and Kuhn. |
| *S. calcitrans* and *S. nigra*, Macq. | *Trypanosoma brucei.* | French Congo. | Bouet and Roubaud. |
| ,, ,, | *T. pecaudi.* | French Sudan. | Bouffard. |
| ,, ,, | *T. cazalboui.* | Sahara. | Bouet and Roubaud. |
| ,, ,, | *T. soudanense.* | ,, | Schat. |
| *Lyperosia exigua*, de Meijere | *T. evansi.* | Java. | Leese. |
| ,, ,, *minuta*, Bezzi | *T. evansi* (?). | India. | |
| *Lyperosia* sp. and *Stomoxys* sp. | *T. evansi.* | Rhodesia. | Montgomery and Kinghorn. |
| *Hæmatobia.* | *T. dimorphon* (?). | — | — |
| *Hæmatobosca.* | — | — | — |
| *Stygeromyia.* | — | — | — |
| *Bdellolarynx.* | — | | |
| *Philæmatomyia.* | | | |

Include blood-sucking species.

**Pupipara.**
Family Hippoboscidæ.

| Organism | Trypanosome / Disease | Locality | Authority |
|---|---|---|---|
| *Hippobosca maculata*, Leach } ,, ,, *rufipes*, v. Olfers | *Trypanosoma theileri* (?). | Transvaal. | Theiler. |
| ,, ,, *rufipes* | Anthrax (?). | Griqualand West. North Africa. | Hutcheon. Ed. and Et. Sergent. |
| *Lynchia maura*, Bigot } ,, ,, *brunnipes* ,, ,, *lividicolor* | *Hæmoproteus columbæ.* ,, | Brazil. | Aragão. |

responsible for the transmission of the large number of parasitic animals that occur in the blood of vertebrates, especially in the tropics. Their great economic importance as carriers of disease agents has become universally recognized during the past twenty years and at the present time it is unnecessary to dwell on this point. In fact there seems to be a tendency for authors to go to the other extreme and credit biting insects with the spread of almost every disease in which the mode of infection remains unknown. Nevertheless, a large number of species of biting-flies have been shewn to be responsible for the spread of various diseases as may be seen from the preceding table, in which are included all biting-flies that are known to carry infections, together with the infection, or infections, which they transmit (Table I).

## CHAPTER IV

### ORTHORRHAPHA NEMATOCERA

*Definition.* As a rule a member of this series may be easily recognized by its long thin body, slender legs and long narrow wings. Moreover the antennæ are long and filiform, being composed of 6 to 15 segments that often bear whorls of hairs, especially in the male. The larvæ are aquatic, or live in decaying organic matter (*e.g. Phlebotomus*).

The Nematocera includes some of the most important biting-flies that carry disease, as the great family of mosquitoes belongs to this group.

*Classification.* Williston divides them into 12 families, of which four are known to include members that either occasionally or habitually feed on blood. In the present work his method of classification has been adopted and the following table includes all the families of the Nematocera. Those which include any members that are known to carry disease are printed in capital letters and will be discussed more fully.

## Synopsis of the Families of Orthorrhapha Nematocera[1].

1 ⎰ Body and wings thickly covered with hairs; flies resembling moths
     (Fig. 20)                    = PSYCHODIDÆ.
     Flies not resembling moths         = 2.

2 ⎰ Wings with a network of fine vein-like creases besides the ordinary
     veins (Fig. 10)                 = *Blepharoceridæ*[2].
     Wings without any additional network of vein-like creases = 3.

3 ⎰ Scutum usually with a V-shaped transverse suture (Fig. 11); wings
     usually with a discal cell         = *Tipulidæ*.
     Scutum without a transverse suture      = 4.

4 ⎰ Wings with a discal cell (Fig. 12)      = *Rhyphidæ*.
     Wings without a discal cell         = 5.

5 ⎰ Antennæ abnormal, apparently consisting of two segments and a
     terminal arista (Fig. 14)          = *Orphnephilidæ*.
     Antennæ normally nematocerous      = 6.

6 ⎰ Posterior edge of wing fringed with scales (Fig 25) = CULICIDÆ.
     Posterior edge of wing not fringed with scales    = 7.

7 ⎰ Minute fragile midges; wings commonly with only three longitudinal
     veins (Fig. 13)                 = *Cecidomyidæ*.
     Not abnormally delicate and fragile; wings usually with numerous
     veins.                           = 8.

8 ⎰ Ocelli present (Fig. 16, *oc*)       = 9.
     Ocelli absent             = 10.

9 ⎰ Coxæ elongate; antennæ usually elongate; *all* the tibiæ end in spurs
     (Fig. 15)                  = *Mycetophilidæ*.
     Coxæ short; antennæ usually shorter than thorax = *Bibionidæ*.

10 ⎰ The costal vein extends all round the wing    = *Dixidæ*.
     The costal vein stops at or near the tip of the wing (Fig. 17) = 11.

11 ⎰ Gnat-like flies with long slender legs; antennæ filiform, often with
     whorls of hairs            = *Chironomidæ*[3].
     Thick-set flies with stout legs; antennæ stout and stiff, hardly longer
     than the head, and never having whorls of hairs; wings remarkably
     broad                      = *Simuliidæ*[3].

---

[1] From Alcock's *Entomology for Medical Officers*, p. 46.

[2] Some of the females belonging to *Curupira* have been suspected of blood-sucking habits.

[3] Signifies that some of the members of these families are known to suck blood.

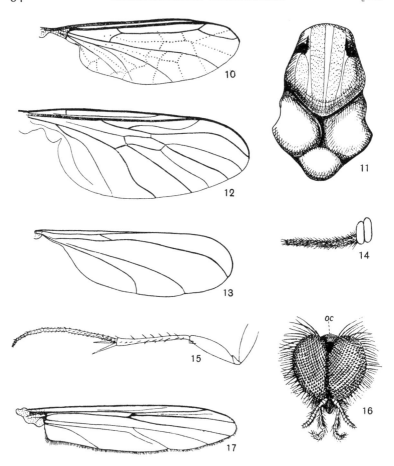

Fig. 10. Wing of *Kelloggina*, a blepharocerid, shewing the network of fine vein-like creases (× 12).

Fig. 11. Thorax of *Tipula*, with **V**-shaped transverse suture on scutum (× 8).

Fig. 12. Wing of *Ryphus* (× 12). The costal vein does not extend beyond the apex of the wing.

Fig. 13. Wing of *Cecidomyia* (× 12). The costal vein extends completely round the wing.

Fig. 14. Antenna of *Orphnephila* (× 80).

Fig. 15. Right hind-leg of *Mycetophilus*, shewing the tibial spurs (× 8).

Fig. 16. Head of *Bibio* (× 12); *oc*, ocelli.

Fig. 17. Wing of *Chironomus* sp. (× 8).

# CHAPTER V

## FAMILY PSYCHODIDÆ (MOTH-FLIES AND SAND-FLIES)

*Definition.* The members of this family are small insects, generally not exceeding 5 mm. in length, which somewhat resemble moths, as the body and wings are thickly covered with hairs, amongst which patches of scales may occur. The wings are unlike those of any other Nematoceran, being oval or lanceloate in form (Fig. 19), and with a somewhat striking venation. The second longitudinal vein branches into three near the base of the wing, and as the transverse veins are very faint, the wing appears to contain nine or ten longitudinal veins without any connections. The antennæ are long, being composed of 16 segments, which often carry whorls of hairs. The larvæ, as a rule, live in decomposing vegetable matter.

The Psychodidæ are cosmopolitan, but are most abundant in tropical and subtropical regions. The species belonging to the genus *Phlebotomus* are the only ones which are known to suck blood habitually.

### *Phlebotomus.*

*General account.* All the members of this genus are small inconspicuously coloured insects, the females of which feed by sucking the blood of vertebrates. In some species the male also sucks blood, and it often possesses mouth-parts resembling those of the female. The flies are commonly known as " Sand-Flies," or, in Southern Europe, " Pappataci Flies," and on account of their voracious habits and the fact that their small size enables them to creep through the meshes of an ordinary mosquito net, they are a source of much annoyance in those parts of the world in which they occur, especially as their bite causes great local irritation. Moreover, the well-known " Pappataci Fever," or " Three-Day Fever," is certainly carried by *P. papatasii*, and probably by other species of the genus, which is, therefore, of considerable importance from a medical point of view.

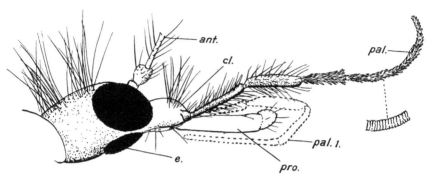

Fig. 18. Head of *Phlebotomus papatasii*; *ant*, antenna; *e*, eye; *cl*, clypeus; *pal*, palpus; *pro*, proboscis. After Newstead.

*Definition.* The genus *Phlebotomus* may easily be distinguished by the following characters :

Psychodidæ in which the mouth is modified for piercing and sucking. The antennæ are long and slender, composed of

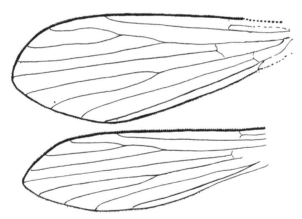

Fig. 19. Wing venation of *Phlebotomus papatasii*; upper, ♀; lower, ♂. After Newstead.

16 segments, and the joints are not markedly constricted. The wings are narrow, covered with hairs, and in repose are

always carried uplifted so that the insect resembles a tiny
moth. The second longitudinal vein branches twice, all three
branches being distinct. The body is hairy. Sexual dimorphism is distinct. The total length never exceeds 3 mm.
and is usually much less.

*Phlebotomus papatasii* is the most important member of
the genus and the following remarks apply especially to this
species.

*Bionomics.* When *P. papatasii* is feeding it lifts its wings
up to an angle of about 45°, this characteristic attitude being
well shewn in Fig. 21. On the slightest disturbance the insect

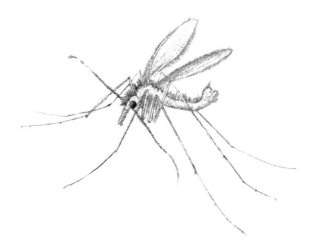

Fig. 20. *Phlebotomus papatasii*, Scop. Male.
After Newstead

moves suddenly to either the right or left by short rapid flights,
somewhat resembling the movements of a flea. If undisturbed
the females rapidly gorge themselves with blood and then
silently fly away to some dark corner. In rooms they usually
hide behind pictures, underneath clothes or in similar places.
In Malta, where they have been studied by Marett and Newstead, their favourite localities during the day seem to be the
numerous small caves and catacombs, and also the interstices
of stone walls. Atmospheric conditions have a marked effect

on the flies, for on still warm nights they are found in large numbers in houses. On the other hand, they rarely appear when cool fresh breezes are blowing, in this respect resembling the common midges of England. The chief breeding places seem to be the crevices between rocks, in loose stone walls, caves, also dark cellars, and especially on the sides of drains kept moist by the occasional splashing of water. Unfortunately, much work remains to be done on this subject, for the task of finding the minute larvæ or pupæ is very difficult,

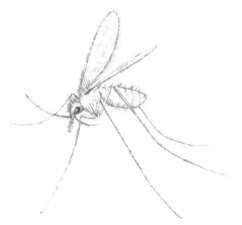

Fig. 21.  *Phlebotomus papatasii*, Scop.   Female.
After Newstead

and little is known about their habits. The difficulty of finding the larvæ is still further increased by their peculiar habit, when exposed to light, of flicking themselves off the surface of the object on which they are resting. The pupæ are even more difficult to detect, for not only are they very minute, but closely resemble the colour of their surroundings. It is therefore not surprising that so little is known about their habits, in spite of the importance of this knowledge from a prophylactic point of view.

The flies are very unequally distributed even in regions that seem to present the same conditions, such as an abundance of stone walls for breeding places. Moreover, some houses are visited much more frequently than others without any apparent reason. In Malta, Newstead found that bedrooms on the first floor facing the sheltered side of the house were much more favoured than those of the opposite side ; and only a single example was ever found in rooms on the second floor. Some persons seem to be immune to the attacks of these insects, as for some reason they have their likes and dislikes with regard to hosts, as well as habitat. It is probable that reptiles constitute the main hosts of these insects, for in West Africa, Roubaud found a lizard covered with gorged females of *P. minutus*. More recently Howlett has brought forward convincing evidence to shew that in India geckos are the chief hosts and are preferred to man.

The flies are especially abundant in the hot season of the year but in tropical countries they may be found at all times. When kept in captivity on wet blotting-paper *P. papatasii* lives but a short time (3–9 days), even though fed on human blood and kept under the most favourable conditions. The life of the adult therefore is probably of but short duration. The females readily oviposit in captivity but often die during the process. From an examination of the ovaries, the number of eggs is found to be from 40 to 50, so that the insect is comparatively little prolific.

*Life-cycle.* After copulation, the female seems to require a feed of blood before being able to lay any eggs. This condition having been fulfilled, the insect then retires to some dark corner and deposits her eggs either singly or in clusters, the total number varying from 30 to 80, according to the species. The act of oviposition is accompanied by very extraordinary movements on the part of the female. The whole process has been described by Newstead in the case of *P. papatasii*. A gravid female was placed into a glass-topped box and supplied with wet blotting-paper, when the insect at once settled on the paper and brought her proboscis into contact with it. After a few seconds she appeared to become intoxicated and collapsed, crossing the middle- and hind-legs behind the abdomen, whilst the front pair remained in their normal position. The abdomen was then raised and fully extended, after which three eggs were laid at short intervals. Each egg was ejected with considerable force to a distance at least three times the length of the abdomen. The whole process occupied about two minutes, after which the insect appeared very fatigued and rested for at least three hours before continuing the egg-laying.

The *eggs* are almost transparent when first laid, and are covered with a thin coating of sticky substance which causes them to adhere to any surface. They are very elongate in form, dark brown, shining, with longitudinal black wavy lines, which are slightly raised and joined by very fine cross-lines. The length of the egg varies from 0·1 to 0·15 mm. (Fig. 22.)

The incubation period is usually from six to nine days, but the eggs are very susceptible to external conditions and will only hatch if kept in a moist atmosphere.

     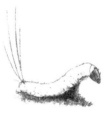

Fig. 22.                              Fig. 23.

Fig. 22.   Freshly extruded egg of *P. papatasii*. After Newstead
Fig. 23.   *P. papatasii*; adult larva. After Newstead.

The *larva* lives in damp earth and is very curious in form. It possesses a large well-marked head with big jaws, the latter being provided with four distinct teeth. The body is covered with toothed spines that may serve as a protection against enemies, and the posterior end bears two pairs of black caudal bristles. The bristles of one pair are almost as long as the body, whilst those of the other pair are short, but increase in length in the later stages (Figs. 7 and 23).

The length of the full-grown larva is about 2·3 mm. In India the larval stage usually lasts from about three weeks to even as long as two months, but its duration depends mainly on the temperature, being much prolonged in cold weather.

The larva closely resembles a caterpillar in its movements ;

it progresses slowly and continually pecks at the stone on which it is placed. The caudal bristles are kept raised and extended in a fan-shaped manner, thus presenting a somewhat characteristic appearance. The larva feeds on semi-decaying vegetable matter and after undergoing a certain number of moults turns into the pupa.

The *pupa* (Fig. 24), which is found on damp earth and under the surface of stones, is remarkable for the large ridges and excrescences on its thorax. The larval skin, with the bristles still attached, usually remains adhering at the caudal extremity.

The fly generally emerges from the pupa after about six to ten days, but as in the other stages this period may be con-

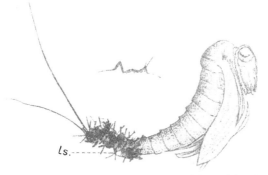

Fig. 24. Pupa of *P. papatasii*; *ls*, larval skin with anal bristles attached. After Newstead.

siderably prolonged by a low temperature. In India, according to Howlett, the life-cycle of the sand-fly varies in duration from a month in the hot weather to six to eight weeks in the cold season, but in Malta Marett found the life-cycle occupied about three months.

*Breeding localities.* Further information with regard to the breeding places of *Phlebotomus* is much to be desired. Captain Marett finds that in Malta the chief localities are the crevices in stone walls and the fissures between rocks in caves.

In Italy Grassi found specimens in dirty cellars and similar dark places containing rubbish of various kinds. He states that the larvæ live in dark and damp places amid all kinds of rubbish ; they prefer underground situations such as cellars and more especially those parts of drains that can only be reached by splashes of dirty water. Although the adult fly is usually excessively abundant in those localities that it infests, no observer has yet succeeded in finding larvæ in any considerable numbers. There are good reasons for believing that one of the breeding places may be the dark and damp inner surfaces of the walls of latrines, and cesspools. The flies are notoriously common in latrines and in the case of a military camp in Herzegovina, Doerr brought forward evidence to shew that in summer the latrines were the only possible breeding places for the swarms of *Phlebotomus* that infested the camp.

*Phlebotomus and disease.* The only disease[1] which is known to be transmitted by members of this genus is the notorious Three-Day Fever, or Pappataci Fever. *P. papatasii* Scopoli is the only species that has been definitely proved to carry the infection, but it is almost certain that *P. minutus* and other members of the genus are equally capable in this respect ; therefore we append a short synopsis of the known species of *Phlebotomus* together with their distribution.

*Synopsis of known species of Phlebotomus.*

*European species[2].*

*A*. Abdominal hairs recumbent.

(1) Integument black. Second segment of palpi slightly longer than third. Legs pale ochreous buff, with ochreous white refulgence. Length of female 2·5 mm.                    *nigerrimus*, Newstead.

---

[1] Since the above account was written Townsend (*Journ. Amcr. Med. Assoc.* vol. 61, p. 1717) has brought forward evidence in support of the view that Verruga Peruviana is transmitted by *Phlebotomus*. These flies were found to be very abundant in the infected districts especially in the Verrugas Canyon. To prove this theory of transmission the author obtained two hairless Mexican dogs. After they had been kept under observation for nearly three months, one of them was inoculated subcutaneously with the ground-up bodies of 20 female *Phlebotomus* collected the night before in the Verrugas Canyon. On the fifth day this dog appeared ill and its blood was found to contain the peculiar endoglobular forms known as Barton's X-bodies, and also nucleated and broken down red cells. On the sixth day a typical nodular eruption was noticed on the right hind-foot and smears from one of the papules shewed bodies resembling *Leishmania*. On the eighth day the dog began to improve. The control dog remained in perfect health.

[2] Modified from Alcock's *Entomology for Medical Officers*.

(2) Integument ochreous. Second segment of palpi one-half the length of the third. Length of female 2 mm., male considerably less.

*minutus*, Rondani.

B. Abdominal hairs erect.

(3) Terminal segment of upper clasper of male hardly half the length of lower clasper. Legs relatively short ; average length of hind-leg 3 mm. Length of female, 1·9–2·2 mm.                *perniciosus*, Newstead

(4) Terminal segment of upper clasper of male slightly longer than lower clasper. Legs relatively long ; length of hind-leg 4 mm. Thorax with a dull red-brown median stripe and a spot on each side. Length of female 2·5–2·65 mm.                *papatasii*, Scopoli.

(5) Resembling the preceding species in every respect except the form of the male claspers, the five spines of the terminal segment of the latter being long and falciform.                *mascittii*, Grassi.

### African species.

P. *papatasii* has been described from Algeria and Tunis and probably occurs throughout the whole of North Africa.

General colour pale-yellow. Wing narrow, about three times as long as broad ; second marginal cell less than a third the length of the wing. Length of female 2 mm. ; male considerably less.                *duboscquii*, Neveu-Lemaire.

Pleuræ clothed with large flat scales like those of mosquitoes. Third segment of palps with a compound group of minute modified spines, spathuliform with short pedicels. Khartoum.                *squamipleuris*, Newstead.

Resembling *minutus* but with shorter and stouter legs. Third to the thirteenth antennal segments bead-like. Gold Coast.

*antennatus*, Newstead.

### Oriental species.

P. *papatasii* is said to occur all over India and P. *minutus* (syn. *babu* Annandale) has also been recorded. In addition the following species have been described :

Head and abdomen brown ; dorsum of thorax dark brown or blackish ; sides of thorax, coxæ, and trochanters yellowish ; legs, antennæ, and palpi grey ; the whole, especially the legs with a silvery sheen. Greatest breadth of wing about a third its length ; greatest length of second marginal cell ("first fork-cell") about a third the length of the wing.

*argentipes*, Annandale.

Uniform grey with strong silvery lights, disk of wings with a bluish iridescence. Greatest breadth of wing not quite a third its length ; greatest length of second marginal cell a little more than a third the length of the wing.

*major*, Annandale.

Thorax, abdomen, and legs (except coxæ and trochanters) brown with a tinge of purple and with silvery lights ; wings purplish, strongly iridescent. Greatest breadth of wing about a third its length ; greatest length of second marginal cell nearly half the length of the wing. South India.

*malabaricus*, Annandale.

Yellowish-grey with silvery lights. Greatest length of wing slightly over one-fourth its length ; greatest length of second marginal cell a little more than a third the length of the wing. Himalayas, between 4000 and 7000 feet.

*himalayensis*, Annandale.

Head and thorax yellowish-brown, abdomen brown with darker glistening hairs; femora yellow with brown tip; tibiæ and tarsi brown with silver sheen. Greatest breadth of wing one-third its length; greatest length of second marginal cell a little more than one-fourth the length of the wing. Batavia.                                                    *perturbans*, Meijere.

### American species.

Yellow, mesonotum brown; legs appear brown in certain lights but are covered with white tomentum; second marginal cell slightly more than twice the length of its petiole. North America.                        *vexator*, Coquillet.

Resembling *vexator*, except that the hairs are mostly yellow, and the second marginal cell is about thrice the length of its petiole. Guatemala.

*cruciatus*, Coquillet.

In female length of head with proboscis, half that of the rest of the body. Wing venation resembling that of *malabaricus*. In the male greatest length of wing 3½ times the greatest breadth. Wings bluntly pointed; hind border not much more strongly arched than the front. Length of second marginal cell three-eighths that of the wing; third marginal, six-elevenths the length. Halteres long and large. Brazil and Peru.                        *rostrans*, Summers.

Dorsal surface of abdomen with numerous scales between the hairs. Palp index 4, 5, 3, 2. Length of body 2 mm. Para.

*squamiventris*, Lutz and Neiva.

Dorsal surface of abdomen without scales. Last segment of palps longer than the others; palp index 4, 2, 3, 5. Length of body about 2 mm. St Paul and Minas.                                              *longipalpis*, Lutz and Neiva.

Dorsal surface of abdomen without scales. General colour brownish-yellow, the upperside darker. Palp index 5, 4, 3, 2.

*intermedius*, Lutz and Neiva.


# CHAPTER VI

## DISEASES CARRIED BY PHLEBOTOMUS

### Pappataci Fever.

*Synonyms.* Sand-Fly Fever; Three-Day Fever; Phlebotomus Fever; Simple Continued Fever; Pink Eye; Sommerfieber; Hundskrankheit; Sommerinfluenza; Soldatenfieber; Endemischer Magencatarrh; Febbre dei tre Giorni; Mal della secca; Febbre estiva; Chitral Fever; Fièvre de Toga.

*History.* This malady seems to have been known for many years in both Italy and India, but was first recognized as a definite disease by Pick in 1886. Taussig, in 1905, noticed that it was connected with the sand-fly and later, in 1908, the researches of Doerr, Franz, and Taussig, clearly demonstrated the nature of this disease and its mode of transmission.

Some authors, especially the French, regard Pappataci Fever as merely a form of dengue, but the febrile symptoms are rather different in the two cases and therefore, for the present, it seems advisable to consider them distinct.

*Distribution.* Pappataci Fever occurs in various parts of Italy and is especially prevalent in Dalmatia, Istria, Herzegovina and various other parts of Austria-Hungary, and has also been recorded from Portugal. It is said to occur in Asia Minor, the Balkan Peninsula, North Africa and the Sudan. The majority of the islands in the Mediterranean seem to be liable to outbreaks, for the disease has been recorded from Corsica, Sicily, Malta, Crete and Cyprus, and probably occurs in most, if not all the islands of the Greek Archipelago. According to Robinson and Blackham the "Seven-Day Fever" of the Peshawur valley is also a variety of Sand-Fly Fever and is carried by *Phlebotomus.* In other parts of India, epidemics probably due to this infection have been observed, but the symptoms in many cases closely approximate those of dengue. The disease is said to occur in China.

*Symptomatology.* In view of the fact that this disease has only recently been distinguished, a short account of the symptoms is included.

Different outbreaks shew considerable variations in the symptoms. The onset of the disease is usually sudden, with febrile symptoms, headache and pains, especially in the extremities. The fever continues for one or two days and usually disappears on the third, fourth, or fifth day, but in some cases may persist as long as seven days. During the attack nervous symptoms are very pronounced ; headache, usually frontal, is constantly present and pains in the back, loins and lower extremities occur in the majority of cases. Muscle pains are frequently present, being chiefly located in the intercostal and lumbar muscles, and the muscles of the calves. On the other hand the joints are very seldom affected and this constitutes one of the means of distinguishing this disease from dengue.

The eyes are injected, especially across the middle of the conjunctivæ, and the bulbi are painful on pressure. The disturbances of the digestive system are very inconstant ; vomiting occurs in about one-third of the cases, usually as an initial symptom. Constipation is the rule when the temperature is high, but later on, diarrhœa often sets in and the liquid stools may contain blood. Epistaxis is a common phenomenon. Various cutaneous eruptions may occur, in the nature of erythema of a morbilliform or multiform character, and a few roseolæ.

The examination of the blood reveals no changes in the number or morphology of the red corpuscles. A pronounced leucopenia has been observed on the first day, and the numbers of leucocytes may fall as low as 1400 per c.mm. on the second day, after which the numbers slowly increase from the third day onwards.

The percentage of polymorphonuclears varies between 80 and less than 50, and Gabbi finds a slight increase of the mononuclears. Eosinophile leucocytes are very scarce, their number being below the normal.

The prognosis is invariably good and the patient's recovery is usually complete within two or three weeks after the beginning of the disease.

In the absence of any knowledge of the causative agent of this disease, the diagnosis can only be based on clinical observations and it is extremely difficult to distinguish between Pappataci Fever and various other febrile diseases. The presence of the transmitting agent may be of some help in establishing the diagnosis, but the discovery of the specific microbe is necessary before this disease can be distinguished with any certainty.

*Mode of infection.* Pappataci Fever is transmitted by the agency of *Phlebotomus papatasii*, the sand-fly. Possibly *P. perniciosus, minutus,* and other species of the genus are also capable of spreading the disease, but up to the present, with the possible exception of Aden[1], no cases have been recorded from localities in which *P. papatasii* is not known to occur.

---

[1] Sand-Fly Fever is said to occur in this region. The only species of *Phlebotomus* hitherto recorded from Aden is *P. minutus.*

Following the bite of an infected fly, there is an incubation period of from 3½ to 7 days, during which the blood of the patient is not infective. Then follows the first day of the attack during which the blood becomes virulent and is capable of infecting any *Phlebotomus* that may feed on it.

The blood loses its infectivity within a very short period, probably not more than 24 hours, and after recovery the patient is immune against any further attacks of the disease.

The flies become infected only if they feed on a patient during the short time that his blood is infective. After ingesting the virus, there is an incubation period of seven to ten days before the insects become infective and beyond this period they may again become non-infective, but experiments on this point are far from complete.

*Causal agent.* Up to the present the causal agent of Pappataci Fever has not been discovered, but it belongs to the group of ultra-microscopic organisms which cause dengue, yellow fever, etc. Its presence in the blood is proved by the fact that the disease may be produced by the inoculation into a non-immune person of blood taken from an infected patient on the first day of the attack. Moreover, the injection of a small quantity of diluted serum filtered through a Chamberland F filter is also followed by a typical attack of fever. The virus is sufficiently resistant to maintain its activity for a week *in vitro*.

It is evident that the fly is a true host for the organism that causes the disease. If the *Phlebotomus* were only infective up to the seventh day after an infective feed, there would be a strong suggestion that the virus was merely retained in the alimentary canal and regurgitated at subsequent meals. This supposition is disproved by the occurrence of a negative phase of about seven days, during which the infective agent of the disease undergoes some development, finally resulting in the fly becoming infective.

*Prophylactic measures.* In view of the limited number of observations on the breeding habits of *Phlebotomus* it is somewhat premature to advance any definite prophylactic measures. If crevices in stone walls and amongst rocks constitute the main breeding places, the task of destroying the immature stages is practically insurmountable.   At present it is only possible to take precautions against being bitten by the insects and the simplest method is the use of repellents.   Major Crawford recommends the following mixture which is said to be a very efficient deterrent : Ol. Anisi, 3 grs. ; Ol. Eucalypti, 3 grs. ; Ol. Terebenth, 3 grs. ; Ung. Acid Borac.

The use of ordinary mosquito nets is of course impossible, as the flies are able to creep through the meshes, but spraying the net with a 1 per cent. solution of formol, or some other repellent, is said to be effective in keeping away these pests. By employing a screen of chiffon or some similar material, it is possible to exclude the flies altogether, but such a method is quite impracticable on warm nights, when the *Phlebotomus* are especially abundant.   A brightly burning lamp appears to attract the flies more than a sleeping human being and is very useful in the absence of a net or punkah.   As they are very sensitive to wind, the use of electric fans in rooms would probably succeed in keeping them away and some such method might well be adopted in the case of patients suffering from Pappataci Fever, for by the careful isolation of all persons suffering from the complaint, the number of cases would be reduced.   As the flies seem to avoid the upper stories of houses it might be advisable to keep patients suffering from the disease in upper bedrooms.

By preventing the flies from feeding on the blood of infected persons it is even possible that the disease might be eradicated, and this is the only method that seems practicable at the present time.

REFERENCES TO LITERATURE ON *PHLEBOTOMUS*
AND PAPPATACI FEVER.

Annandale, N. (1910).   The Indian Species of Papataci Fly (*Phlebotomus*).   *Rec. Ind. Mus.* vol. IV. pp. 35–52.   With 3 plates.
Birt, C. (1910).   Phlebotomus fever in Malta and Crete.   *Journ. R.A.M.C.* vol. XIV. pp. 142–159 and 236–258.
—— (1910).   Sand-fly fever in India.   *Journ. R.A.M.C.* vol. XV. pp. 140–147.

Crawford, G. S. (1909). On the beneficial results of recent sanitary work in Malta. *Brit. Med. Journ.* vol. II. pp. 383–385.

Doerr, Franz and Taussig (1909). *Das Pappatacifieber.* Leipzig and Wien : Franz Deuticke.

Franca, C. (1913). *Phlebotomus papatasii* (Scopoli) et Fièvre à Pappataci au Portugal. *Bull. Soc. Path. Exot.* vol. VI. pp. 123–124.

Gabbi (1910). Sulla febbre dei tre giorni o febbre da pappataci. *Pathologica,* vol. II. pp. 546–550.

Grassi, B. (1907). Ricerche sui flebotomi. *Mem. d. Soc. Ital. d. Scienze,* Ser. 3 a, vol. XIV. pp. 353–394, with 4 plates.

—— (1908). Intorno ad un nuovo flebotomo. *Att. R. Accad. Linc.* Ser. 5 a, vol. XVII. pp. 681–682.

Howlett, F. M. (1909). Indian Sandflies. *Trans. Bombay Med. Congr.* Ser. 3, pp. 239–242.

—— (1913). The Natural Host of *Phlebotomus minutus. Ind. Journ. Med. Research,* vol. I. pp. 34–38.

Leger, M. and Seguinard, J. (1912). Fièvre de Pappataci en Corse. *Bull. Soc. Path. Exot.* vol. V. pp. 710–713.

Lutz and Neiva (1912). Contribuição para o Conhecimento das Especies do Genero Phlebotomus existentes no Brazil. *Mem. Inst. Oswaldo Cruz.* vol. IV. pp. 84–95.

Marett, P. J. (1910). Preliminary report on the investigation into the breeding-places of the sand-fly in Malta. *Journ. R.A.M.C.* vol. XV. pp. 286–291.

—— (1911). The life-history of *Phlebotomus. Ibid.* vol. XVII. pp. 13–29, with 1 plate.

Newstead, R. (1911). The papataci flies (*Phlebotomus*) of the Maltese Islands. *Bull. Entomol. Research,* vol. II. pp. 47–48.

—— (1912). Notes on *Phlebotomus*, with Descriptions of New Species. Part I. *Ibid.* vol. III. pp. 361–367.

Robinson and Blackham (1912). Sand-flies and Sand-Fly Fever on the North-West Frontier of India. *Journ. R.A.M.C.* vol. XIX. pp. 447–452.

Seidelin, H. (1912). Pappataci Fever. *Yellow Fever Bull.* vol. II. pp. 74–84.

Summers, Sophia L. M. (1913). A Synopsis of the Genus *Phlebotomus. Journ. Lond. School Trop. Med.* vol. II. pp. 104–116.

# CHAPTER VII

## FAMILY CULICIDÆ (GNATS OR MOSQUITOES)

### General Account.

*Definition.* The Culicidæ are slender flies easily distinguished from all other Nematocera by the presence of a row of scales on the posterior margin of the wings. In addition, the long projecting proboscis, and the plumose antennæ of the males are characteristic features.

**External anatomy.** The head is small and subspherical; the occiput is always more or less covered with scales of various forms. The eyes are large and reniform and may, or may not, meet in the middle line; in the living insect they are often brilliantly coloured, but in preserved specimens these colours usually fade. Ocelli are absent. The antennæ are long and slender, composed of 14 or 15 segments; the basal segment is large, round, and is sometimes provided with scales. The second segment fits into a depression at the apex of the first, and the remaining segments are all more or less elongated cylinders. Just above the base, or in the middle, of each segment arises a whorl of long thick hairs, which are somewhat scanty in the female, but in the male are so thick-set as to give the antenna the appearance of a bottle-brush; in addition, the last two segments of the male antenna are nearly always more elongated and nearly bare.

The mouth-parts consist of the following appendages :

(i)  A pair of mandibles, each of which is an extremely delicate chitinous blade adapted for piercing the skin. In the male the mandibles are absent (Figs. 26 and 27).

(ii)  The first pair of maxillæ, generally known simply as the maxillæ, are extremely fine stylets usually longer than the mandibles. In the male the maxillæ are sometimes rudimentary. From the outer side of the base of each maxilla, arises a maxillary palp, the form of which varies according to the sex.

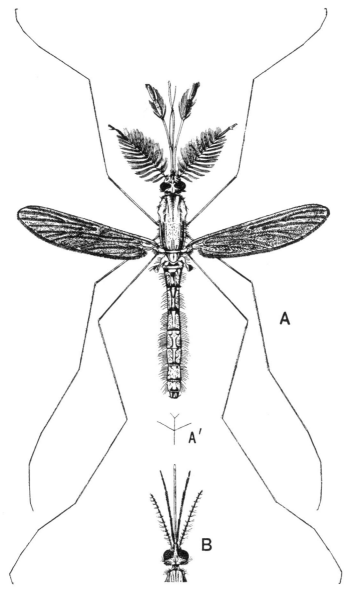

Fig. 25. *Anopheles maculipennis*. A, enlarged view of male; A', diagram of ditto to shew the natural size; B, head of female. Modified from Nuttall and Shipley.

In *Anopheles* the palps are five-jointed and as long as the proboscis in both male and female ; in the female *Culex* they are very short three- to four-jointed structures, whilst in the male *Culex* they are five-jointed and at least as long as in *Anopheles* ; in *Aëdes* the palps are short in both sexes.

(iii)  The second maxillæ are united together to form the labium, which ensheaths all the other mouth appendages with the exception of the palps, and the whole structure is generally known as the proboscis.  It consists of a soft dorsally-grooved rod which bears a pair of small labellæ at the distal extremity.

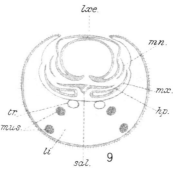

Fig. 26.    Transverse section through about the middle of the proboscis of a female *Anopheles maculipennis* shewing the relative position of the parts when at rest.    Two tracheæ (*tr*) and two pairs of extensor and flexor muscles (*mus*) are seen in the labium.    After Nuttall and Shipley. Lettering as in Fig. 27.

Each of the latter represents the distal segment of the two-jointed second maxillæ, the proximal segments of which are completely fused together.  The labellæ serve to guide the piercing organs of the mosquito.  The cavity of the labium is hollow and it is within this space that the embryos of *Filaria bancrofti* and *F. immitis* come to rest after leaving the thoracic muscles or Malpighian tubules of an infected mosquito.  The labium is covered by a thin cuticle and the filariæ escape by rupturing this membrane when the insect feeds.

In addition to the paired appendages mentioned above, there are two very important median structures.

(iv)  The labrum, or upper lip, which is united with the epipharynx, is an incomplete tube, in cross-section appearing something like an Ω ; the slit-like opening is placed ventrally. At its distal extremity the labrum of the female narrows to a sharp point, whilst in the male the tip is truncated.

(v)  The hypopharynx arises just above the base of the labium and in the female is shaped " like a two-edged sword." When applied to the labrum it closes the ventral slit and the two structures together form a suctorial tube.   In the male the hypopharynx is frequently fused with the labium and is

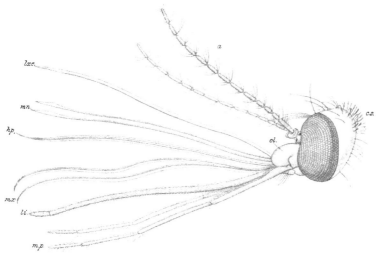

Fig. 27.   Side view of the head of a female *Anopheles maculipennis*, × about 26, with the various mouth-parts separated, but in the relative position in which they lie when enclosed in the groove of the labium.   After Nuttall and Shipley.

  *a*, antennæ ; *cl*, clypeus ; *cs*, cephalic scales ; *hp*, hypopharynx ; *li*, labium ; *lxe*, labrum + epipharynx ; *mn*, mandibles ; *mp*, maxillary palps ; *mx*, first maxillæ.

never adapted for piercing.  In both male and female the thickened ventral part of the hypopharynx is traversed by the median salivary groove, ending at the distal extremity.

The relative position of the mouth-parts is well shewn in the accompanying diagram (Fig. 27).

The thorax is by far the largest of the three divisions of the body, being some 12–15 times as large as the head, and

4–6 times as large as the abdomen. The major portion is taken up by the mesothorax, which forms the chief region of the mid-body. Its dorsal element, the scutum, is a large plate projecting slightly over the head ; posteriorly it is bounded by a curved narrow thickening of the integument known as the scutellum, which often bears conspicuous rows of hairs. Behind this comes the post-scutellum, or metathorax, a triangular plate which overlaps part of the first abdominal segment. The presence or absence of hairs and scales on the post-scutellum is of generic importance.

At each side of the thorax are two large spiracles, respectively pro- and meso-thoracic in origin (Fig. 4).

The six legs are each composed of the typical insect parts, viz. the coxa, trochanter, femur, tibia and tarsus, the last of which is five-jointed and ends in a pair of claws. The four proximal joints are often covered with scales. The first joint of the tarsus is long and hairy and its proportionate length with the tibia is of specific value. The shape of the claws varies according to the sex ; in the female they are equal and simple or may have a single tooth ; in the male those of the fore-legs are usually unequal and toothed.

The wings are long and narrow and while at rest lie flat over the abdomen. The venation is very characteristic, there being six distinct longitudinal veins and two prominent fork-cells, and the costal vein extends completely round the edge of the wing (Fig. 28).

The auxiliary vein is distinct, sometimes extending beyond the middle of the wing. The second, fourth, and fifth longitudinal veins are furcate.

The hind margin of the wings is fringed with a row of hairs or scales and in addition all the veins are more or less covered with scales. The shape and arrangement of these scales varies in different groups and is the chief basis of Theobald's classification.

On the under surface, at the base of the wing, is a curious stridulating organ, consisting of a complex system of chitinous bars, by means of which two ridged surfaces are made to rub against each other when the wings vibrate (Fig. 28). It is probable that this organ is responsible for some of the characteristic buzzing of the mosquito.

Each halter consists of a short chitinous rod arising from a basal plate and ending in a rounded knob. The concave basal plate and a knob at the base of the halter are covered with small papillæ, and Shipley and Wilson have suggested that by these two surfaces rubbing against each other when the halter vibrates, a faint note may be produced.

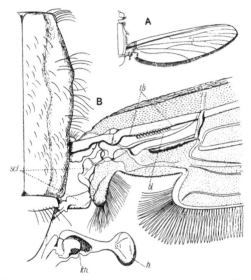

Fig. 28.    View of under surface of the base of the wing of *Anopheles maculipennis*, shewing stridulating organ.    After Shipley and Wilson.

A, right half of thorax with right wing.   The shaded portion indicates the area which bears the stridulating organ.   B, the stridulating organ, highly magnified.   *bl*, ridged blade; *h*, haltere; *kn*, knob; *scl*, sclerites; *tb*, toothed bar.

The abdomen consists of eight segments, each composed of a dorsal chitinous plate, the tergum, and a ventral chitinous plate, the sternum, between which is a soft membrane, the pleuron.   On each side are six abdominal stigmata opening in segments two to seven inclusive.   The surface of the abdomen may be covered either with scales or hairs.   The terminal segment is bilobed and in the male each lobe terminates in a long chitinous claw, the clasper.

**Internal anatomy.** The internal anatomy of the Culicidæ is very constant and the following description of *Anopheles maculipennis* will apply, with but slight modifications, to any other member of the family. This example has been selected since it has been minutely described by Nuttall and Shipley, from whose account the present description is largely taken.

(*a*) *Digestive organs.* According to the above-mentioned authors the alimentary canal may be divided into eleven parts as follows : mouth ; buccal cavity ; pharynx or pumping organ ; œsophagus, with which are connected three diverticula, two dorsal and one ventral ; œsophageal valve ; mid-gut ; ileum ; colon ; rectum ; and anus.

The *mouth* is that region where the various mouth-parts coalesce and is of no special interest. The *buccal cavity* extends from the mouth to a valvular arrangement situated at the commencement of the pharynx. It is lined with chitin throughout, that of the floor being much stouter than that of the roof, which forms a kind of soft palate capable of being raised or depressed by means of muscles. Accordingly the size of the buccal cavity can be increased by these means and it may at times assist in suction. At the junction of the buccal cavity and pharynx is situated a valvular apparatus, formed by a double row of chitinous hairs attached to the ventral surface. These hairs, in addition to acting as a valve, may also serve as a kind of filter and keep out large particles.

The *pharynx*, or pumping organ, extends from this valve to the commencement of the œsophagus, and consists of a thick-walled tube composed of three longitudinal, chitinous plates, conjoined by a fold of chitin at their margins. The lumen of the tube is triangular in shape, and powerful muscles, arising from each of the three chitinous plates and attached to the exoskeleton, serve to separate the walls and increase the capacity of the pharynx. By means of the powerful pharyngeal muscles, which almost fill the head of the mosquito, the insect is enabled to suck up liquids into its pharynx, and after the relaxation of the muscles the walls contract again, by virtue of the elasticity of the chitinous supporting plates. Any ingested liquid is thus forced out of

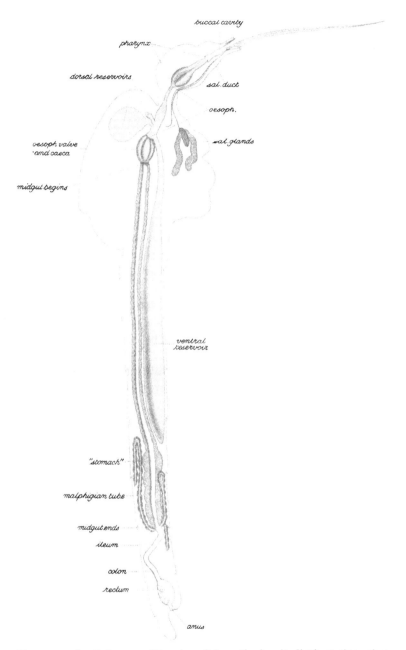

buccal cavity

pharynx

dorsal reservoirs

sal. duct

oesoph.

sal. glands

oesoph valve
and caeca

midgut begins

ventral
reservoir

"stomach"

malphigian tube

midgut ends

ileum

colon

rectum

anus

Fig. 29.  *Anopheles maculipennis.*  Schematic longitudinal section of a
female insect shewing the relations of the various parts of the alimentary
canal to each other, and to the exoskeleton, also the salivary glands of
one side with their duct joining the common duct, which is prolonged into
the hypopharynx.  The ventral reservoir is filled, the stomach contracted.
One of the dorsal reservoirs is cut off near to where it joins the œsophagus.
After Nuttall and Shipley.

the pharynx into the next region of the alimentary canal. The pharynx of the female mosquito is both larger and stronger than that of the male, this being the result of the more voracious habits of the former.

The *œsophagus* is a short, circular tube, extending from the posterior end of the tri-radiate pharynx to the œsophageal valve.

Into its posterior end, about on the level of the origin of the first pair of legs, open the three œsophageal diverticula. The largest of these is the ventral diverticulum opening into the œsophagus by means of a single median pore and extending backwards beneath the alimentary canal as far as the sixth or seventh segment. The other two dorso-lateral diverticula are much smaller and open one on each side of the œsophagus.

The function of these sacs is still far from being settled, for although Nuttall and Shipley have shewn that food material is passed into them, yet it is doubtful whether their chief function is to serve as reservoirs.

The sacs generally contain small bubbles of carbon dioxide and also larger or smaller numbers of a small round fungus belonging to the Entomophtoraceæ.

The presence of these bubbles in the sacs has caused certain authors to suppose that there was some connection between them and the tracheal system, whilst others, noticing the rhythmic contractions of the ventral sac, have supposed that it was an accessory pumping apparatus. The main function of the diverticula is probably to assist in the feeding of the mosquito and the manner in which this is affected will be described later (*vide* habits).

The *œsophageal valve* is homologous with the proventriculus of many insects, and serves as a valve between the œsophagus and the mid-gut. It is little more than a slight invagination of the intestinal wall surrounded by a very thick sphincter muscle. Six small protuberances, the remnants of the cæcal appendages of the larva, can usually be seen in the walls of the valve.

The *mid-gut* is the only part of the alimentary canal that is not lined with chitin and consequently the only part in which any food absorption takes place. Commencing at the œsophageal valve it consists of a straight tube expanded posteriorly, extending to about the posterior limit of the sixth segment. The expanded posterior region is commonly termed the " *stomach* " and this term may conveniently be retained; it is in this hinder region of the mid-gut that the malarial parasite develops. The wall of the mid-gut is surrounded by both longitudinal and circular muscle layers and the latter throw the surface into a series of folds so that this region of the alimentary canal has an annulated appearance. The mid-gut is extremely well supplied with tracheæ, which branch in such a manner that the whole surface is covered with fine air-capillaries. The interior is lined by a layer of large cubical cells, some of which are secretory in function.

The *ileum* commences at the junction of the Malpighian tubules with the mid-gut ; it is a thin-walled tube lined with chitin raised up in the form of ridges. It passes insensibly into the *colon*, which is merely a straight tube opening suddenly into the large oval *rectum*. The latter contains six large ovoid papillæ which, considerably diminish the size of the chamber. These rectal papillæ are abundantly supplied with tracheæ and their function is possibly respiratory.

The rectum narrows just before the anus, which opens in the last segment of the body, immediately beneath the genital aperture. It is guarded by two short lateral papillæ.

The *Malpighian tubules* are five in number, opening into the alimentary canal at the junction of the mid- and hind-gut. The wall of each tubule is composed of large secretory cells abundantly supplied with tracheæ. These cells are excretory in function, for the Malpighian tubules often contain uric acid and other waste nitrogenous products.

The Malpighian tubules are frequently the haunt of protozoal parasites, the lumen of the tubes being a common place in which to find insect flagellates.

The *salivary apparatus*; commencing with the opening at the tip of the hypopharynx, it consists of the following parts : a median groove, or " salivary gutter," extending from the tip to the base of the hypopharynx. This groove is arched over by thin chitinous lamellæ and therefore serves the purpose of a duct. At the base of the hypopharynx is the salivary receptacle or pump, connecting the salivary groove with the common salivary duct. The pump is somewhat drum-like in form, its membrane being moved by muscles by means of which the saliva is first pumped out of the glands and then down the salivary groove to the tip of the hypopharynx. The salivary pump is situated beneath the floor of the buccal cavity. From its posterior end a median, common salivary duct extends backwards until it reaches the commencement of the pharynx, at which point it branches into two. These secondary ducts run side by side along the ventral wall of the neck into the thoracic cavity, where they diverge and each branches into three smaller ducts. Each of the latter terminates in a salivary gland, there being three glands on each side.

These three salivary glands are at first arranged in the form of a triangle but subsequently their position changes and the gland which at first occupies a dorsal position comes to lie in between the other two glands. It is usually known as the "central gland" and differs both in size and structure from the other two, known as the "lateral glands."

The size of the glands varies according to the size of the insect but is always greater in the females than in the males. The dimensions of the glands of an average-sized female are as follows : length of lateral glands, 880 μ ; length of central gland, 510 μ ; width of glands, 85 μ. In the male the large glands only measure about 200 μ in length by 50 μ in breadth.

The salivary glands are of very great importance from a parasitological point of view, since the infective sporozoites of malaria congregate within the cells of these organs and are passed out with the salivary secretion. Therefore by a microscopical examination of these glands it is possible to find out whether or not a mosquito is infected.

The structure of the three glands is similar, each consisting of an elongated sac the lumen of which is surrounded by a single layer of secretory cells, but they differ somewhat in their finer details. The acinus of each of the lateral glands is more or less filled with an abundant secretion, which also fills the secretory cells to such an extent that their nuclei are forced to the periphery. Moreover, these cells are granular in appearance, in contradistinction to those of the central gland, which are clear  The lumen of the central gland is much smaller than that of each lateral gland, and the clear secretion almost entirely fills the cells.

This central gland has long been supposed to be the source of the irritating substance which is inoculated when a mosquito begins to feed, and accordingly is still commonly known under the name of " Poison-Gland." Schaudinn, however, has shewn that its secretion produces no effect when injected into the skin and the irritation following a bite is due to the entrance into the wound of a fungus, which is derived from the œsophageal diverticula.

(b) *The reproductive organs.* The genital organs of the female consist of a pair of lobulated masses containing numerous eggs in various stages of development. From each a short wide duct leads into a common oviduct opening to the exterior in the eighth segment. Into the common duct open three short seminal receptacles and also a cement-gland. The function of the latter is probably to secrete a protective coating for the eggs.

The male genital organs consist of a pair of minute testes situated in the eighth segment. From each arises a simple tube, the vas deferens, and the two unite just before the opening to the exterior, forming a common ejaculatory duct. The latter ends in a short penis and the external aperture, situated on the ninth segment, is guarded by an elaborate arrangement of claspers, or gonapophyses, that are of some importance from a classificatory point of view. The spermatozoa are stored, and also complete their development, in two receptaculæ seminales, opening one on each side into the vasa deferentia immediately before their junction.

(c) *The respiratory system.* This consists of two large tracheæ running longitudinally one on each side of the body and giving off branches to all the internal organs. Each main longitudinal trunk is connected by means of short branches with the stigmata, or breathing pores, of which there are two pairs of large thoracic, situated on the mesothorax and meta-thorax respectively, and six pairs of abdominal, on the second to the seventh segments.

(d) *The circulatory system.* As in the majority of insects the circulatory system consists of a dorsal tube or heart contained within a pericardium. The heart is provided with valves and by its rhythmic contractions the blood, which bathes all the organs, is kept circulating round the body.

(e) *The nervous system.* This consists of a double ventral nerve-cord uniting a series of ganglia, one to each segment. The anterior or cephalic ganglion, situated in the head and supplying nerves to the appendages of this region, is remarkable for its large size in comparison with that of the insect. From this ganglion the ventral nerve-cords pass one on each side of the œsophagus, to unite in an infra-œsophageal ganglion. The double ventral nerve-cord continues posteriorly from this ganglion and in each segment, except the last, is enlarged into a segmental ganglion.

**Life-cycle.** The life-cycle of all species of mosquitoes may be briefly outlined in a few words. The female, after being fertilized, deposits her eggs on, or near, the surface of some water. After a short interval these hatch out giving rise to young aquatic larvæ, which grow until they reach a certain size and then pupate. The resulting pupa is actively motile and swims about in the water as vigorously as the larva. After a comparatively short existence the anterior dorsal region of the pupa splits and the adult insect emerges.

*The egg.* The number of eggs laid by the female varies considerably, from 40 to 100 (*A. maculipennis*), up to as many as 400 (*Culex pipiens*). The eggs may occur singly, as in the case of *Anopheles* and *Stegomyia*, or adhere together forming boat- or raft-shaped masses, as in *Culex* and many other Culi-cinæ, and being provided with air-chambers, they invariably float on the surface of the water. The shape of the eggs is different in each genus; those of *Anopheles* are boat-shaped with a distinct float at the sides, growing broader in the middle (Fig. 31, A, B), whilst those of *Culex* are fusiform (Fig. 30). In the great majority of mosquitoes the eggs are laid on the

surface of the water and the larvæ hatch out after two or three
days.

In *Aëdes* and *Psorophora,* however, the eggs are laid singly,
in most cases not upon the surface of water, but in such situations that the egg lies dormant for some time awaiting favourable conditions for the development of the larvæ.   In Northern

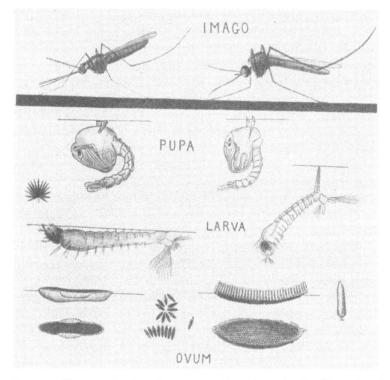

Fig. 30.   Diagram shewing the corresponding stages in the life-cycle of
   *Anopheles* (on the left) and *Culex* (on the right).   From a wall diagram
   drawn by Professor Nuttall.

regions it seems that some of the eggs, although they may be
repeatedly submerged, will not hatch until they have been
frozen, and it is by means of these eggs that the mosquitoes
manage to persist through the winter.

*The larva.*   So far as known the larvæ of all mosquitoes are
entirely aquatic in habit.   The larva possesses a distinct head

provided with strong mandibles adapted for biting. The shape
of the head varies in different families, being long and narrow
in the majority of Anophelinæ and large and broad in the
Culicinæ. The thorax is broad and its three segments are
fused together to form a single mass. The abdomen is long
and slender, and is composed of nine distinct segments. The
anus opens at the apex of the terminal segment and is surrounded by four, more or less well-developed, tracheal gills.
The respiratory system consists of two main longitudinal
tracheæ opening on the dorsal surface of the eighth abdominal
segment, either by two separate apertures in a hollow at the
base of a papilla (as in the Anophelinæ) or at the apex of a
distinct breathing tube or syphon of varying length (as in the
Culicinæ). The presence or absence of this structure furnishes
an easy method of distinguishing the larvæ of Anophelines from
those of the Culicines.

Moreover, it is possible to distinguish different genera and
even species by means of the larval characters, such as the
arrangements of the hairs on the segments, the form of the
mandibles and other head appendages, the shape of the
syphon, etc.

The larva progresses in the water by means of energetic
wriggling movements, but the larvæ of Culicines are generally
more active than those of the Anophelines. Moreover, in the
latter, because of the situation of the respiratory apertures,
and the presence of the palmate hairs, the larvæ float horizontally under the surface of the water, and closely resemble
bits of floating sticks. The Culicine larvæ merely bring the
tip of the breathing syphon in contact with the surface film
of the water and then hang downwards so that their bodies
make an angle with the surface of the water. This position
is also partly due to the heavy jaws and head, which weigh
down the anterior end. The difference in the attitude assumed
by the larvæ when at the surface of the water is very
characteristic and constitutes one of the simplest methods of
distinguishing between Anophelines and Culicines at this stage
of development (Fig. 30).

The larvæ may be either herbivorous or carnivorous. As a

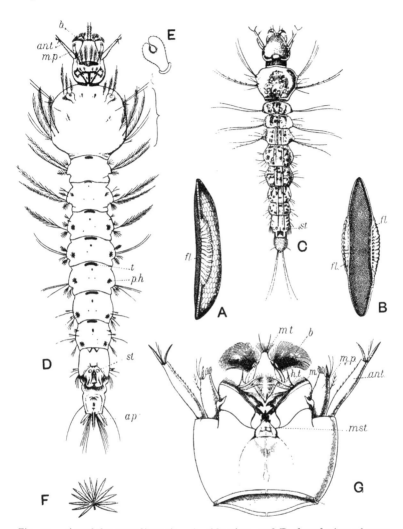

Fig. 31. *Anopheles maculipennis*. A, side view, and B, dorsal view of egg;
C, young larva, and D, fully-grown larva ; E, flabellum or flap overhanging
the base of certain thoracic hairs ; F, a palmate hair ; G, ventral view of
head of fully-grown larva. After Nuttall and Shipley. Lettering :
*ant*, antenna ; *ap*, anal papillæ ; *b*, brush ; *fl*, float ; *h*, stout hairs of
mandible which arrange the brush ; *m*, hooked hairs at edge of maxilla ;
*mp*, palp of maxilla ; *mst*, the " under-lip," or metastoma ; *mt*, median
tuft of hairs ; *ph*, palmate hair ; *st*, stigma.

general rule they feed on algæ, but many species swallow any kind of minute object that may be in the water. By means of the mouth-brushes (Fig. 31, G, b) currents are set up towards the mouth, and any small particles are carried with the stream and swallowed. Certain larvæ (e.g. Culex pipiens) seem to thrive best when the water is charged with animal refuse, whilst the larvæ of Psorophora, Lutzia and some other genera are actively predacious, feeding upon other mosquito larvæ.

When food is abundant and the temperature favourable the larva grows rapidly and may become full-grown in little more than a week. The duration of the larval stage, however, is extremely variable, for the larvæ of some species (e.g. Wyeomyia smithii) can live for nearly a year without any food. The duration is also greatly prolonged by low temperatures and it is probable that some species pass through the winter in the larval form.

During its growth the larva moults four times, the last of these moults giving rise to the pupa.

The pupa is also aquatic, and swims actively through the water, though of course it is unable to take in any food, the appendages of the head and thorax of the future fly being enclosed in a common chitinous covering. The pupa respires by means of a pair of appendages on the thorax, the respiratory trumpets, or horns (Fig. 8, tr). These trumpets communicate with the anterior pair of thoracic spiracles and when the pupa is at the top of the water they break through the surface film and thus admit air to the spiracles. The pupa is kept floating at the surface by means of a pair of fan-like tufts of hairs, situated on the dorsal surface of the first abdominal segment. The abdomen is composed of nine distinct segments; the eighth bears at its apex a pair of large chitinous plates, the paddles or fins. The shape of the trumpets and paddles varies in different species but these characters are of no generic value.

The duration of the pupal stage as a rule does not exceed more than two or three days, but as in the case of the other stages may be prolonged by low temperatures. Towards the end of this period the pupa becomes inflated with air and when the adult is about to emerge it gradually straightens its abdomen and floats almost horizontally on the surface of the water. The thoracic region then splits longitudinally and the adult mosquito gradually draws itself out of the skin and after a few minutes is able to fly away.

## BIOLOGY OF THE ADULT MOSQUITO.

*Food-habits.* Although the females of a large number of species of mosquitoes habitually feed on blood, the habit is by no means universal throughout the family, as practically all the males and a considerable number of the females feed on various plant juices. Some species, *e.g. Stegomyia fasciata*, attack man much more readily than others. The majority of the Culicinæ seem to be mainly parasitic on birds.

Mosquitoes are very susceptible to heat and cold, for during the winter they never bite except on occasional warm days. The reaction to heat is so striking that this is probably one of the main reasons of their being attracted towards warm-blooded animals and other warm objects. Howlett has shewn that hungry female mosquitoes (*Anopheles* and *Culex*) will bite viciously at a test-tube of boiling water, or even of hot copper sulphate solution. In the latter case the insects could be observed to thrust their proboscides into the crust of copper sulphate that had crystallized on the outside of the tube. It is possible that the blood-sucking habit may have been derived from what was originally a simple thermotropism (attraction by heat). A large number of mosquitoes feed only at night, but *Stegomyia fasciata* and most of the northern species, and also those inhabiting jungle, feed during the day-time

*The method of feeding.* When a female mosquito commences to feed, the tip of the labrum is placed against the surface, and then the sharp maxillæ and mandibles are thrust into the skin. The labrum is then forced into the wound and thus the whole six stylets of the proboscis enter the skin, being guided by the labium. The latter is doubled back as the mouth-parts enter deeper into the host.

The subsequent processes can only be conjectured from experiments on mosquitoes under artificial conditions, but are probably as follows.

After piercing the skin the insect begins to pass its salivary secretion along the groove in the labrum. The function of this secretion is, however, quite unknown. Meanwhile the amount of carbon dioxide in the tracheæ of the insect increases considerably owing to its proximity to the body of its host and as a result the muscular contractions are considerably augmented. The effect of this increase in the muscular contractions is to cause compression of the œsophageal diverticula, and their contents, consisting of bubbles of carbon dioxide and also of a fungus, are forced into the œsophagus and forwards through the proboscis into the wound caused by the bite. The lumen of the proboscis, buccal cavity and œsophagus is thus filled with carbon dioxide, derived from the diverticula, and this gas is supposed to retard the coagulation of the blood. The fungus, which is also extruded from the diverticula, enters the skin and is the cause of the great irritation and local swelling that often follow the bite of a mosquito. The association of this fungus with the mosquito constitutes one of the most interesting cases of commensalism hitherto described. The fungus is present in the egg, larva and pupa, and can always be found in the œsophageal diverticula of freshly emerged mosquitoes. In this region it multiplies on the food which is taken into the diverticula, and during its growth produces bubbles of carbon dioxide. When the mosquito feeds, the majority of the fungi and the bubbles of carbon dioxide are extruded, but the few remaining fungi rapidly grow on the blood which passes into the diverticula during the meal, and thus more carbon dioxide is produced. Schaudinn shewed that the inoculation of the salivary glands of the mosquito into the skin did not produce any effect, whereas the inoculation of the contents of the ventral diverticulum was followed by the formation of an irritant swelling resembling that caused by the bite of a mosquito. These results have also been confirmed by Major Williams, I.M.S., whilst working in the Quick Laboratory, Cambridge.

*Colour.* Mosquitoes, like all other blood-sucking insects, have a decided preference for dark colours and avoid lighter shades. Nuttall found that dark blue and dark red were the

most attractive colours to *Anopheles maculipennis*, whilst
yellow, white, and orange seemed to repel the insects. His
experiment is of sufficient interest to be reproduced in detail :
    " To test the influence of colour a number of pasteboard
boxes were taken, which measured 20 by 16 cms. and had a
depth of 10 cms. The boxes were lined with cloth, having a
slightly roughened surface, to which the insects could com-
fortably cling. All of the fabrics had a dull—not shiny—
surface, and each box was lined with cloth of a different colour.
The boxes were placed in rows upon the floor and upon each
other in tiers, the order being changed each day after the
observations had been made. The interior of the boxes was
moderately illuminated by light reflected from the surface of
the white tent. On 17 days during a month beginning with
the middle of June, we counted the number of flies which had
accumulated in the boxes. Counts were actually made on
17 sunny and cloudy days, and with the following result

| Colour of box | Number of *A. maculipennis* counted in each box during 17 days |
|---|---|
| Navy blue | 108 |
| Dark red | 90 |
| Brown (reddish) | 81 |
| Scarlet | 59 |
| Black | 49 |
| Slate grey | 31 |
| Dark green (olive) | 24 |
| Violet | 18 |
| Leaf green | 17 |
| Blue | 14 |
| Pearl grey | 9 |
| Pale green | 4 |
| Light blue (forget-me-not) | 3 |
| Ochre | 2 |
| White | 2 |
| Orange | 1 |
| Yellow | 0 |
| | 512 |

    " It is evident, therefore, that white or khaki-coloured
clothing is the most suitable in regions where mosquitoes are
troublesome."

*Sound.* We have already referred to the stridulating apparatus described by Shipley and Wilson, by means of which the insect emits a sound whilst flying. Certain males seem to be very susceptible to notes resembling the hum of the female and the insects have been noticed to swarm around instruments emitting particular notes. At Grantchester, near Cambridge, where *Anopheles maculipennis* and *Culex pipiens* are fairly common, the writer has noticed that these insects may be aroused to activity by the sound of a piano or violin.

Howard was informed by Mr A. De P. Weaver, that while engaged in some experiments in harmonic telegraphy, in which a musical note of a certain pitch was produced by electrical means, he found that when the note was raised to a certain number of vibrations per second, all mosquitoes, not only in the same room but also from other parts, would congregate near the apparatus and would be precipitated from the air with considerable force. He therefore covered a large surface with sticky fly-paper and after sounding the note for a few seconds caught all the mosquitoes in the vicinity.

*Habitat and modes of dissemination.* As a rule mosquitoes do not wander more than one or two hundred yards from their breeding places (see page 72). Nevertheless, occasionally migratory flights have been noticed during which the insects travelled many miles. Such a mode of dissemination, however, is certainly very rare and generally mosquitoes are spread by human agency. Ships and trains are both responsible for the introduction of species into fresh localities, as the females may remain in the holds of ships or in the carriages of trains for several days, and thus be carried hundreds of miles. The occurrence of certain species at scattered seaports in various parts of the world shews that this mode of dissemination has been of considerable importance in the past, when ships carried unprotected tanks of water.

*Resting position.* When at rest an Anopheline can generally be distinguished from a Culicine by the attitude of the body and the legs. Anophelines usually rest with the proboscis pointing towards the surface, and as the proboscis and the rest of the body are in a straight line, the insect has a very characteristic appearance and seems to be standing on its head. On the other hand, in the Culicinæ the proboscis forms an angle with the rest of the body and therefore the insect has a hump-backed appearance; moreover, it generally rests with its body parallel to the surface, or with the posterior extremity bent towards the surface. These differences in the position of rest, whilst being useful for the recognition of living mosquitoes, are by no means constant, as *Anopheles* sometimes settles in the same manner as *Culex*. The differences between the two positions are well shewn in Fig. 30.

*Hibernation.* In cold regions mosquitoes generally pass through the winter in the egg stage, but in addition some of the females hibernate in dark corners. During last winter several females of *A. maculipennis* and *Theobaldia annulata* hibernated at the top of a wardrobe in the author's bedroom at Grantchester, disappearing after the warm weather in April. In tropical countries mosquitoes generally hibernate during the dry season, when all the breeding pools disappear. In addition, however, some of their eggs may remain in the mud at the bottom of dried pools and develop when these are again filled with water.

*Longevity.* There are very few observations on the longevity of mosquitoes, but the length of life of the female seems to be far greater than that of the male. Those females which hibernate may live for nearly a year, but in confinement Anophelines have not been kept alive for more than about a month. In the case of *Aëdes* Knab has found that the female may live for at least three months, and *Stegomyia* has been kept alive for 154 days.

*Mating habits.* In many species, *e.g. Culex pipiens*, the males form large swarms, to which the females seem to be attracted. The latter, however, merely fly to the swarm in order to secure a mate, and as soon as this is effected the pair at once drops out of the swarm. This habit of forming swarms is not entirely confined to the male sex, for swarms of females have been observed side by side with those of males. Copulation may be accomplished either on the wing, as in the case of *Stegomyia fasciata*, or whilst resting, and is generally of but short duration.

*Flight.* Although long flights have been recorded in isolated cases, there is little doubt that as a rule the flight of mosquitoes is very limited, rarely exceeding a quarter of a mile. From a prophylactic point of view, the distance they are capable of travelling is of great importance, for in most countries it is only possible to keep circumscribed areas free from mosquitoes, and if the insects were able to travel any considerable distance these areas would be continually invaded by mosquitoes from the surrounding country. It is known that this does not happen to any marked degree, but occasionally long flights have been recorded suggesting that under some conditions the Culicidæ may travel considerable distances. The majority of such flights seem to be of a migratory nature and the cause of them is unknown. The most authentic accounts all come from America, where the salt-marsh species belonging to the genus *Aëdes* are certainly capable of travelling five to ten miles, whilst distances of as much as 40 miles have been recorded. Such flights, however, must be regarded as very exceptional and, from a prophylactic point of view, may be disregarded.

*Enemies.* In the section on the methods of destruction of these insects, we shall have occasion to refer again to some of the natural enemies of the mosquitoes. The greatest mortality takes place amongst the immature stages, which are exposed to the attacks of countless enemies. In fact the observations of Nicholls and others have shewn that the larvæ of mosquitoes are practically unable to exist in permanent waters, as the latter contain such large numbers of predaceous aquatic animals, such as fish, dragon-fly larvæ, beetles, etc. The importance of fish in destroying larvæ is now generally recognized, but unfortunately in many cases it is rather difficult to employ this means of destruction, as the mosquitoes can breed in small pools of water where fishes cannot live.

The bladder-worts, *Utricularia*, capture various animals in their small bladders, and in this way considerable numbers of the larvæ may be destroyed, as the plants will grow in stagnant pools. In addition another insectivorous plant, *Aldrovanda vesiculosa*, a member of the sundew family, captures mosquito larvæ, its leaves closing quickly on any animal that touches them.

The larvæ are sometimes destroyed by fungi and bacteria, but these groups of organisms are neither of them very important enemies.

Both the adult insect and its immature stages are parasitized by various species of Protozoa and also by nematodes and trematodes. Insect enemies are responsible for the destruction of enormous numbers of mosquitoes. The larvæ of Hydrophilidæ and Dytiscidæ devour large numbers of larvæ,

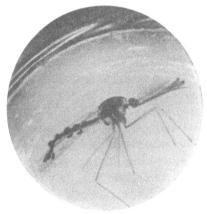

Fig. 32. *Anopheles maculipennis* ♂ captured in Cambridge, shewing acarine parasites attached to the body. (From a photograph taken by Professor Nuttall.)

and one *Dytiscus* larva has been known to destroy 434 mosquito larvæ in two days. Whirligig beetles (Gyrinidæ) are also great enemies of the larvæ, and no *Anopheles* has a chance in any water inhabited by them. Similarly the various species of aquatic Hemiptera destroy the larvæ and also emerging imagoes, or females laying their eggs. Dragon-flies in the adult stage feed on other flying insects, and in their immature stages devour mosquito larvæ, etc. Their voracious habits, in all stages, are notorious, and they must destroy enormous numbers of Culicidæ along with other Diptera. Some of the most formidable natural enemies of the mosquito larvæ are to be found amongst the family Culicidæ itself. The predaceous and cannibalistic larvæ of *Psorophora, Lutzia, Megarhinus,* etc., readily attack larvæ either of their own, or other species. The larva of *Lutzia* is so effective that in Rio de Janeiro it has been employed to destroy the larvæ of the more dangerous *Stegomyia fasciata.* The immature stages of many other aquatic Diptera also prey on the Culicidæ.

Various predaceous Diptera, especially the Empididæ, capture mosquitoes along with other insects ; a blood-sucking fly, *Simulium,* has been observed to kill mosquitoes by sucking the blood out of them. A most curious case, however, is that of an Anthomyid fly, *Lispa sinensis,* which has been seen to catch and eat the larvæ of mosquitoes in Hongkong. A Dolichopodid fly of Panama also attacks the larvæ in a similar manner.

Mites have frequently been seen attached to the bodies of both the adult and immature stages of mosquitoes. In some regions, *e.g.* Uganda, as many as 50 per cent. of the mosquitoes may be attacked. The presence of these mites, however, does not seem to affect seriously the health of the host, though no doubt it may be weakened. Spiders undoubtedly destroy large numbers of mosquitoes, and are amongst the most efficient natural enemies of the adult insects. The jumping spiders of the genus *Salticus* are very common in houses in the tropics, and are a most valuable aid in the destruction of both mosquitoes and flies.

Newts and the aquatic larvæ of salamanders readily devour mosquito larvæ, and the latter are rarely found in pools inhabited by these batrachians.

In India the common gecko lizard destroys large numbers of Culicidæ in houses, and therefore should be encouraged as it is quite harmless.

Birds and bats, however, must be regarded as the most important vertebrate enemies of the adult mosquitoes. The smaller insectivorous birds, night-hawks, swifts and swallows, all devour enormous numbers of Diptera. More than 600 insects, mostly mosquitoes, have been counted from the stomach of an American swift (*Chætura pelagica*). In addition aquatic and shore-birds eat considerable numbers of the larvæ. At least nine species of shore-birds, mostly phaloropes and sand-pipers, are known to eat mosquitoes, and any such birds should be strictly protected.

### REFERENCES.

Howard, L. O. (1902). *Mosquitoes.* New York: McClure, Phillips and Co.

Howard, L. O., Dyar, H. G. and Knab, F. (1912). *The Mosquitoes of North and Central America and the West Indies.* Carnegie Institute of Washington. Publication No. 159. (Contains complete references to literature on the subject.)

Howlett, F. M. (1910). The Influence of Temperature upon the Biting of Mosquitoes. *Parasitology*, vol. III. pp. 479–484.

Imms, A. D. (1907–8). On the Larval and Pupal Stages of *Anopheles maculipennis*, Meigen. *Journ. of Hygiene*, vol. VII. pp. 291–318, and *Parasitology*, vol. I. pp. 103–133.

Nicholls, Lucius (1912). Some observations on the Bionomics and Breeding-places of *Anopheles* in Saint Lucia, West Indies. *Bull. Entomol. Research*, vol. III. pp. 251–268.

Nuttall, G. H. F. and Shipley, A. E. (1901–1903). The Structure and Biology of *Anopheles*. *Journ. of Hygiene*, vol. I. pp. 45–77, 269–276 and 451–484; vol. II. pp. 58–84; vol. III. pp. 166–215.

Schaudinn (1904). Generations- und Wirtswechsel bei Trypanosomen und Spirochæten. *Arb. a. d. Kaiserlichen Gesundheitsamte*, vol. XX. pp. 387–438.

Shipley, A. E. and Wilson, E. (1902). On a possible stridulating organ in the Mosquito (*Anopheles maculipennis* Meigen). *Trans. Roy. Soc. Edin.* vol. XL. pp. 367–372.

Theobald, F. V. (1901–10). *A monograph of the Culicidæ of the World.* London: Brit. Mus. Vols. I–V.

# CHAPTER VIII

CULICIDÆ (MOSQUITOES) *continued*.  CLASSIFICATION

The most recent classification of the Culicidæ is that given by Edwards, and is as follows.

*Family.* CULICIDÆ.
  *Sub-family.* CULICINAE. (Ordinary mosquito with long proboscis.)
    1.  Tribe.  Anophelinæ.
    2.  Tribe.  Megarhininæ.

3. Tribe. Culicinæ

= Metanotopsilæ $\left\{\begin{array}{l}\text{Culicinæ}\\ \text{Aedinæ}\\ \text{Uranotæninæ}\end{array}\right\}$ of Theobald.

4. Tribe. Sabethinæ

= Metanototrichæ $\left\{\begin{array}{l}\text{Trichoprosoponinæ}\\ \text{Dendromyinæ}\end{array}\right\}$ of Theobald.

*Sub-family.* CHAOBORINÆ. (Midge-like mosquitoes without piercing proboscis.)

= Corethra. Meigen.
= Sayomyia. Coquillet.

*Sub-family.* DIXINÆ. (No piercing proboscis.)

## TRIBE I. ANOPHELINÆ.

Female palps as long as the proboscis. Male palpi clubbed.
Scutellum simple and bar-shaped.

Larva without respiratory tube.

According to Theobald and others adopting his views the Anophelinæ consist of some 20 or more genera distinguished by differences in scale structure. The general nature of this subdivision and the more important genera are shewn in the following scheme :

I. No true scales[1] on either thorax or abdomen.

*a.* Upright head scales are narrow and rod-like *Stethomyia.* Theobald.

*b.* Upright head scales are of ordinary expanded type.

(*a*) Wing scales moderately broad, widest in the middle.
Without prothoracic tuft .. .. *Anopheles* Meigen.
With prothoracic tuft .. .. *Patagiamyia.* James.

(*b*) Wing scales narrow, widest towards free end
*Myzomyia.* Blanchard.

(*c*) Wing scales inflated .. .. .. *Cycloleppteron.* Theobald.

II. No true scales dorsally on either thorax or abdomen, but there is a tuft of scales ventrally on the penultimate abdominal segment. *Myzorhynchus* Blanchard.

---

[1] A very useful distinction has been made by James between *true* and *false* scales. True scales, besides being broader, have striations which can readily be counted. False scales, which correspond roughly to the *hair-like scales* of Theobald, shew only indistinct striations which are too indefinite to be counted.

III. Thorax covered with true scales.

*a.* No scales on abdomen.
Head scales of ordinary type  ..  ..  *Pyretophorus*. Blanchard.
Head scales rather flattened  ..  ..  *Myzorhynchella*. Theobald.
*b.* Scales on last few segments of abdomen only
*Nyssorhynchus*. Blanchard.
*c.* Many scales on abdomen but no lateral tufts
*Neocellia*. Theobald.
*d.* Lateral scale tufts as well as other scales on the abdomen.
*Cellia*. Theobald.

In addition there are genera represented by only one or two species. Thus there is *Feltinella* Theobald, near *Patagiamyia*, for *F. pallidopalpi* Theo. (basal lobes of male genitalia jointed); and *Lophoscelomyia* Theo. for *L. asiatica* Leicester, a peculiar species with scale tufts on the femora, also related to *Patagiamyia*. Near *Myzomyia* come *Pseudomyzomyia* Theo., for *P. rossii* Giles[1], and *Neomyzomyia* Theo., for *N. elegans* James. *Kerteszia* Theo., for *K. boliviensis* Theo., and *Manguinhosia* Cruz, for *M. lutzi* Cruz, are also genera without scales on the thorax, but with scales on the last segments of the abdomen. Both are of new world distribution. Near *Neocellia*, but with a complete row of ventral scale tufts, is *Christophersia* James, for *Ch. kochii* Dönitz, and near *Nyssorhynchus*, but with outstanding scales on the antenna, is *Calvertina* Ludlow, for *C. lineata* Ludlow. Very peculiar genera are *Christya* Theo., for *C. implexa* Theo., an immense *Anopheles* with long lateral tufts of hair-like scales on the abdomen, *Chagasia* Cruz, for *C. fajardoi* Cruz, a species with *Culex*-like attitude, and *Arribalzagia* Theo., for *A. maculipes* Theo., and two other species of elaborately ornamented and very large Anophelines from Brazil. The genus *Bironella* Theo., for *B. gracilis* Theo., a species known only from a single male specimen, has very short forked cells. It is not quite certain, however, that it is an Anopheline.

Edwards sinks all these genera excepting *Bironella* under *Anopheles* Meigen, maintaining that the differences in scale

[1] *M. rossii* Giles is the type species of *Myzomyia*. Therefore the formation of a genus *Pseudomyzomyia* having *M. rossii* as the type species is not allowable.

structure are insufficient upon which to found genera. In this case the Anophelinæ are considered as represented by a single genus (*Anopheles* Meigen, type species *A. maculipennis* Meigen) containing some hundred or more species.

These conflicting views regarding nomenclature make it very difficult at present to treat of the systematic arrangement of this sub-family. The most that can be done is to give some classified tabulation of the species based on their more conspicuous characters, and to indicate as far as possible groups of species corresponding to a particular scale structure and hitherto given generic rank. In this respect use has been made of the general scheme of the natural affinities of the Anophelinæ given by Christophers. In this scheme the Anophelinæ are subdivided into three main natural divisions, the relation of these divisions to the genera already mentioned being as follows :

A.  Protoanopheles.
   *Stethomyia.*
   *Anopheles, Patagiamyia* and *Lophoscelomyia.*
   *Myzorhynchus, Cyclolepteron, Arribalzagia* and *Notonotricha* (Coquillet).
B.  Deuteroanopheles.
   *Myzomyia* and *Pyretophorus.*
   *Pseudomyzomyia.*
   *Nyssorhynchus, Neocellia* and *Cellia.*
C.  Neoanopheles.
   *Neomyzomyia,* etc.

In the following table the known species of Anophelinæ are arranged in the form of a synoptic table. In this table 12 groups more or less readily differentiated both by general characters and by scale structure are given. The species which compose these groups often so closely resemble one another that they differ only in a few minute details, a generalized description serving for the chief characters of all the species in the group. The chief characters of any species, therefore, to a large extent can be gleaned from the table, but for a full description of each species the present space is inadequate, and systematic works on the Culicidæ must be consulted.

A second table is given shewing all described species of *Anopheles*, with their synonymy if necessary, and their relation as far as is known to the transmission of malaria.

## *Dichotomous Table shewing Natural Grouping of Species of Anophelinæ.*

1. Costa has less than four main dark spots .. .. .. .. 2
   Costa has at least four main dark spots .. .. .. .. 6
2. Costa without any pale interruption even at apex .. .. 3
   Costa with at least one pale interruption .. .. .. .. 4
3. Female palps with second segment disproportionately long
                             Group  1.  (*Stethomyia.*)
   Female palps of ordinary Anopheline type
                             Group  2.  (*Anopheles.*)
4. No true scales on mesothorax .. .. .. .. .. 5
   Mesothorax with true scales .. Group 5. (*Arribalzagia.*)
5. Wing veins without mixed dark and light scales
                             Group  3.  (*Patagiamyia.*)
   Wing veins with mixed dark and light scales
                             Group  4.  (*Myzorhynchus.*)
6. Not more than three dark spots on sixth vein .. .. .. 7
   More than three dark spots on sixth vein Group 12. (*Neomyzomyia.*)
7. Terminal segment of female palps considerably less than half length of
       penultimate segment .. .. .. .. .. .. 8
   Terminal segment at least half length penultimate .. .. 9
8. Mesothorax without true scales .. Group 6. (*Myzomyia.*)[1]
   Mesothorax with true scales .. Group 7. (*Pyretophorus.*)[1]
9. Mesothorax not clothed with true scales Group 8. (*Pseudomyzomyia.*)[1]
   Mesothorax covered with true scales .. .. .. .. 10
10. Abdomen without lateral tufts .. .. .. .. .. 11
    Abdomen with lateral tufts .. .. Group 11. (*Cellia.*)
11. Palps very shaggy as in *Myzorhynchus* Group 10. (*Myzorhynchella.*)
    Palps not so shaggy .. .. .. Group 9. (*Nyssorhynchus.*)

## *Table shewing Detailed Tabulation of Species of Anophelinæ.*

# A.  Protoanopheles.

Number of main dark costal spots is less than four. Junctions of cross-veins with longitudinal veins and bifurcations of second and fourth veins dark scaled.

A'. Costa devoid of any pale areas even at apex of wing.

    **Group 1.**  Female palps with the second segment disproportionally long, segments three and four both being short.
      (*Stethomyia.* Theobald. Type species *S. nimba.* Theo.)
        *General characters of groups.*
          *Appearance.* Attitude *Culex*-like, legs thin and slender. Palps long and thin.

---

[1] *Vide,* however, remarks on the type species of these genera and nomenclature.

*Markings.*   Wings.   Unspotted.

            Palps.   Unbanded.

            Legs.    Entirely unornamented.

*Scale structure.*   Head scales narrow and linear, not expanded as in all other *Anopheles*.   No scales on pro-thorax, mesothorax or abdomen.

*Species.*

     *A. nimba.*   Theobald.

     *A. aitkeni.*   James.

     *A. culiciformis.*   James and Liston.

     *A. corethroides.*   Theobald.

*Synonymy.*

     *A. pallida.*   Ludlow = *A. aitkeni* (James).

     *A. fragilis.*   Theobald = *A. aitkeni* (James).

     *A. treacheri.*   Leicester = *A. aitkeni* (James).

Differentiation of species.

Thorax adorned.

   Silvery median and lateral lines    ..   *A. nimba.*

   No silvery lines ..    ..    ..    ..   *A. corethroides.*

Thorax not adorned.

   Anterior forked cell very long ..    ..   *A. aitkeni.*

   Anterior forked cell not unusually long   *A. culiciformis.*

**Group 2.**   Second segment of female palps not disproportionately long, terminal segment not less than half length of penultimate (orthodactylous).

     (*Anopheles* Meigen, *sensu.* James. Type species *A. maculipennis.* Meigen.)

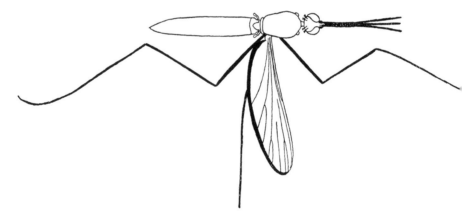

Fig. 33.   *Anopheles bifurcatus.*   (Group 2.)

*General characters of group.*

     *Appearance.*   Attitude *Anopheles*-like. Mostly large species with thin palps and slender limbs.

*Markings.* Wings devoid of any pale spots (except *A. crucians* and *A. eiseni*).

*Palps.* Unbanded (except in *A. smithii* and faint bands in *A. immaculatus*).

*Legs.* Unornamented except for pale areas at tibio-femoral and tibio-tarsal joints. Tarsi unbanded.

*Scale structure.* Head scales expanded. No prothoracic tuft. No scales on mesothorax or abdomen. Wing scales moderately broad.

*Species.*
- *A. maculipennis.* Meigen.
- *A. bifurcatus.* Linnæus.
- *A. plumbeus.* Haliday.
- *A. algeriensis.* Theobald.
- *A. barianensis.* James and Liston.
- *A. barberi.* Coquillet*.
- *A. immaculatus.* James.
- *A. smithii.* Theobald.
- *A. eiseni.* Coquillet.
- *A. crucians.* Wiedemann.

\* *Cœlodiazesis barberi.* Coquillet.

*Synonymy.*

*C. bifurcatus.* Meigen
*A. quadrimaculatus.* Say  } = *A. maculipennis.* Meigen.
*A. annulimanus.* Van der Wulp

*C. claviger.* Fabricius  } = *A. maculipennis.* Meigen.
*A. grisescens.* Stephens  or *A. bifurcatus.* Linn.

*A. atropos.* Dyar and Knab
*A. occidentalis.* Dyar and Knab } = ? *A. maculipennis.* Meigen.

*C. trifurcatus.* Fabricius
*A. villosus.* Desvoidy } = *A. bifurcatus.* Linnæus.
*A. walkeri.* Theobald

*A. nigripes.* Stæger = *A. plumbeus.* Haliday.
*A. ferruginosus.* Wied. = *A. crucians.* Wied (?).

*Differentiation of species.*

A. Wings without pale spots on any of the veins.
Dark spots at cross-veins and bifurcations .. *A. maculipennis.*
Wings uniformly dark without any spots.

  (i) *Palps unbanded.*
  Petiole of first forked cell more than ⅓ length of cell.
    Thorax with pale but not white streak anteriorly.
      Abdomen with yellow hairs .. .. *A. bifurcatus.*
      Abdomen with brown hairs .. .. *A. algeriensis.*
      Abdomen with black and white hairs .. *A. barianensis.*
    Thorax with white streak .. .. .. *A. nigripes.*
  Petiole of first forked cell ⅓ length of cell .. *A. barberi.*

  (ii) *Palps banded.*
  Banding indistinct, light mosquito .. .. *A. immaculatus.*
  Banding narrow but distinct, dark mosquito *A. smithii.*

B.  Wings with some pale areas.
        Hind tibiæ with broad, white, apical band        *A. eiseni.*
        Hind tibiæ without broad band    ..    ..    *A. crucians.*

A″.  Costa shews at least one pale interruption.

(*a*)  *No true scales on mesothorax.*

**Group 3.**  Wing veins do not shew any conspicuous admixture of dark
and light scales.

(*Patagiamyia.*  James.  Type species *A. gigas.*  Giles.)

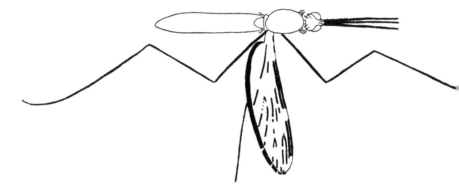

Fig. 34.  *Anopheles* (*Patagiamyia*) *gigas.*  (Group 3.)

*General characters of group.*

*Appearance.*  Attitude *Anopheles*-like.  Usually rather large Ano-
            phelines of brownish colour.

*Markings.*  Wings spotted.  Dark costal spots may be distinct and
            well separated by pale areas but there are not four
            main dark spots.
            Palps.  Unbanded or with four narrow bands including
            pale apex.
            Legs.  Knee spots present.  Tarsi unbanded or banded,
            but not conspicuously.  Except for a white band on
            femur present in some species no other ornamentation
            of legs.

*Scale structure.*  Head scales expanded.  No prothoracic tuft.  No
            true scales on mesothorax.  Abdomen may or
            may not have scales on last few segments of
            abdomen, but some scales are usually present,
            especially in male.

*Species.*

A. *gigas.* Giles.
A. *simlensis.* James and Liston.
A. *punctipennis.* Say.
A. *formosus.* Ludlow.
*A. *pallidopalpi.* Theobald.
**A. *lindesayi.* Giles.
**A. *lindesayi* var. *maculata.* Theobald.
**A. *asiatica.* Leicester.
**A. *wellingtonianus.* Alcock.
A. *atratipes.* Skuse.
A. *franciscanus.* McCracken.
A. *perplexans.* Ludlow.
A. *pseudopunctipennis.* Theobald.
*Feltinella.* Theobald. Type species *F. pallidopalpi.*
**Lophoscelomyia.* Theobald. Type species *L. asiatica.* Leicester.

*Synonymy.*

A. (*Culex*) *hyemalis.* Filch = *A. punctipennis.* Say.
*Lophomyia.* Giles = *Lophoscelomyia.* Theobald.

*Differentiation of species.*

Costa with large prominent dark spots.
Palps not banded  ..   ..   ..   ..  *A. gigas.*
Palps banded.
  Tarsi banded.

                             *A. simlensis.*
                             *A. formosus.*

  Tarsi unbanded.
    Fringe spots present at all vein endings
                           *A. pseudopunctipennis.*
                           *A. franciscanus.*

    Fringe spots absent
                           *A. punctipennis.*
                           *A. pallidopalpi.*

    One fringe spot present  ..   ..  *A. perplexans.*
Costa with narrow interruptions only.
  Femur with broad white band.
    Ruff of scales on femur.
      White band apical  ..   ..   ..  *A. asiatica.*
      White band not apical   ..   ..  *A. wellingtonianus.*
    No ruff of projecting scales  ..   ..  *A. lindesayi.*
  Femur without pale band   ..   ..  *A. atratipes.*

**Group 4.** Wing scales with conspicuous admixture of dark and light
    scales.
  (*Myzorhynchus.* Blanchard. Type species *M. sinensis.* Wied.)
  *General characters of group.*
    *Appearance.* Large species, black or nearly so. *Anopheles*-attitude
      strongly developed. Palps markedly shaggy.

                                  6—2

*Markings.*   Wings dark with minute pale interruptions on costa
usually only two in number, one at apex and one at
junction of subcosta with costa. Sixth vein has two
conspicuous dark spots, the scales forming which
aggregated. Light spots on upper surface of wing
not in all cases reproduced below.

Palps.   Unbanded or with four narrow pale bands
including pale apex.

Legs.   Knee spots, banded tarsus, and in some cases
further ornamentation.

*Scale structure.*   Head scales expanded. Prothoracic tuft present.
No scales on mesothorax. May or may not be
scales on terminal portion of abdomen. A tuft
of scales usually present on ventral surface of
penultimate abdominal segment. Wing scales
very broad.

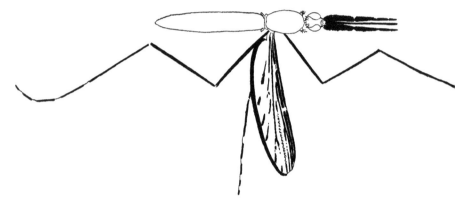

Fig. 35.   *Anopheles (Myzorhynchus) barbirostris.* (Group 4.)

*Species.*

A. *barbirostris.* Van der Wulp.
A. *pseudobarbirostris.* Ludlow.
A. *bancroftii.* Giles.
A. *umbrosus.* Theobald.
A. *albotæniatus.* Theobald.
A. *strachani.* Theobald.
A. *sinensis.* Wiedemann.
A. *sinensis* var. *indiensis.* Theobald.
A. *pseudopictus.* Grassi.
A. *paludis.* Theobald.
{ A. *paludis* var. *similis.* Theobald.
{ A. *mauritianus.* Grandpré.
*A. *grabhamii.* Theobald.

* *Cycloleppteron.* Theobald.   Type species *C. grabhamii.* Theobald.

*Synonymy.*

A. *vanus.* Walker  
A. *annularis.* Van der Wulp  
A. *jesoënsis.* Tsuzuki       = *A. sinensis.* Wied.  
A. *plumiger.* Dönitz  
A. *minutus.* Theobald  

A. *uigerrimus.* Giles        } = *A. sinensis* var. *indiensis.*  
A. *nigerrimus.* James and Liston }     Theobald.  

A. *separatus.* Leicester      } = ? *A. sinensis.* Wied.  
A. *peditæniatus.* Leicester }  

A. *brachypus.* Dönitz = (?) *A. sinensis.* Wied.  
A. *alboannulatus.* James and Liston = *A. albotæniatus.* Theobald.  
A. *paludis* var. *similis.* Theobald = *A. mauritianus.* Grandpré.  
A. *mauritianus.* Grandpré = (?) *A. paludis.* Theobald.  

A. *coustani.* Laveran  
A. *ziemani.* Van Grünberg   } = *A. mauritianus.* Grandpré.  
A. *tenebrosus.* Dönitz  

A. *pictus.* Loew      } = *A. pseudopictus.* Grassi.  
A. *pictus.* Ficalbi }  

*Differentiation of species.*

A. Wing scales not inflated (*Myzorhynchus*).  
    Tip of hind tarsus not white.  
    Palpi not banded.  
    Hind tarsal points narrowly banded.  
      No fringe spots .. .. .. .. *A. strachini.*  
      One fringe spot .. .. .. .. *A. umbrosus.*  
      Two fringe spots.  
        Legs not mottled .. .. .. *A. barbirostris.*  
        Legs mottled .. .. .. *A. pseudobarbirostris.*  
      Several fringe spots .. .. .. *A. bancroftii.*  
    Hind tarsi broadly banded .. .. .. *A. albotæniatus.*  
    Palpi banded.  
      Wing fringe with one pale spot .. *A. sinensis.*  
      Wing fringe unspotted .. .. .. *A. pseudopictus.*  
B. Wing scales inflated (*Cycloleppteron*) .. .. *A. grabhamii.*

(b) *Mesonotum with true scales.*

**Group 5.** Costa with broad pale interruptions.

    (*Arribalzagia.* Theobald. Type species *A. maculipes.* Theobald.)  
    *General characters of group.*  
      *Appearance.* Large highly ornamented species.  
      *Markings.* Wings prominently spotted, but with three main dark spots only. Small accessory spots present in addition to those at base of costa. Pale spots on upper surface of wing in many cases not represented beneath. Sixth vein with more than two spots.  
      *Palps.* Four pale bands.  
      *Legs.* Speckled and ornamented.

*Scale structure.* Heavily scaled species. Head scales expanded. Prothorax with tufts. Mesothorax with broad scales. Abdomen with scales and lateral tufts.

*Species.*

  *A. maculipes.* Theobald.
  *A. pseudomaculipes.* Chagas.
  *A. malefactor.* Dyar and Knab.
  \*A. *mediopunctatus.* Theobald.
  \*A. *intermedium.* Chagas.

\* *Notonotricha.* Coquillet. Type species *N. mediopunctatus.*

## B.  Deuteroanopheles.

Number of main dark costal spots, four. Not more than three dark spots on sixth vein. Junctions of cross-veins with longitudinals and bifurcations of second and fourth veins the seat of light interruptions (except *Myzorhynchella*).

B′.  Female palps with terminal segment considerably less than half penultimate. Tarsi not broadly banded. Tips of hind-legs not white.

**Group 6.**  Mesothorax without true scales.
  (*Myzomyia.* Blanchard[1].)

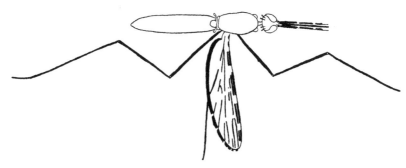

Fig. 36.  *Anopheles (Myzomyia) listoni.* (Group 6.)

---

[1] The type species of *Myzomyia* is *M. rossii* Giles, but this species does not conform to the characters of *Myzomyia* as now usually understood. Group 6, therefore, though it contains most of the well-known *Myzomyiæ* (*A. funesta, A. listoni,* etc.) cannot correctly be described as *Myzomyia,* which name ought to be retained for whatever group *M. rossii* represents. Similarly, the name *Pseudomyzomyia* proposed by Theobald for *M. rossii* is incorrect.

*General characters of group.*

*Markings.*  Small brownish species.  Wings with four main dark costal spots.  Middle spot not completely broken (*i.e.* shewing double interruption on first longitudinal as in *A. maculatus.*  Theobald).  Sixth vein with two or fewer dark spots (except *A. albirostris* Theobald, which has three).  Fringe spots usually absent at sixth vein and often deficient at other vein endings.

*Palps.*  Three pale bands, the apical one including the whole of the apical segment[1].

*Legs.*  Knee spots and sometimes narrow and inconspicuous tarsal banding, but no other ornamentation.

*Scale structure.*  Head scales expanded.  No prothoracic scale tufts.  Mesothorax without true scales.  Abdomen without scales.  Wing scales narrow.

*Species.*

 *A. funesta.*  Giles.
 *A. funesta* var. *subumbrosa.*  Theobald.
 *A. funesta* var. *umbrosa.*  Theobald.
 *A. listoni.*  Liston.
 *A. rhodesiensis.*  Theobald.
 *A. culicifacies.*  Giles.
 *A. nili.*  Theobald.
 *A. turkhudi.*  Liston.
 *A. hispaniola.*  Theobald.
 *A. albirostris.*  Theobald.
 *A. hebes.*  Dönitz.
 *A. flavicosta.*  Edwards.
 *A. impunctus.*  Dönitz.
 *A. longipalpis.*  Theobald.
 *A. pyretophoroides.*  Theobald.
 *A. azriki.*  Patton.
 *A. d'thali.*  Patton.
 *A. jehafi.*  Patton.

*Synonymy.*

 *A. listoni.*  Giles  ⎫
 *A. turkhudi.*  Giles  ⎬ = *A. culicifacies.*  Giles.
 *A. indica.*  Theobald ⎭
 *A. leptomeres.*  Theobald = (?) *A. culicifacies.*  Giles.
 *A. kumassii.*  Chalmers = *A. funesta.*  Giles.
 *A. umbrosa.*  Edwards (nom. preoc.) = *A. funesta* var. *umbrosa.* Theobald.
 *A. fluviatilis.*  Stephens and Christophers.  MSS. ⎱ = *A. listoni.*
 *A. christophersi.*  Theobald ⎰ Liston.
 *A. christophersi* var. *alboapicalis.*  Theo. = *A. albirostris.*  Theo.
 *A. albirostris.*  Theo. = (?) *A. aconita.*  Dönitz.
 *A. formosaensis.*  Tsuzuki = (?) *A. aconita* var. *cohæsa.*  Dönitz.
 *A. impunctata.*  Dönitz-Blanchard = *A. impunctus.*  Dönitz.
 *A. pictus.*  Macdonald = *A. hispaniola.*  Theobald.
 *A. cruzii.*  Dyar and Knab = *A. lutzi.*  Theobald.

---

[1] In *A. turkhudi* and *A. hispaniola* the tip is dark.

*Differentiation of species.*

Proboscis unbanded.
  Apex of palps pale.
    Fringe spots present at all veins except sixth.
      Tarsal banding distinct though not conspicuous.
        Third longitudinal light    ..    ..    ..    *A. funesta.*
        Third longitudinal dark    ..    ..    ..    *A. funesta* var.
                                              *umbrosa.*
      Tarsal banding absent or very narrow and indistinct
                                      *A. listoni.*
    Fringe spots absent or present only at two or three veins.
      Palps with three pale bands.
        No fringe spots  ..    ..    ..    ..    ..    *A. rhodesiensis.*
        Two fringe spots ..    ..    ..    ..    ..    *A. culicifacies.*
      Palps with pale apex only    ..    ..    ..    *A. nili.*
  Apex of palps dark.
    Black apex narrow    ..    ..    ..    ..    ..    *A. turkhudi.*
    Black apex broader    ..    ..    ..    ..    ..    *A. hispaniola.*
Proboscis with apical half white ..    ..    ..    ..    *A. albirostris.*
                                            *A. aconita.*

**Group 7.**    Mesothorax with blue scales.

(*Pyretophorus* [1].    Blanchard.)

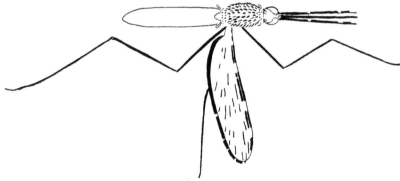

Fig. 37.    *Anopheles* (*Pyretophorus*) *neavei*.    (Group 7.)

*General characters of group.*

  *Appearance.*    Mostly rather light brown species with notably long and thin palps.

  *Markings.*    Wings with four dark spots usually not completely broken.    Wing fringe spots most frequently absent from sixth vein.

            Palps.    With three bands or four.    Sometimes with dark apex.

            Legs.    Free from speckling or marked banding of tarsus.

[1] Though most of the members of the genus *Pyretophorus* are included here, this generic name cannot be employed, as *P. costalis* Loew, the type species, clearly belongs to a separate group.

*Scale structure.* Head scales expanded. No prothoracic tuft. Mesothorax scaled. Abdomen completely devoid of
scales.

*Species.*

A. *superpictus.* Grassi.
A. *nursei.* Theobald.
A. *nigrifasciatus.* Theobald.
A. *cleopatræ.* Willcocks. MSS.
A. *cardamitisi.* Newstead and Carter.
A. *distinctus.* Newstead and Carter.
A. *distinctus* var. *melanocosta.* Newstead and Carter.
A. *palestinensis.* Theobald.
A. *cinereus.* Theobald.
A. *sergentii.* Theobald.
A. *jeyporensis.* James.
A. *myzomyfacies.* Theobald.
A. *chaudoyei.* Theobald.
A. *transvaalensis.* Carter.
A. *minimus.* Theobald.
A. *pitchfordi.* Power.
A. *arabiensis.* Patton.
A. *austenii.* Theobald.

*Synonymy.*

A. *nursei.* Theobald = (?) A. *nigrifasciatus.* Theobald variety
A. *chaudoyei.* Billet = A. *chaudoyei.* Theobald.

*Differentiation of species.*

Palps with one broad pale band.
  Apex of palps light.
    Third costal spot not completely broken.
      Sixth vein with two dark spots    ..    ..   A. *sergentii.*
      Sixth vein with three dark spots.
        Costal spots more or less confluent    ..   A. *distinctus*
        Costal spots distinct.
        Tarsi not banded.

|  |  |
|---|---|
| Very similar species .. .. | .. { A. *nursei.* / A. *cleopatræ.* / A. *palestinensis.* / A. *minimus.* |
| Fore and hind tarsi banded .. | .. A. *cinereus.* |
| All tarsi banded .. .. .. | .. { A. *cardamatisi.* / A. *superpictus.* |

  Apex of palps dark.
    Tarsi not banded .. .. .. .. .. A. *nigrifasciatus.*
    Tarsi not banded.
      Three dark lines on mesonotum .. .. A. *myzomyfacies.*
      Two dark lines on mesonotum .. .. A. *chaudoyei.*
Palps with two broad pale bands .. .. .. A. *austenii.*

B″.  Apical segment of female palps at least half length of penultimate.  Tarsi broadly banded.

(a)  *Mesothorax not completely clothed with true scales.*

**Group 8.**

(*Pseudomyzomyia.* Theobald[1].  *Myzomyia.* Blanchard.  Type species, *Ps. rossii.* Giles.)

*General characters of group.*

*Appearance.*  Light fawn to moderately dark species.  Palps rather shaggy.

*Markings.*  Wings with light areas much developed.  Costa with four main dark spots.  Third spot completely broken.  Sixth vein with two dark spots.  Fringe spots at all veins.

Palps.  Three light bands, the apical one including whole of last segment.

Legs.  Tarsi banded.  May be speckled.  Tips of hind tarsi not white.

*Scale structure.*  Head scales expanded.  No prothoracic tufts.  Mesothorax mostly with narrow hair-like scales.  Abdomen with some scales on last segment, especially in male.

*Species.*

A. *rossii.*  Giles.

A. *indefinata.*  Ludlow.

A. *ludlowi.*  Theobald.

A. *mangyana.*  Banks.

*Synonymy.*

A. *mangyana.*  Banks=(?) A. *ludlowi.*  Theobald.

A. *vagus.*  Dönitz=A. *rossii.*  Giles.

A. *rossii* var. *indefinata.*  Ludlow=A. *indefinata.*  Ludlow.

*Differentiation of Species.*

Legs not speckled.

| Apical palpal band very broad | .. | .. | A. *indefinata.* |
| Apical band not so broad | .. | .. | A. *rossii.* |

Legs speckled.

| Large species | .. | .. | .. | A. *ludlowi.* |
| Smaller species | .. | .. | .. | A. *mangyana.* |

(b)  *Mesothorax completely clothed with true scales.*
*Abdomen without lateral tufts.*

**Group 9.**  Palps moderately shaggy only.  Bifurcations of second and fourth veins both sites of pale interruptions.  Head scales as in majority of Anophelines.

(*Nyssorhynchus.*  Blanchard[2].)

---

[1] *Vide* footnote to Group 6, on page 86.

[2] Here again there is confusion in the nomenclature.  The type species of *Laverania* Theobald (=*Nyssorhynchus* Blanchard) is A. (*Cellia*) *argyrotarsis.* The well-known group of so-called *Nyssorhynchus*, therefore, is incorrectly so called.

*General characters of group.*

*Appearance.* Highly ornamented species. Tips of hind tarsi always white.

*Markings.* Wings clearly spotted.  Fringe spots at all vein endings. Sixth vein with three spots.

*Palps.* With three bands.

*Legs.* With white hind tarsi often speckled.

*Scale structure.* Head scales expanded.  Mesothorax covered with scales. Abdomen with some scales.

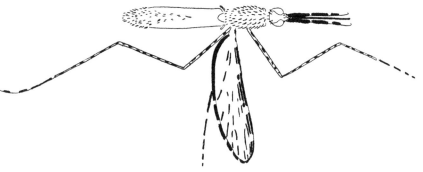

Fig. 38.  *Anopheles (Nyssorhynchus) maculatus.*  (Group 9.)

*Species.*

A. *fuliginosus.*  Giles.
A. *nivipes.*  Theobald.
A. *freeræ.*  Banks.
A. *philippinensis.*  Ludlow.
A. *fowleri.*  Christophers.
A. *jamesii.*  Theobald.
A. *pretoriensis.*  Theobald.
A. *maculipalpis.*  Giles.
A. *maculatus.*  Theobald.
A. *theobaldi.*  Giles.
*A. *willmori.*  James.
*A. *stephensi.*  Theobald.
A. *costalis.*  Loew.
A. *costalis* var. *melas.*  Theobald.
A. *pseudocostalis.*  Theobald.
A. *merus.*  Dönitz.
A. *marshallii.*  Theobald.
†A. *kochii.*  Dönitz.
A. *karwari.*  James and Liston.
A. *ardensis.*  Theobald.
A. *aureosquamiger.*  Theobald.

* *Neocellia.*  Theobald.  Type species *A. willmori.*  James.
† *Christophersia.*  James.  Type species *A. kochii.*  Dönitz.

††*A. lineata.* Ludlow.
 *A. flava.* Ludlow.
 *A. waponi.* Edwards.
 *A. tibani.* Patton.

†† *Calvertina.* Ludlow. Type species *A. lineata.* Ludlow.

*Synonymy.*

*A. gambiæ.* Giles ⎫
*A. gracilis.* Dönitz ⎭ =*A. costalis.* Loew.

*A. jamesii.* Liston ⎫
*A. leucopus.* Dönitz ⎭ =*A. fuliginosus.* Giles.

*A. dudgeoni.* Theobald=*A. willmori.* James.
*A. indica.* Theobald=*A. willmori* var. James.

*A. pseudowillmori.* Theobald. ⎫
*A. willmori.* Leicester         ⎬ =*A. maculatus.* Theobald.
*A. willmori.* Watson           ⎭

*A. maculipalpis.* James and Liston ⎫ =*A. maculipalpis* var.
*A. indiensis.* Theobald            ⎭   *indiensis.* Theo.

*A. nigrans.* Staunton=*A. karwari.* James.
*A. halli.* James=*A. kochii.* Dönitz.

*A. intermedia.* Rothwell ⎫
*A. metaboles.* Theobald  ⎭ =*A. stephensi.* Theobald.


*Differentiation of species.*

A.  Tips of hind tarsi white.
 Palps with not more than one broad band.

  (*a*)  Legs not speckled.
   White band at junction of first and second tarsal segment.
                                    ⎧ *A. fuliginosus.*
    Very closely related species ..    ..    .. ⎨ *A. nivipes.*
                                    ⎨ *A. freeræ.*
                                    ⎩ *A. philippinensis.*
   No white band at junction of first and second tarsal segments
                                          *A. fowleri.*

  (*b*)  Legs speckled.
   Palpi with speckling in addition to bands  ..  *A. maculipalpis.*
   Palps without speckling.
    Three tarsal segments pure white  ..  .. *A. jamesii.*
    Two tarsal segments pure white  ..  .. *A. pretoriensis.*
   Palps with two broad bands.
    Two tarsal segments altogether white  ..  .. *A. theobaldi.*
    One tarsal segment only altogether white.
     Scales on last few segments of abdomen  .. *A. maculatus.*
     Scales on all segments ..  ..  ..  .. *A. willmori.*
   Palp with more than two broad bands.
    Palps with five white bands   ..  ..  .. *A. kochii.*
    Palps with four white bands   ..  ..  .. *A. karwari.*

B.　Tips of hind tarsi not white.
　　Apical band of palps only broad.
　　　First tarsus not spotted.
　　　　Fringe spots narrow.
　　　　　Femur speckled　　　..　　..　　..　　..　*A. costalis.*
　　　　　Femur not speckled　..　　..　　..　　..　*A. pseudocostalis.*
　　　　Fringe spots broad　　　..　　..　　..　　..　*A. merus.*
　　　First tarsus spotted　　　　..　　..　　..　　..　*A. ardensis.*
　　Two palpal bands broad.
　　　A few scales on abdomen　　　..　　..　　..　*A. marshallii.*
　　　Many scales on abdomen ..　　..　　..　　..　*A. stephensi.*

Group 10.　Palps markedly shaggy.　Bifurcations of second and fourth
　　　　　veins (one or both) dark scaled.　Head scales flattened.
　　(*Myzorhynchella.*　Theobald.　Type species *M. nigra.*　Theobald.)
　　　*General characters of group.*
　　　　*Appearance.*　Black species.　Palps shaggy.
　　　　*Markings.*　Costa with four main dark spots, the light interruptions
　　　　　　in some cases bridged by dark on first longitudinal.
　　　　　　Palps.　Unbanded or with four bands.
　　　　　　Legs.　May be ornamented.
　　　*Scale structure.*　Head scales flattish.　Prothoracic tuft present.
　　　　　　　Mesothorax scaled.　Abdomen free from scales.
　　　*Species.*
　　　　　*A. nigra.*　Theobald.
　　　　　*A. lutzi*[1].　Cruz.
　　　　　*A. parva.*　Chagas.
　　　　　*A. nigritarsis.*　Chagas.
　　　　　*A. tibiomaculata.*　Neiva.
　　　　　*A. gilesa.*　Neiva.

　　　　　　(c)　*Abdomen with lateral scale tufts.*
Group 11.
　　(*Cellia.*　Theobald.　Type species *A. pharoensis.*　Theobald.)

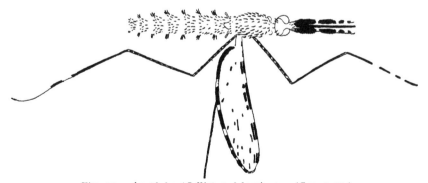

Fig. 39.　*Anopheles (Cellia) pulcherrimus.*　(Group 11.)

[1] There are three species of *A. lutzi*, of which *A. (Myzomyia) lutzi* Theobald
was first so named.　*A. (Myzorhynchella) lutzi* Cruz, therefore, requires
renaming if generic distinctions between the Anophelinæ are dropped.

*General characters of group.*

    *Markings.* Costa with four main dark spots.   Fringe spots at all veins.

    Palps.   With four light bands.

    Legs.   Ornamented.

    *Scale structure.*   Head scales expanded.   Prothorax may have a few scales or a tuft.   Mesothorax covered with scales.   Abdomen with scales and lateral scale tufts.

*Species.*

| | |
|---|---|
| *A. argyrotarsis.*  Desvoidy. | *A. pharoensis* var. *alba.*  Ventrillon. |
| *A. albimanus.*  Wied. | *A. bigotii.*  Theobald. |
| *A. jacobi.*  Hill and Haydon. | *A. gorgasi.*  Dyar and Knab. |
| *A. cincta.*  Newstead and Carter. | *A. squamosa.*  Theobald. |
| *A. pulcherrima.*  Theobald. | *A. squamosa* var. *arnoldi.*  Newstead |
| *A. pharoensis.*  Theobald. | and Carter. |

*Synonymy.*

*A. albipes.*   Theobald
*A. cubensis.*   Agramonte
*A. tarsi-maculatus.*   Goeldi   $\Big\} = A.$ *albimanus.*   Wied.
*A. argyrotarsis.*   Theobald
*A. albitarsis.*   Arribalzaga $= A.$ *argyrotarsis.*   Desvoidy.
*A. albofimbriata.*   Giles $= A.$ *pharoensis.*   Theobald.
*A. bozasi.*   Neveu-Lemaire $= (?) A.$ *pharoensis.*   Theobald.
*A. braziliensis.*   Chagas $= (?) A.$ *argyrotarsis.*   Desvoidy.
*A. punctipennis.*   Bigot. MSS. $= A.$ *bigotii.*   Theobald.
*A. squamosa arnoldi.*   Stephens and Christophers $= A.$ *squamosa* var. *arnoldi.*   Stephens and Christophers.

*Differentiation of species.*

Tips of all legs pale.
    Metatarsus with distinct bands    ..    ..    ..  *A. cincta.*
    Metatarsus with flecks of white only ..    ..    ..  *A. jacobi.*
Tips of hind-legs only pale.
  (*a*)  Three segments of hind tarsus altogether white.
    Apex of abdomen dark    ..    ..    ..  *A. argyrotarsis.*
    Apex of abdomen whitish grey    ..    ..  *A. braziliensis.*
  (*b*)  Three segments of hind tarsus white except for small dark band on last segment    ..  *A. albimanus.*
  (*c*)  One segment only of hind tarsus white.
    Femora and tibiæ mottled  ..    ..    ..    ..  *A. pharoensis.*
    Femora and tibiæ not mottled  ..    ..    ..  *A. bigotii.*
Tips of hind-legs not pale ..    ..    ..    ..    ..  *A. squamosa.*

## C.   Neoanopheles.

Costa with four main dark spots.   Sixth vein with more than three dark spots.   Junctions of cross-veins with longitudinal veins and bifurcations of second and fourth veins the seat of pale interruptions.

**Group 12.**

(*Neomyzomyia.*  Theobald.   Type species *A. elegans.* James.)

*General characters of group.*

*Markings.*   Wings with a large number of spots on veins.   Third
   longitudinal with several dark and light areas.   Sixth
   vein may have five or six dark spots.
      Palps.   With well-marked white bands.
      Legs.   Speckled and ornamented.
*Scale structure.*   Prothorax usually with scale tuft.

*Species.*

| | | |
|---|---|---|
| *A. elegans* [1]. James. | *A. punctulata.* | Dönitz. |
| *A. annulipes.* Walker. | *A. tessellatus.* | Theobald. |
| *A. masteri.* Skuse. | *A. natalensis.* | Hill and Haydon. |
| *A. deceptor.* Dönitz. | *A. watsoni.* | Leicester. |

*Synonymy.*

   *A. ceylonica.*   Newstead and Carter=(?) *A. tessellatus.* Theobald.
   *A. leucosphyrus.*   Dönitz=(?) *A. elegans.* James.
   *A. muscivus.*   Skuse=*A. annulipes.* Walker.
   *A. ocellatus.*   Theobald=*A. punctatus.* Dönitz.
   *A. punctulatus.*   Theobald=*A. tessellatus.* Theobald.
   *A. punctulata.*   James=*A. tessellatus.* Theobald.
   *A. thorntonii.*   Ludlow=(?) *A. tessellatus.* Theobald.

*Peculiar Anophelines not placed in Table.*

*A. jajardoi.*   Lutz (*Chagasia,* Cruz).
*A. boliviensis.*   Theobald (*Kerteszia,* Theobald).
*A. lutzi.*   Cruz (*Manguinhosia,* Cruz).
*A. gracilis.*   Theobald (*Bironella,* Theobald).
*A. implexa.*   Theobald (*Christya,* Theobald).
*A. lineata.*   Ludlow (*Calvertina,* Ludlow).
*A. brunnipes.*   (? *Nyssorhynchus.*) Theobald.
*A. christyi.*   (? *Nyssorhynchus, Neocellia.*) Newstead and Carter.
*A. lutzi.*   (? *Myzomyia.*) Theobald.
*A. wellcomei.*   (? *Anopheles.*) Theobald.
*A. pseudosquamosa.*   (? *Cellia.*) Newstead and Carter.

*Insufficiently described or doubtful Species.*

| | |
|---|---|
| *A. annulipalpis.* Arrib. | *A. maculicosta.* Becker. |
| *A. annulipes.* Arrib. | *A. martini.* Laveran. |
| *A. antennatus.* Becker. | *A. multicolor.* Camboulin. |
| *A. cohæsus.* Doune [2]. | *A. pursati.* Laveran. |
| *A. error.* Theobald=(no species). | *A. stigmaticus.* Skuse. |
| *A. farauti.* Laveran. | *A. subpictus.* Grassi. |
| *A. formosaensis* II. Tsuzuki [2]. | *A. vincenti.* Laveran. |
| *A. neiriti.* Ventrillon. | |

[1] *Neomyzomyia* Theobald.
[2] According to Kinoshita, *A. cohæsus* and *A. formosaensis = A. listoni.*

TABLE II. *The known species of Anophelines, with thei*
*their habitat and connectio*

| Species and Synonyms | Present group tabulation and generic synonymy | Distribution |
|---|---|---|
| 1. *A. aconita* Dönitz [3] .. .. | 6. (*Myzomyia*) .. Malay .. .. | |
| 2. *A. aconita* var. *cohæsa* Dönitz [4] .. | 6. (*Myzomyia*) .. Malay .. .. | |
| 3. *A. aitkeni* James [1a] (1903) .. | 1. (*Stethomyia*) .. India, Malay .. | |
| 4. *A. albimana* Wiedemann [1] .. | 11. (*Cellia*) .. S. & C. America .. | |
| 5. *A. albipes* Theobald [2] .. .. | 11. (*Cellia*) .. W. Indies, S. America | |
| 6. *A. albirostris* Theobald [6] .. .. | 6. (*Myzomyia*) .. Malay, etc. .. .. | |
| 7. *A. albitarsis* Arribalzaga [3] .. | — | — |
| 8. *A. alboannulatus* James & Liston [4] | 4. (*Myzorhynchus*) | Malay .. .. |
| 9. *A. albofimbriata* Giles (1904) .. | 11. (*Cellia*) .. | Egypt .. .. |
| 10. *A. albotæniatus* Leicester [2] .. | 4. (*Myzorhynchus*) | Malay .. .. |
| 11. *A. algeriensis* Theobald [6] (1903) .. | 2. (*Anopheles*) .. | N. Africa .. |
| 12. *A. annularis* Van der Wulp [4] .. | 4. (*Myzorhynchus*) | Malay .. .. |
| 13. *A. annulimanus* Van der Wulp [2] .. | 2. (*Anopheles*) .. | — |
| 14. *A. annulipalpis* Arrib. [1] .. .. | — | Argentine .. .. |
| 15. *A. annulipes* Walker [3] .. .. | 12. (*Nyssorhynchus*) | Australia .. .. |
| 16. *A. annulipes* Arrib. [1] .. .. | — | Argentine .. .. |
| 17. *A. antennatus* Becker .. .. | — | — |
| 18. *A. ardensis* Theobald [11] .. .. | 10. (*Pyretophorus*) .. | Natal .. .. |
| 19. *A. argyrotarsis* Desvoidy [1] .. | 11. (*Cellia*) .. | West Indies, S. America, etc. .. |
| 20. *A. arabiensis* Patton .. .. | ? 10. .. .. | Aden .. .. |
| 21. *A. arnoldi* Stephens & Christophers | 11. (*Cellia*) .. | Transvaal .. .. |
| 22. *A. asiatica* Leicester [1] .. .. | 3. (*Lophoscelomyia*) | Malay .. .. |
| 23. *A. atratipes* Skuse [1] .. .. | 3. (*Pyretophorus*) .. | Australia .. .. |
| 24. *A. atropos* Dyar & Knab [2] .. | 2. (*Anopheles*) .. | N. America .. .. |
| 25. *A. aureosquamiger* Theobald [14] .. | 10. (*Nyssorhynchus*) | Transvaal .. .. |
| 26. *A. aurivostris* Watson .. .. | — | — |
| 27. *A. austenii* Theobald [10] .. .. | 7. (*Pyretophorus*) .. | Angola .. .. |
| 28. *A. azriki* Patton .. .. .. | 6. (*Myzomyia*) (?) | Aden .. .. |
| 29. *A. bancroftii* Giles [4b] .. .. | 4. (*Myzorhynchus*) | Australia .. .. |
| 30. *A. barberi* Coquillet [4] (1903) .. | 2. (*Anopheles*) .. | — |
| 31. *A. barbirostris* Van der Wulp [4] .. | 4. (*Myzorhynchus*) | India, Malay, China |
| 32. *A. barianensis* James & Liston [4] (1911) .. .. .. .. | 2. (*Anopheles*) .. | India .. .. |
| 33. *A. bellator* Dyar & Knab [2] .. | 6. (*Myzomyia*) (?) | |
| 34. *A. bifurcatus* Linnæus [2] (1758) .. | 2. (*Anopheles*) .. | Europe .. .. |
| 35. *A. bifurcatus* Meigen [1] .. .. | 2. (*Anopheles*) .. | Europe .. .. |
| 36. *A. bigotii* Theobald [2] .. .. | 11. (*Cellia*) .. | Chili .. .. .. |
| 37. *A. bisignata* .. .. .. .. | 6. (*Myzomyia*) .. | — |
| 38. *A. boliviensis* Theobald [12] .. | (*Kerteszia*) .. | S. America .. |
| 39. *A. bozasi* Neveu-Lemaire [3] .. | 11. (*Cellia*) .. | N. Africa .. .. |
| 40. *A. brachypus* Dönitz .. .. | 4. (*Myzorhynchus*) | Malay .. .. |

| ransmission experiments. :ycle observed of— r. Malignant tertian, .q. Quartan ; f z, to zygote stage, nd s, to sporozoite stage | Observations regarding transmission in nature. (z) Zygote and (s) Sporozoite stage observed | Epidemiological evidence of transmission | Remarks |
|---|---|---|---|
| — | — | — | =*A. albirostris* Theobald (?). |
| — | — | — | =*A. formosaënsis* II Tsuzuki. |
| — | — | Daniels, ( + )? Christophers ( + ) ? | Forest and jungle species biting by day like a *Stegomyia*. |
| arling, s.t. s), m.t. (s) | Darling, (t) .. | — | Commonest carrier in Central and Tropical S. America. 70 % of those fed by Darling became infected. |
| — | — | — | =*A. albimana* Wied. |
| :aunton, m.t. | Staunton, (z) .. | James, Staunton, ( + ) | Important carrier in Malay. |
| — | — | — | =*A. argyrotarsis.* |
| — | — | — | =*A. albotæniatus.* |
| — | — | — | =*A. pharoënsis.* |
| — | Ed.& Et.Sergent, (s) | — | Important carrier in Algeria (littoral). |
| — | — | — | =*A. sinensis* Wied. |
| — | — | — | =*A. maculipennis* Wied. |
| inoshita, л.т. | — | — | Common Australian species. |
| — | — | — | — |
| ·arling, (f) | Darling, m.t. (?), (z) | — | — |
| — | Patton, (s) .. | — | Important carrier in Aden Hinterland. =*A. squamosa* var. *arnoldi* Newstead and Carter. |
| — | — | — | — |
| — | — | — | =? *A. albirostris* Theobald. |
| — | — | — | — |
| tephens & Christophers m.t. | Doubtful (Christophers) | — | — |
| — | — | Unlikely to carry in nature owing to distribution | Hill species. 8000 ft. |
| ·rassi, (t) .. | Grassi, (t) .. | — | Common English *Anopheles*. =*A. maculipennis* Meigen. |
| — | — | — | — |
| — | — | — | =*A. sinensis* (?). |

H. B. F.

| Species and Synonyms | Present group tabulation and generic synonymy | Distribution |
|---|---|---|
| 41. A. braziliensis Chagas .. .. | 11. (Cellia) .. | S. America .. .. |
| 42. A. brunnipes Theobald [17] .. | ? (Nyssorhynchus) | Angola .. .. |
| 43. A. cardamitisi Newst. & Carter [1] | 7. (Pyretophorus) .. | Greece .. .. |
| 44. A. ceylonica Newst. & Carter [1] .. | 12. — | Ceylon .. .. |
| 45. A. chaudoyei Theobald [6] .. | 7. (Pyretophorus) .. | Algeria, etc. .. .. |
| 46. A. chaudoyei Billet .. .. .. | — | — |
| 47. A. christophersi Theobald [4] .. | — | — |
| 48. A. christophersi var. alboapicales Theobald [17] .. .. .. | — | — |
| 49. A. christyi Newst. & Carter [2] .. | 11. (Neocellia) .. | Uganda .. .. |
| 50. A. cincta Newst. & Carter [1] .. | 11. (Cellia) .. | West Africa .. .. |
| 51. A. cinereus Theobald [2] .. .. | 7. (Pyretophorus) .. | Africa .. .. |
| 52. A. claviger Fabricius .. .. | — | — |
| 53. A. cohæsus Doune .. .. .. | — | — |
| 54. A. corethroides Theobald [14] (1907) | 1. (Stethomyia) .. | Australia .. .. |
| 55. *A. costalis Loew [2] .. .. .. | 10. (Pyretophorus) .. | Africa .. .. |
| 56. A. costalis var. melas Theobald [6] | 10. (Pyretophorus) .. | Africa .. .. |
| 57. A. coustani Laveran [2] .. .. | — | — |
| 58. A. crucians Wied. [2] (1828) .. | 2. (Anopheles) .. | N. America .. .. |
| 59. A. cruzii Dyar and Knab [1] .. | — | — |
| 60. A. cubensis Agramonte .. .. | — | — |
| 61. A. culicifacies Giles [3] .. .. | 6. (Myzomyia) .. | India .. .. |
| 62. A. culiciformis James & Liston [4] (1904) .. .. .. .. | 1. (Stethomyia) .. | India .. .. |
| 63. A. deceptor Dönitz [2] .. .. | 12. ( ) | Malay .. .. |
| 64. A. distinctus Newst. & Carter [2] .. | 7. (Pyretophorus) .. | Rhodesia .. .. |
| 65. A. distinctus var. melanocosta Newst. & Carter [2] .. | 7. (Pyretophorus) .. | Rhodesia .. .. |
| 66. A. d'thali Patton .. .. .. | 6. (Myzomyia) (?) | Aden .. .. |
| 67. A. dudgeoni Theobald [16] .. .. | 11. (Neocellia) .. | — |
| 68. A. eiseni Coquillet [3] (1902) .. | 2. (Anopheles) .. | C. America .. .. |
| 69. A. elegans James [1a] .. .. | 12. (Neomyzomyia) | — |
| 70. A. error Theobald [2] .. .. | (Aldrichia) .. | |
| 71. A. fajardoi Lutz [1] .. .. .. | (Chagasia) .. | Brazil .. .. |
| 72. A. farauti Laveran [3] .. .. | — | — |
| 73. A. ferruginosus Wied. [2] .. .. | — | — |
| 74. A. flava Ludlow [5] .. .. .. | 10. (Nyssorhynchus) | — |
| 75. A. flavicosta Edwards [1] .. .. | ? | Nigeria .. .. |
| 76. A. fluviatilis Stephens & Christophers MSS. .. .. .. | — | — |
| 77. A. formosaënsis I Tsuzuki .. .. | 6. (Myzomyia) .. | Formosa .. .. |
| 78. A. formosaënsis II Tsuzuki .. | ? | Formosa .. .. |
| | 3. (Patagiamyia) .. | Formosa .. .. |
| 79. A. formosus Ludlow [6b] .. .. | | |
| 80. A. fowleri Christophers [1] .. .. | 10. (Nyssorhynchus or Neocellia) | India .. .. |

| Transmission experiments. Cycle observed of— T. Malignant tertian, s.T. Simple tertian, Q. Quartan ; f z, to zygote stage, and s, to sporozoite stage | Observations regarding transmission in nature. (z) Zygote and (s) Sporozoite stage observed | Epidemiological evidence of transmission | Remarks |
|---|---|---|---|
| — | — | — | $=A. argyrotarsis$ (?). |
| — | — | — | — |
| — | — | — | $=A. tessellatus$ Theobald. |
| — | — | Billet, ( + )  .. | Common *Anopheles* in oases, **breeding** in saline waters. |
| — | — | — | $=A. chaudoyei$ Theobald. |
| — | — | — | $=A. listoni$ Liston. |
| — | — | — | $=A. albirostris.$ |
| — | — | — | — |
| — | — | — | $= \begin{cases} A. maculipennis \text{ Meigen.} \\ A. bifurcatus \text{ Linnæus.} \end{cases}$ |
| — | — | — | — |
| oss, Annett & Austen s.T. Q. M.T. | Ross, Stephens & Christophers, etc. (s) | — | Active and common transmitter in Tropical Africa. |
| — | — | — | $=A. mauritianus$ Grandpré. |
| — | — | — | $=A. (Myzomyia) lutzi$ Theobald. |
| — | — | — | $=A. albimana$ Wied. |
| tephens & Christophers, s.T. Q. M.T. | Stephens & Christophers, (s) | — | Commonest Indian carrier. |
| — | — | — | — |
| — | — | Patton, ( + ?) .. | — |
| — | — | — | $=A. willmori$ James. |
| — | — | — | Forest species in Andamans (**Christophers**), ? any part in transmission. |
| — | — | — | $=$no species. |
| — | — | — | $=A. crucians$ (?). |
| — | — | — | $=A. listoni$ Liston. |
| suzuki, M.T. s) | Tsuzuki (s) | Tsuzuki, ( + ) .. | $=A. aconita$ var. *cohæsa* Dönitz (?). |
| suzuki, M.T. s) | Tsuzuki (s) | Tsuzuki, ( + ) .. | — |
| — | — | — | — |

| Species and Synonyms | Present group tabulation and generic synonymy | Distribution |
|---|---|---|
| 81. *A. fragilis* Theobald [8] .. .. | — | — |
| 82. *A. franciscanus* McCracken [1] .. | ? (*Anopheles*) .. | California, etc. .. |
| 83. *A. freeræ* Banks [1] .. .. .. | 10. (*Nyssorhynchus*) | Philippines .. .. |
| 84. *A. fuliginosus* Giles [4a] .. .. | 10. (*Nyssorhynchus*) | India, etc. .. .. |
| | | |
| 85. *A. funesta* Giles [2] .. .. .. | 6. (*Myzomyia*) .. | Africa .. .. |
| | | |
| 86. *A. funesta* var. *subumbrosa* Theobald [6] .. .. .. .. | 6. (*Myzomyia*) .. | Africa .. .. |
| 87. *A. funesta* var. *umbrosa* .. .. | 6. (*Myzomyia*) .. | Africa .. .. |
| 88. *A. funesta* var. *neiriti* Blanchard .. | 6. (*Myzomyia*) .. | Africa .. .. |
| 89. *A. gambiæ* Giles [4b] .. .. | — | — |
| 90. *A. gigas* Giles [3] .. .. .. | 3. (*Patagiamyia*) | India .. .. |
| | | |
| 91. *A. gilesi* Neiva .. .. .. | 9. (*Myzorhynchella*) | Brazil .. .. |
| 92. *A. gorgasi* Dyar and Knab .. | 11. (*Cellia*) .. | C. America .. .. |
| 93. *A. grabhamii* Theobald .. .. | 4. (*Cycloleppteron*) | W. Indies, S. America |
| 94. *A. gracilis* Theobald [12] .. .. | (*Bironella*) .. | — |
| 95. *A. gracilis* Dönitz .. .. | — | — |
| 96. *A. grisescens* Stephens [2] .. .. | — | — |
| 97. *A. halli* James [3a] .. .. .. | — | — |
| 98. *A. hebes* Dönitz [3] .. .. .. | 6. (*Myzomyia*) .. | East and S.W. Africa |
| 99. *A. hispaniola* Theobald [6] .. .. | 6. (*Myzomyia*) .. | N. Africa, Spain .. |
| | | |
| 100. *A. (C.) hyemalis* Fitch .. .. | | |
| 101. *A. immaculatus* James [1] (1902) .. | 2. (*Anopheles*) .. | India .. .. |
| 102. *A. implexa* Theobald [7] .. .. | (*Christya*) .. | Africa .. .. |
| 103. *A. impunctus* Dönitz .. .. | 6. (*Myzomyia*) .. | Egypt .. .. |
| 104. *A. indefinata* Ludlow [4] .. .. | — | — |
| | | |
| 105. *A. indica* Theobald [14] .. .. | 10. (*Neocellia*) .. | India .. .. |
| 106. *A. indica* Theobald [2] .. .. | 6. (*Myzomyia*) .. | India .. .. |
| 107. *A. indiensis* Theobald [14] .. | 10. (*Nyssorhynchus*) | India .. .. |
| 108. *A. indiensis* .. .. .. | 4. (*Myzorhynchus*) | India .. .. |
| 109. *A. intermedia* Rothwell .. .. | — | India .. .. |
| 110. *A. intermedium* Chagas .. .. | 5. (*Cycloleppteron, Notonotricha*) | Brazil .. .. |
| 111. *A. jacobi* Hill and Haydon .. .. | 11. (*Cellia*) .. | Natal .. .. |
| 112. *A. jamesii* Theobald [2] .. .. | 10. (*Nyssorhynchus*) | India .. .. |
| 113. *A. jamesii* Liston .. .. .. | — | — |
| 114. *A. jehafi* Patton .. .. .. | — | — |
| 115. *A. jesoënsis* Tsuzuki .. .. | — | Formosa, etc. .. |
| 116. *A. jeyporensis* James [1] .. .. | 7. (*Pyretophorus*) .. | India .. .. |
| 117. *A. harwari* James & Liston .. | 10. (*Nyssorhynchus*) | India, Malay .. |
| | | |
| 118. *A. kochii* Dönitz [1] .. .. | — | — |
| | | |
| 119. *A. kumassii* Chalmers .. .. | — | — |
| 120. *A. leptomeres* Theobald [6] .. .. | — | — |
| 121. *A. leucopus* Dönitz [1] .. .. | — | — |

| ransmission experiments. Cycle observed of— r. Malignant tertian, T. Simple tertian, Q. Quartan; z, to zygote stage, nd s, to sporozoite stage | Observations regarding transmission in nature. (z) Zygote and (s) Sporozoite stage observed | Epidemiological evidence of transmission | Remarks |
|---|---|---|---|
| — | — | — | — |
| — | — | — | — |
| ephens & hristophers, T. (z) Q. (z). | Adie, (s) .. .. | — | Not an active carrier as far as known. Adie found only 1 in 200 infected. |
| oss, Annett Austen, T. Q. Daniels, M.T. | Stephens & Christophers, (s); sometimes 50 % infected | — | Active and important common carrier in Tropical Africa. |
| — | — | — | — |
| — | — | — | *vide A. neiriti* Ventrillon [1]. |
| — | — | — | $=A.$ *funesta* Giles. |
| — | — | Improbable acting as carrier owing to distribution | Hill species. |
| — | — | — | — |
| — | — | — | — |
| — | — | — | $=A.$ *costalis* Loew. |
| — | — | — | $=A.$ *maculipennis* or *A. bifurcatus*. |
| — | — | — | $=A.$ *hochii* Dönitz. |
| — | Ed. & Et. Sergent, (T) (s) | — | Common carrier, Algeria and S. Spain. |
| — | — | — | $=A.$ *punctipennis* Say. |
| — | — | — | — |
| — | Negative in Andamans (Christophers) | — | — |
| — | — | — | $=A.$ *willmori* James var. |
| — | — | — | $=A.$ *culicifacies* Giles. |
| — | — | — | $=A.$ *maculipalpis* var. *indiensis* Theo. |
| — | — | — | $=A.$ *sinensis* var. *indiensis* Theobald. |
| ruz, (T) .. | — | — | $=A.$ *stephensi* Liston. |
| — | — | — | — |
| — | — | — | $=A.$ *fuliginosus* Giles. |
| — | — | — | $=A.$ *cinereus* (?) (Theobald). |
| — | — | — | $=A.$ *sinensis*. |
| — | — | Staunton (suspected) Daniels, ( + ) probable | — |
| — | — | — | $=A.$ *funesta* Giles. |
| — | — | — | $=A.$ *culicifacies* Giles (?). |
| — | — | — | $=A.$ *fuliginosus* Giles. |

| Species and Synonyms | Present group tabulation and generic synonymy | Distribution |
|---|---|---|
| 122. A. leucosphyrus Dönitz [1] .. .. | 12. (Neomyzomyia) | Malay, etc. .. .. |
| 123. A. lindesayi Giles [4a] .. .. | 3. (Patagiamyia) | India .. .. |
| 124. A. lindesayi var. maculata Theobald [17] .. .. .. .. | 3. (Patagiamyia) | India .. .. |
| 125. A. lineata Ludlow .. .. .. | (Calvertia) .. | Philippines .. .. |
| 126. *A. listoni Liston [1] .. .. .. | 6. (Myzomyia) .. | India .. .. |
| 127. A. listoni Giles .. .. .. | — | — |
| 128. A. longipalpis Theobald [6] .. | 6. (Myzomyia) .. | Central Africa .. |
| 129. *A. ludlowi Theobald [6] .. .. | 8. (Pseudomyzomyia) | Malay .. .. |
| 130. A. lutzi Cruz .. .. .. .. | 9. (Myzorhynchella) | Brazil .. .. |
| 131. A. lutzi Cruz .. .. .. .. | (Manguinhosia) | Brazil .. .. |
| 132. *A. lutzi Theobald .. .. .. | ? (Myzomyia ?) .. | Brazil .. .. |
| 133. *A. maculatus Theobald [2] .. .. | 10. (Nyssorhynchus) | India .. .. |
| 134. A. maculicosta Becker .. .. | — | — |
| 135. A. maculipalpis Giles [4b] .. .. | 10. (Nyssorhynchus) | China .. .. |
| 136. A. maculipalpis James & Liston .. | — | — |
| 137. *A. maculipalpis var. indiensis Theobald .. .. .. .. | 10. (Nyssorhynchus) | India .. .. |
| 138. *A. maculipennis Meigen [2] (1818) .. | 2. (Anopheles) .. | Europe, America .. |
| 139. A. maculipes Theobald [6] .. .. | 5. (Arribalzagia) .. | Brazil .. .. |
| 140. †A. malefactor Dyar and Knab [1a] .. | 5. (Arribalzagia) .. | Brazil .. .. |
| 141. A. mangyana Banks [1] .. .. | — | — |
| 142. A. marshallii Theobald [6] .. .. | 10. (Pyretophorus) .. | Mashonaland .. |
| 143. A. martini Laveran [3] .. .. | — | Cambodia .. .. |
| 144. A. mauritianus Grandpré .. .. | 4. (Myzorhynchus) | Mauritius, Madagascar |
| 145. A. masteri Skuse [1] .. .. .. | 12. (Nyssorhynchus) | Australia .. .. |
| 146. A. mediopunctatus Theobald [6] .. | 5. (Cycloleppteron) | Brazil .. .. |
| 147. A. merus Dönitz .. .. .. | — | Africa .. .. |
| 148. A. metaboles Theobald [4] .. .. | — | — |
| 149. A. minimus Theobald [2] .. .. | 7. (Pyretophorus) .. | China .. .. |
| 150. A. minutus Theobald [6] .. .. | — | — |
| 151. A. multicolor Cambouln .. .. | — | — |
| 152. A. muscivus Skuse [1] .. .. | — | — |
| 153. A. myzomyfacies Theobald [14] .. | 7. (Pyretophorus) .. | Algeria .. .. |
| 154. A. natalensis Hill & Haydon .. | 2. (Myzorhynchus ?) | Natal .. .. |
| 155. A. nigerrimus Giles [4a] .. .. | — | — |
| 156. A. nigerrimus James & Liston [4] .. | — | — |
| 157. A. nigra Theobald [14] .. .. | 9. (Myzorhynchella) | Brazil, etc. .. .. |
| 158. A. nigrans Staunton .. .. | — | — |
| 159. A. nigrifasciatus Theobald [14] .. | 7. (Pyretophorus) .. | India .. .. |
| 160. A. nigripes Stæger .. .. .. | — | — |
| 161. A. nigritarsis Chagas [1] .. .. | 9. (Myzorhynchella) | Brazil .. .. |
| 162. A. nili Theobald [9] .. .. | 6. (Myzomyia) .. | Africa .. .. |

| Transmission experiments. Cycle observed of— r.T. Malignant tertian, Q. Quartan; T. Simple tertian, z, to zygote stage, and s, to sporozoite stage | Observations regarding transmission in nature. (z) Zygote and (s) Sporozoite stage observed | Epidemiological evidence of transmission | Remarks |
|---|---|---|---|
| — | — | — | Hill species. |
| inoshita, (T) | Stephens & Christophers, (s) | — | Active and important carrier in certain terai tracts in India. |
| — | — | —. | =A. culicifacies Giles. |
| — | Christophers, (z) M.T. | Christophers (carrier in Andamans) | Important salt-swamp breeding and littoral malaria carrier. |
| — | — | Lutz, (T)  .. | Forest carrier, breeding in bromelias, etc. |
| aunton, M.T. | Watson (N. willmori Watson = N. maculatus), Staunton | — | Common terai species, India. Common carrier, Malay States (referred to as N. willmori by Watson). |
| — | — | — | =A. maculipalpis var. indiensis Theo. |
| ephens & hristophers, .T. (z) | Robertson, Liston, Bentley, (s) | — | Common carrier in N.W. Terai. |
| rassi, etc. | Grassi, etc.  .. | — | Common carrier in Europe and North America. |
| arling, (F) | — | — | Not concerned in transmission as Panama (Darling). |
| — | — | — | =A. ludlowi Theobald (?). |
| — | — | Laveran, (+) | — |
| — | — | Ross. Doubtful carrier not actively transmitting in Mauritius | Probably = A. paludis Theobald |
| ruz, (T)  .. | — | — | — |
| — | — | — | =A. stephensi Liston. |
| — | — | — | =A. sinensis. |
| — | — | — | =A. annulipes Walker. |
| — | Ed. Sergent, (s)  .. | — | — |
| — | — | — | =A. sinensis. |
| — | — | — | =A. sinensis. |
| — | — | — | =A. karwari James. |
| — | — | — | =A. plumbeus Haliday. |
| — | — | — | — |

| Species and Synonyms | Present group tabulation and generic synonymy | Distribution |
|---|---|---|
| 163. A. nimba Theobald [6] (1903) .. | 1. (Stethomyia) .. | Brazil, etc. .. |
| 164. A. nivipes Theobald [8] .. .. | 10. (Nyssorhynchus) | Malay .. .. |
| 165. A. nursei Theobald [14] .. .. | 7. (Pyretophorus) .. | India .. .. |
| 166. A. ocellatus Theobald .. | — | — |
| 167. A. occidentalis Dyar & Knab .. | — | — |
| 168. A. palestinensis Theobald [6] .. | 7. (Pyretophorus) .. | Palestine, Cyprus .. |
| 169. A. pallida Ludlow .. .. | — | — |
| 170. A. pallidopalpi Theobald [14] .. | 3. (Feltinella) .. | Sierra Leone .. |
| 171. A. paludis Theobald [1] .. .. | 4. (Myzorhynchus) | — |
| 172. A. paludis var. similis Theobald [6] | — | — |
| 173. A. parva Chagas [1] .. .. .. | 9. (Myzorhynchella) | Brazil .. .. |
| 174. A. peditæniatus Leicester [2] .. | — | |
| 175. A. perplexans Ludlow .. .. | 3. (Anopheles) .. | N. America .. .. |
| 176. A. pharoënsis Theobald [2] .. | 11. (Cellia) .. | Egypt .. .. |
| | | |
| 177. A. pharoënsis var. alba Ventrillon .. | 11. (Cellia) .. | |
| 178. A. philippinensis Ludlow [1] .. | 10. (Nyssorhynchus) | Philippines .. . |
| 179. A. pictus Loew [1] .. .. | — | |
| 180. A. pictus Ficalbi [2] .. .. .. | — | |
| 181. A. pictus Macdonald .. .. | — | |
| 182. A. pitchfordi Power .. .. .. | 7. (Pyretophorus) .. | Africa .. . |
| 183. A. plumbeus Haliday (1828) .. | 2. (Anopheles) .. | Europe .. . |
| 184. A. plumiger Dönitz [1] .. .. | — | — |
| 185. A. pretoriensis Theobald [6] .. | 10. (Nyssorhynchus) | Transvaal .. . |
| 186. A. pseudobarbirostris Ludlow [2] .. | 4. (Myzorhynchus) | Philippines .. . |
| 187. A. pseudocostalis Theobald [17] .. | 10. (Pyretophorus) .. | Africa .. . |
| 188. A. pseudomaculipes Chagas [1] .. | 5. (Arribalzagia) .. | Brazil .. . |
| 189. A. pseudopictus Grassi [1] .. .. | 4. (Myzorhynchus) | Europe .. . |
| 190. *A. pseudopunctipennis Theobald [3] | 3. (Anopheles) .. | N. America .. . |
| | | |
| 191. A. pseudosquamosa Newst. & Carter [2] .. .. .. .. .. | (Cellia) .. | Rhodesia .. . |
| 192. A. pseudowillmori Theobald [17] .. | — | — |
| 193. A. pulcherrima Theobald [4] .. | 11. (Cellia) .. | India .. . |
| 194. †A. punctipennis Say [1] .. .. | 3. (Patagiamyia) .. | N. America .. . |
| | | |
| 195. A. punctipennis Bigot MSS. .. | — | — |
| 196. A. punctulata Dönitz [1] .. .. | 12. (Cellia) .. .. | East Indies, etc. . |
| 197. A. pursati Laveran [3] .. .. | — | — |
| 198. A. pyretophoroides Theobald [14] .. | 6. (Myzomyia) .. | Transvaal .. . |
| 199. A. quadrimaculatus Say [2] .. | — | — |
| 200. A. rhodesiensis Theobald [2] .. | 6. (Myzomyia) .. | Africa .. . |
| 201. †A. rossii Giles [1] .. .. .. | 8. (Pseudomyzomyia) | India, China . |
| | | |
| 202. A. rossii var. indefinata Ludlow [4] | — | — |
| 203. A. separatus Leicester .. .. | 4. (Myzorhynchus) | Malay .. . |
| 204. A. sergentii Theobald [14] .. .. | 7. (Pyretophorus) .. | Algeria .. . |
| 205. A. simlensis James [4] .. .. | 3. (Patagiamyia) .. | India .. . |

| Transmission experiments. Cycle observed of— T. Malignant tertian, s.T. Simple tertian, Q. Quartan; f z, to zygote stage, and s, to sporozoite stage | Observations regarding transmission in nature. (z) Zygote and (s) Sporozoite stage observed | Epidemiological evidence of transmission | Remarks |
|---|---|---|---|
| — | — | — | — |
| — | — | — | Possibly=A. nigrifasciatus var. |
| — | — | — | =A. punctulatus Dönitz. |
| — | — | — | =(?) A. maculipennis. |
| — | — | — | =A. aitkeni James (?). |
| — | — | — | =A. mauritianus Grandpré. |
| — | — | — | =A. sinensis. |
| ewstead, Dutton & Todd, (T) | — | — | — |
| — | — | — | =A. pseudopictus Grassi. |
| — | — | — | =A. pseudopictus Grassi. |
| — | — | — | =A. hispaniola. |
| — | — | — | =A. sinensis. |
| — | — | — | — |
| ruz, (T) .. | — | — | — |
| arling, M.T. (s) | — | — | Only slightly concerned in transmission in Canal Zone (Darling). 12·9 % of those fed by Darling became infected. |
| — | — | — | =A. maculatus. |
| irschberg, (F) | — | — | — |
| — | — | — | =A. bigotii. |
| — | — | Laveran, (+) | — |
| — | — | — | =A. maculipennis (American). |
| tephens & Christophers, . M.T. | James, Stephens & Christophers, (F); Bentley, Staunton | Little relation | Apparently transmit very little, if at all, in nature, though commonest Indian species. |
| — | — | — | =A. indefinata Ludlow. |
| — | — | — | =? A. sinensis. |
| — | — | Unlikely to be transmitter from distribution. | Hill species. |

| Species and Synonyms | Present group tabulation and generic synonymy | Distribution |
|---|---|---|
| 206. *A. sinensis* Wiedemann [2] .. .. | 4. (*Myzorhynchus*) | India, China, Malay |

| | | |
|---|---|---|
| 207. *A. smithii* Theobald [10] (1905) .. | 2. (*Anopheles*) .. | Sierra Leone .. |
| 208. *A. squamosus* Theobald [2] .. | 11. (*Cellia*) .. | Africa .. .. |
| 209. *A. squamosus* var. *arnoldi* Newst. & Carter [2] .. .. .. | 11. (*Cellia*) .. | Africa .. .. |
| 210. *A. stephensi* Liston [1] .. .. | 10. (*Nyssorhynchus, Neocellia*) .. | India .. .. |
| 211. *A. stigmaticus* Skuse [1] .. .. | — | Australia .. .. |
| 212. *A. strachani* Theobald [14] .. .. | 4. (*Myzorhynchus*) | W. Africa .. .. |
| 213. *A. subpictus* Grassi .. .. .. | — | India .. .. |
| 214. *A. superpictus* Grassi [1] .. .. | 7. (*Pyretophorus*) .. | Europe .. .. |
| 215. *A. tarsimaculatus* Gœldi .. .. | 11. (*Cellia*) .. | S. America .. |

| | | |
|---|---|---|
| 216. *A. tenebrosus* Dönitz .. .. | — | — |
| 217. *A. tessellatum* Theobald [2] .. .. | 12. — | Malay .. .. |
| 218. *A. theobaldi* Giles [3] .. .. | 10. (*Nyssorhynchus*) | India .. .. |

| | | |
|---|---|---|
| 219. *A. thorntonii* Ludlow (1904) .. | — | — |
| 220. *A. tibani* Patton .. .. .. | — | Aden .. .. |
| 221. *A. tibiomaculata* Neiva [1] .. .. | 9. (*Myzorhynchella*) | Brazil .. .. |
| 222. *A. transvaalensis* Carter .. .. | 7. (*Pyretophorus*) .. | Transvaal .. .. |
| 223. *A. treacheri* Leicester .. .. | — | — |
| 224. *A. trifurcatus* Fabricius [1] .. .. | — | — |
| 225. *A. turkhudi* Liston [1] .. .. | 6. (*Myzomyia*) .. | India .. .. |

| | | |
|---|---|---|
| 226. *A. umbrosa* Edwards [1] .. .. | 6. (*Myzomyia*) .. | Africa .. .. |
| 227. *A. umbrosus* Theobald [6] .. .. | 4. (*Myzorhynchus*) | Malay .. .. |

| | | |
|---|---|---|
| 228. *A. unicolor* .. .. .. .. | (*Myzomyia*) .. | — |
| 229. *A. vagus* Dönitz [3] .. .. | — | — |
| 230. *A. vanus* Walker [4] .. .. | — | — |
| 231. *A. villosus* Desvoidy [1] .. .. | — | — |
| 232. *A. vincenti* Laveran [1a] .. .. | — | — |
| 233. *A. walkeri* Theobald [2] .. .. | — | — |
| 234. *A. watsonii* Edwards [1] .. .. | 10. (*Nyssorhynchus*) | Nigeria .. .. |
| 235. *A. watsonii* Leicester [2] .. .. | 12. — | Malay .. .. |
| 236. *A. wellcomei* Theobald [9] .. .. | (*Anopheles*) .. | — |
| 237. *A. wellingtonianus* Alcock .. .. | 3. (*Patagiamyia, Myzorhynchus*) | — |
| 238. *A. willmori* James .. .. .. | 10. (*Nyssorhynchus*) | India .. .. |
| 239. *A. willmori* var. *maculosa* James .. | 10. (*Nyssorhynchus*) | India .. .. |
| 240. *A. willmori* Leicester .. .. | — | — |
| 241. *A. ziemani* Van Grunberg .. .. | — | — |

| ransmission experiments. ycle observed of— :. Malignant tertian, T. Simple tertian, Q. Quartan; z, to zygote stage, id s, to sporozoite stage | Observations regarding transmission in nature. (z) Zygote and (s) Sporozoite stage observed | Epidemiological evidence of transmission | Remarks |
|---|---|---|---|
| uzuki, Q, & thers Kinohita, s.t. .m.t.=F | — | — | — |
| — | — | — | — |
| — | — | — | — |
| ephens & hristophers | Liston, (t); Bentley, (t) | — | Important and active carrier. Carries in towns owing to power of breeding in cisterns, wells, etc. |
| — | — | — | — |
| — | — | — | — |
| — | Grassi, (t); Bignami & Bastianelli, (t) | — | — |
| arling, m.t. z) | — | — | =(?) A. albimana. Considered distinct by Dyar and Knab. 60 % of those fed by Darling became infected. |
| | | | =A. mauritianus. |
| ephens & hristophers, .t. (z) Q.(z) | — | — | Probably transmits in terai and other parts of India. |
| | — | — | =A. tessellatum. |
| — | — | — | — |
| — | — | — | — |
| — | — | — | =A. aitkeni James. |
| — | — | — | =A. bifurcatus Linnæus. |
| tephens & hristophers, t. (z) | — | Gill. Large numbers in very malarious spot | Probably transmits. |
| taunton, m.t. (f) | — | Watson considers to be carrier | — |
| — | — | — | =A. rossii Giles. |
| — | — | — | =A. sinensis Wied. |
| — | — | — | =A. bifurcatus Linnæus. |
| — | — | — | =A. bifurcatus Linnæus. |
| — | — | — | — |
| — | — | — | — |
| — | — | — | — |
| — | Adie (Mrs), (s) .. | — | Carrier in terai country. |
| — | — | — | =A. maculatus Theobald. |
| — | — | — | =A. mauritianus Grandpré. |

### TRIBE 2. MEGARHININÆ.

Proboscis with the apical half much thinner than the basal, and bent downwards at an angle with it. Scutellum evenly rounded. Wings long and narrow ; fork cells both very short, but with the first much shorter than the second. Large species completely clothed with flat, more or less metallic, scales, usually blue or green. Larvæ predaceous ; adults not bloodsuckers. The Megarhininæ are popularly known as Elephant mosquitoes owing to their enormous size. None of the species have been shewn to be directly concerned in the spread of disease, but the predaceous larvæ of some species play an important rôle in keeping down the number of other species of mosquitoes. *T. immisericors* (Walker), the common Elephant mosquito of India and Burmah, for example, in the larval stage is generally found living on the larvæ of *Stegomyia*. The two chief genera are *Megarhinus* and *Toxorhynchites*, the former of new world and the latter of old world distribution.

### TRIBE 3. CULICINÆ.

Thorax more or less rounded ; metanotum without bristles ; scutellum more or less distinctly trilobed. Larvæ with air tube and median ventral brush on anal segment (after the first stage).

This sub-family includes over 600 species and, next to the Anophelinæ, is the most important from the point of view of the transmission of disease. Theobald in his monograph recognizes nearly 100 genera, arranged as follows :

Palpæ of male long   .. .. .. .. .. *Culicinæ.*
Palpæ of male short.
    First forked cell of wing long .. .. .. *Aëdinæ.*
    First forked cell of wing very short .. .. *Uranotæninæ.*

In addition certain peculiar forms have been given the rank of a sub-family by Theobald. In other respects having the characters of Culicinæ, but differing in having a seventh vein on the wing with scales, is Heptaphlebomyinæ. Also resembling Culicinæ, but having a very long second segment of the antenna, is Deinoceratinæ.

Edwards divides the Culicinæ into two main groups :

(1) *Culex* group. Eggs laid in masses ; last segment of female abdomen broad, immovable ; claws of female never toothed.

Genera : *Culex, Tæniorhynchus, Ædomyia, Theobaldia, Uranotænia.*

(2) *Aëdes* group. Eggs laid singly ; last segment of female abdomen narrow, usually completely retracted into the penultimate ; claws of female, at least on the four anterior legs, nearly always toothed.

Genera : *Mucidus, Psorophora, Janthinosoma, Ochlerotatus, Stegomyia, Aëdes.*

The following scheme is that of Edwards, giving the chief characters of the more important genera.

### Table of Genera of Culicinæ (Edwards).

1. Claws of female toothed .. .. .. ·.. .. .. 2
   Claws of female simple .. .. .. .. .. .. 5
2. Posterior cross-vein slightly beyond mid cross-vein ; legs shaggily scaled ; female palpi half as long as proboscis .. .. .. .. *Mucidus.*
   Posterior cross-vein before mid cross-vein ; legs not shaggily scaled ; female palpi not half as long as proboscis .. .. .. .. .. .. 3
3. Male palpi with two apparent joints .. .. *Banksinella.*
   Male palpi with three apparent joints .. .. .. .. 4
4. Last two joints of male palpi thin, about equal in length ; black and white species ; head all flat-scaled .. .. .. .. .. .. *Stegomyia.*
   (Includes *Stegomyia, Desvoidya, Leicesteria, Scutomyia* and *Kingia* of Theobald.)
   Last two joints of male palpi more or less thickened, especially the penultimate, which is longer than the terminal ; not usually black and white species, head not usually flat-scaled above .. *Ochlerotatus.*
   (Includes *Acartomyia, Ædimorphus, Andersonia, Bathosomyia, Cacomyia, Culicada, Culicelsa, Danielsia, Duttonia, Ecculex, Finlaya, Gilesia, Gualteria, Inimetoculex, Lepidoplatys, Lepidotomyia, Leslieomyia, Molpemyia, Myxosquamus, Neopecomyia, Pecomyia, Phagomyia, Polyleptiomyia, Protoculex, Protomacleaya, Pseudoculex, Pseudograbhamia, Pseudohowardina, Pseudoskusea, Reedomyia, Stegoconops, Stenoscutus,* of Theobald and others.)

5. Eighth segment of female abdomen slender, retractile ; male resembling a *Stegomyia* .. *Howardina*.

Eighth segment of female abdomen broad truncate (except in *Mimomyia*), not retractile .. .. .. 6

6. Head without any flat scales in the middle above ; proboscis never swollen at tip .. .. .. .. .. 7

Head with at least a row of flat scales round the eye margins, usually almost entirely clothed with flat scales ; proboscis often swollen at tip .. .. .. .. .. .. .. .. .. 13

7. Wing scales very broad and dense .. .. .. .. 8

Wing scales not very broad .. .. .. .. .. 9

8. Male palpi as long as proboscis, thin last joint very short .. .. .. .. .. .. *Mansonioìdes*.

Palpi similar in both sexes, very short ; middle femora with a tuft of scales at the tip .. *Ædomyia*.

9. Fork cells very short ; wings nearly bare ; male palpi two-jointed .. .. .. .. *Mimomyia*.

(Includes *Boycia, Conopomyia, Hispidimyia, Ludlowia, Mimomyia, Radioculex*, of Theobald, etc.)

Fork cells not very short ; male palpi three-jointed .. .. .. .. .. .. .. .. 10

10. Metatarsus of hind-legs distinctly shorter than the tibia ; male palpi long, the last two joints swollen .. .. .. .. .. .. .. .. 11

Metatarsus of hind-legs at least as long as the tibia, male palpi thin .. .. .. .. .. .. .. 12

11. Penultimate joint of male palpi thicker and somewhat longer than terminal one, usually yellow species .. .. .. .. .. .. *Tæniorhynchus*.

(Includes *Tæniorhynchus* and *Mansonia* of Theobald.)

Penultimate joint of male palpi thinner but not longer than terminal one ; not yellow species ; cross-veins almost in a line .. .. .. *Theobaldia*.

12. Male palpi longer than proboscis, last two joints curved upwards .. .. .. .. .. *Culex*.

(Includes *Aporoculex, Heptaphlebomyia, Lasioconops, Leucomyia, Lutzia, Maillotia, Melanoconion, Microculex, Oculeomyia*, and *Trichopronomyia* of Theobald.)

Male palpi shorter than proboscis, straight .. *Protomelanoconion*.

13. A row of small flat scales round the eyes ; basal joint of male palpi with a row of projecting scales ; otherwise like *Culex* .. .. .. *Culiciomyia*.

(Includes *Culiciomyia, Trichorhynchus, Neomelanoconion*, and *Pectinopalpus* of Theobald.)

Head mostly or entirely flat-scaled in middle .. .. .. 14

14. Proboscis not swollen at tip ; fork cells not very short .. .. .. .. .. .. .. .. 15

Proboscis swollen at tip or fork cells very short, first shorter than second .. .. .. .. .. 17

15. Lateral vein scales with apices simple, ♂ antennæ
    plumose         ..      ..      ..      ..      ..      ..      ..      16
    Lateral vein scales with apices dentate, ♂ antennæ
    pilose          ..      ..      ..      ..      ..      ..      *Hodgesia.*
16. Medium-sized species, pale palpi thin, almost
    without hairs and slightly shorter than the
    proboscis ..    ..      ..      ..      ..      ..      *Eumelanomyia.*
    Very small species, male palpi short like those of
    the female      ..      ..      ..      ..      ..      *Micraëdes.*
17. Fork cells very short, first shorter than second      ..      ..      18
    Fork cells not very short, first not shorter than
    second          ..      ..      ..      ..      ..      ..      ..      ..      19
18. Lateral vein scales absent ; male palpi long, two-
    jointed, apical one swollen ; fore and mid-claws
    of male unequal, toothed      ..      ..      ..      *Mimomyia.*
    Lateral vein scales present, broad ; male palpi
    very short ; male claws not toothed, the front
    pair small and equal      ..      ..      ..      ..      *Uranotænia.*
    (Includes *Uranotænia, Pseudouranotænia, Anisocheleomyia, Pseudo-*
    *ficalbia* of Theobald.)
19. Proboscis not hairy      ..      ..      ..      ..      *Ingramia.*
                (=*Dasymyia.*   Leicester.)
    Proboscis with long hairs ..      ..      ..      ..      *Harpagomyia.*
                (=*Malaya.*   Leicester.)

Of the genera noted above some are more important than
others, both as regards the number of species and their relation
to disease transmission.

*Mucidus* (seven species).   The larvæ are predaceous and, like those of the
    *Megarhininæ,* feed on other mosquito larvæ.   Species of *Mucidus* have a
    very striking " mouldy " appearance, due to the long outstanding scales
    on the legs, etc.   Not one of the species has been noted as concerned in
    the transmission of disease.
*Banksinella* (five species).   Some species at least suck human blood with
    avidity.   No species has been proved to transmit any disease.
*Stegomyia* and *Kingia* (over 40 species).   Mosquitoes of the genus *Stegomyia*
    are medium-sized, brilliantly banded and marked with black and silvery
    white.   The head is entirely covered with flat appressed scales and all
    lobes of the scutellum likewise carry broad flat scales.

The following is Theobald's table for the differentiation of
the species of *Stegomyia,* with some additional ones described
since his work was published.

## *Genus* STEGOMYIA *Theobald* (1910).

### A.  Proboscis banded.

a.  Legs basally banded.
    Thorax brown, with scattered creamy-white scales
                                *annulirostris.*  Theobald.
    Thorax black, with narrow-curved golden scales
                                *periskeleta.*  Giles.
aa.  Legs with basal and apical banding.
    Forelegs with no bands ; mid with apical and basal bands on first
    tarsal and second tarsal ; hind with basal bands.
    Thorax white in front, with a brown eye-like spot on each side.
                                *thomsoni.*  Theobald.

### AA.  Proboscis unbanded

β.  Legs basally banded.
  γ.  Abdomen basally banded.
    Thorax with one median silvery-white line   *scutellaris.*  Walker.
    Thorax similar, but two white spots near where line ends
                                *gebeleinensis.*  Theobald.
    Thorax with a white line on each pleuron in addition to a median
    silvery-white line   ..   ..  *pseudoscutellaris.*  Theobald.
    Thorax with two median yellow lines and lateral curved silvery
    lines   ..   ..   ..   ..   ..  *fasciata.*  Fabricius.
    Thorax with two short median lines and a white patch on each
    side  ..   ..   ..   ..   ..   ..  *nigeria.*  Theobald.
    Thorax with large lateral white spots in front, smaller ones by
    wings, two narrow median yellow lines, and two posterior sub-
    median white lines   ..   ..   ..   ..  *lilii.*  Theobald.
    Thorax with a white W-shaped area in front, a prolongation
    curved on each side enclosing a brown eye-like spot
                                *W-alba.*  Theobald.
    Thorax with white frontal median spot, two large lateral spots,
    a small one in front of the wings, a narrow median white line
    and narrow sub-median ones on posterior half.  Last two hind
    tarsi white   ..   ..   ..   ..  *wellmanii.*  Theobald.
    Thorax brown, with broad white line in front extending laterally
    towards wings, where they swell into a large patch, a white line
    on each side just past wing roots.  Last two hind tarsi white
                                *desmotes.*  Giles.
    Thorax with silvery-white spot on each side in front, small one
    over root of wings, and white over their base.  *Last two hind
    tarsi white*   ..   ..   ..   ..  *pseudonigeria.*  Theobald.
    Thorax with two lateral white spots, front one the largest, small
    median one near head, two yellow median lines, a short silvery
    one on each side before scutellum   ..  *simpsoni.*  Theobald.
    Thorax with a silvery-white scaled area in front and another each
    side in front of wings   ..   ..  *argenteomaculata.*  Theobald.

Thorax with median yellowish-white line, a silvery patch on each
side in front of wings, extending as a fine yellow line to scutellum,
and another silvery spot before base of each wing
*poweri*. Theobald.
Thorax with small grey scaled area in front of roots of wings and
three short creamy lines behind   ..   *minutissima*. Theobald.
Thorax ? (denuded).   Abdomen black ;   fifth segment with
yellow basal band ;   sixth, unbanded ;   seventh, two median
lateral white spots ;   eighth, two basal lateral white spots ;
second hind tarsal nearly all white   ..   *dubia*. Theobald.
Thorax dark brown ;   abdomen with dark scales and basal
ochraceous bandings well-marked on segments 2, 3, 4 and 5
*quasinigritia*. Ludlow.
Thorax dark brown.   Abdomen dark brown, with brilliant lateral
white spots, sometimes extending across tergum as basal bands
*nigritia*. Ludlow.
γγ.  Abdomen unbanded.
Third hind tarsal nearly all white.
Thorax with two lateral white marks directed upwards
*africana*. Theobald.
Thorax with white spot in front and another in front of each wing
*apicoargentia*. Theobald.
First hind tarsal all white, second basally white, last two dark.
Thorax chestnut-brown with a broad patch of white scales on each
side in front and a median pale line   ..   *terrens*. Walker.
First hind tarsal with very small basal white spot ;   second tarsal
mostly white, other segments black   ..   *pollinctor*. Graham.
ββ.  Legs with white lines as well as basal bands.
Thorax brown with white lines ;   abdomen with basal bands
*grantii*. Theobald.
βββ.  Fore and mid-legs with apical bands ;   hind basal.
Fourth tarsal of hind-legs nearly all white
*mediopunctata*. Theobald.
Mid metatarsi with basal pale banding, base and apex of hind,
also base of first tarsal ..      ..      ..   *assamensis*. Theobald.
Basal two-thirds of hind femora white, metatarsus and first three
tarsal joints with basal white bands   ..   *imitator*. Leicester.
ββββ.  Fore and mid-legs unbanded ;   hind femora white basally and at apex.
Thorax black scaled in female and golden scaled in the male.
Abdomen unbanded dorsally but banded ventrally with large
square pearly white spots laterally   ..   *dissimilis*. Leicester.
βββββ.  Legs unbanded.
δ.  Abdomen basally banded.
Thorax, front half white, rest bronzy-brown
*pseudonivea*. Theobald.
Thorax deep brown, with scattered golden scales, shewing two
dark eye-like spots ;   head white, dark on each side and behind
*albocephala*. Theobald.
Thorax brown, with golden stripes ;   abdomen with narrow basal
bands fifth and sixth segments only ..   *auriostriata*. Banks.

δδ.  Abdominal banding indistinct.
    Thorax with broad silvery-white patch on each side in front
                                  *albolateralis.*  Theobald.
δδδ.  Abdomen unbanded.
    Thorax, six silvery spots  ..    ..  *argenteopunctata.*  Theobald.
    Thorax with dark-brown narrow curved scales.  Scutellum with
        very marked meridian lobe    ..    ..  *hatiensis.*  Carter.
δδδδ.  Abdomen with apical white lateral spots.
    Thorax unadorned, except for pale scaled lines internally
                                  *punctolateralis.*  Theobald.
    Abdomen with basal white lateral spots.
    Thorax with two pale indistinct median parallel lines and two
        silvery lateral spots ..    ..    ..    *minuta.*  Theobald.
    Thorax unadorned.
    White spot mid head  ..    ..    ..  *tripunctata.*  Theobald.
    No white spot    ..    ..    ..    *amesii.*  Ludlow.
    Thorax brownish-black with dark bronze scales.  Abdomen clad
        with purple-black scales and white triangular lateral spots
                                  *fusca.*  Leicester.
δδδδδ.  Abdomen with silvery apical lateral spots on all segments except
        first two    ..    ..    ..  *tasmaniensis.*  Strickland.

## AAA.  Proboscis yellow basally, dark apically.

Abdomen with apical pale bands  ..    ..*crassipes.*  Van der Wulp.

## AAAA.  Proboscis with median interrupted white lines on basal half.

Head black, anterior margin grey  ..  *albomarginata.*  Newstead.

*Desvoidya* (five species).  Large mosquitoes active by day like *Stegomyia*,
small with silvery venter, but less ornamented than *Stegomyia*.
*Leicesteria* (ten species).  Resembling *Desvoidya*, but the female pupæ are
half the length of the proboscis.
*Ochlerotatus.*  This genus as reconstructed by Edwards is an important one
from the large number of different forms included.  Of the original genera
now sunk under *Ochlerotatus*, many contain but few species, and have not
been shewn to play any part in disease transmission.
*Culicada* is a genus represented by many species and especially occurs in
North America and Europe.
*Howardina* (seven species).  The best known species in this genus is the
common *H. sugens* (*Scutomyia* Meigen=*Stegomyia* Meigen).
*Grabhamia* (twenty-eight species).  There are a large number of common species
of this genus which usually have a characteristic floury appearance.
They are of active bloodsucking habits.
*Mansonioides* (three species).  These have an even more pronouncedly floury
or " pepper and salt " appearance.
*Aedomyia* and *Numomyia.*  These are now domestic species, having no relation to any disease.  Many do not, under ordinary circumstances, feed
upon man.

*Tæniorhynchus* and *Mansonia*. Mosquitoes of the genus *Mansonia* are especially characteristic of swamp country, and occur in enormous numbers in many parts of Tropical Africa and elsewhere. They are concerned in the transmission of Filariasis.

*Theobaldia*. Large gnats common in the temperate zone.

*Culex* (several hundred species). *Culex pipiens*=common English gnat. *Culex fatigans*=commonest mosquito of tropics acting as transmitting agent of Filariasis. It is also the definitive host of *Plasmodium præcox*, the malarial parasite of birds. *Culex concolor* as a larva has actively cannibal habits, and plays an important part in keeping down the numbers of the common *C. fatigans* and its near allies.

*Culiciomyia*, and other genera of little importance as carriers, etc.

TRIBE 4. SABETHINÆ.

The members of this tribe are not known to carry any disease.

PUBLICATIONS OF IMPORTANCE IN CONNECTION WITH NOMENCLATURE AND SYSTEMATIC WORK ON CULICIDÆ.

The numbers in brackets refer to the data given in the Table o species of *Anopheles* (pp. 96–107).

The asterisks mark recent and important papers, or those in which recognized species of *Anopheles* are described.

Agramonte (1900). *El progresso medico*, x. p. 460.
Arribalzaga [1] (1878). *El naturalista Argentino.*
— [2] (1883). *Bol. Acad. nac. d. Ciencias*, IV.
* — [3] (1891). *Rivista del Museo de la Plata (Culicidæ).*
*Bancroft (1908). *Annals of the Queensland Museum*, No. 8.
*Banks (1906). *Philippine Journal of Science*, vol. I. No. 9.
Becker (1903). *Mitteilungen aus dem Zool. Mus. in Berlin*, II. p. 68.
*Blanchard [1a] (1901) [1b] (1905). *Les moustiques, histoire naturelle et médicale.* Paris.
* — [2] (1901). *Compt. rend. Soc. Biol.* vol. LIII. p. 1045.
* — [3] (1902). *Ibid.* vol. LIV, p. 793.
*Bourroul (1904). *Mosquitos do Brasil.* Bahia.
Camboulin (1902). *C. R. Acad. Sc.* CXXXV. p. 704.
*Carter [1] (1910). *The Entomologist*, vol. XLIII. p. 237.
*Chagas [1]. In *Peryassu.*
Chalmers [1] (1900). *Lancet.*
— [2] (1905). *Spolia Zeylandica*, II. 8, p. 169.
*Christophers [1] (1911). *Paludism*, No. 2.
Coquillet [1] (1896). *Canadian Entom.* XXVIII.
* — [2] (1900). *U.S. Depart. Agric., Div. Entom. Circular*, Second Series, No. 40.
* — [3] (1902). *New York Entom. Soc. (Journal)*, vol. X. p. 191.

\*Coquillet [4] (1903).  *Canadian Entom.* xxxv.
\* —— [5] (1900).  *U.S. Depart. of Agric., Bureau of Entom.* Tech.
   Ser. No. 11.
Cruz [1] (1906).  *Brazil Medico,* xx. 20, p. 199.
\* —— [2] (1908).  In *Peryassu.*
Desvoidy [1] (1827).  *Mém. d. l. Soc. d'Hist. Nat. de Paris,* III. p. 411.
—— [2] (1828).  *Ibid.* vol. IV.
\*Dönitz [1] (1901).  *Insekten Börse,* XVIII.
\* —— [2] (1902).  *Zeits. f. Hygiene,* XLI. p. 15.
\* —— [4] (1903).  *Ibid.* XLIII. p. 215.
\*Dyar and Knab [1a] (1907).  *Journ. New York Entom. Soc.* xv. p. 198.
\* —— [1b] (1909).  *Proc. of the U.S. Nat. Museum,* xxxv. p. 53.
\* —— [2].  *Proc. Biol. Soc. Washington,* XIX. p. 160.
\*Edwards [1] (1911).  *Bull. Entom. Research,* II. part 2, p. 141.
\* —— [2] (1911).  *Ibid.* II. part 3, p. 241.
\* —— [3] (1912).  *Ibid.* III. part 1, p. 1.
\* —— [4] (1912).  *Ibid.* III. part 3, p. 241.
Fabricius [1] (1775).  *Systema entomologica,* etc.
—— [2] (1777).  *Genera insectorum.*
—— [3] (1781).  *Species insectorum,* etc.
—— [4] (1877).  *Mantissa insectorum,* etc.
—— [5] (1794).  *Entomologia systematica emendata et aucta.*
—— [6] (1805).  *Syst. Antliatorum,* etc. 6, p. 35.
Ficalbi [1] (1896).  *Bull. Soc. Entom. Ital.* XXVIII.
\* —— [2] (1899).  *Ibid.* XXXI.
Fischer [1] (1812).  *Mém. Soc. Impériale Nat. Moscou,* IV. p. 167.
Fitch (1885).  *New York State Museum,* 2nd Entom. Report.
\*Giles [1] (1899).  *Jour. Trop. Medicine,* II. p. 62.
\* —— [2] (1900).  *Liverpool School of Trop. Med.,* Memoir II.
\* —— [3] (1901).  *Entom. Monthly Mag.* XII. p. 196.
\* —— [4a] (1900) [4b] (1902).  *Handbook of Gnats or Mosquitoes.*
   London.
\* —— [5] (1904).  *A Revision of the Anophelinæ* (supp. to handbook).
\*Goeldi (1905).  *Os mosquitos no Para.*  Para.
\*Grandpré [1] (1900).  *Planters' Gazette Press.*  Port Louis.
—— [2] (1902).  *Zool. Anz.* xxv. No. 677, 21 July.
\*Grassi [1] (1899).  *Atti Accad. d. Lincei,* Ser. 5, Memor. III.
Grünberg (1905).  *Zool. Anz.* XXIX. p. 377.
Haliday [1] (1828).  *Zool. Journal,* XII.
—— [2] (1833).  *Entom. Magazine,* I.
—— [3] (1839).  *Annals of Natural History.*
\*Hill and Haydon (1907).  *Annals of the Natal Gov. Museum.*
\*Howard (1901).  *Mosquitoes; how they live,* etc.  New York.
\* —— Dyar and Knab (1912).  *The mosquitoes of North and Central
   America and the West Indies.*  Publ. 159.  Carnegie Inst. Washington.
\*James [1] (1902).  *Sci. Memoirs Med. and San. Departs. of Gov. of
   India,* No. 2

*James [1a]. In *Theobald*, vol. III.
* —— [2] (1910). *Records of the Indian Museum*, IV. No. 5.
* —— [3] (1910). *Paludism*, No. 1.
*James and Liston [4a] (1904) [4b] (1911). *The Anopheline Mosquitoes of India*. Calcutta.
Kertész (1904). *Állattan Közl.* III.
Laveran [1a] (1901). *C. R. Soc. Biol.* XXIII. p. 993.
—— [1b] (1901). *Ibid.* LIII.
—— [2] (1902). *Archiv d. Parasit.* VI. p. 359.
—— [3] (1902). *C. R. Soc. Biol.* LIV. p. 907.
*Leicester [1] (1904). *The Entomologist*, XXXVII. p. 13.
* —— [2] (1908). *Studies from the Instit. for Med. Research (Federated Malay States)*, vol. III.
Linnæus [1] (1746). *Fauna Suecica.*
—— [2] (1735). *Systema Naturæ.*
*Liston [1] (1901). *Indian Med. Gazette*, XXXVI. pp. 361, 441.
—— [2] (1901). *Bombay Med. and Phys. Soc.* V. No. 8.
Loew [1] (1845). *Dipterologische Beiträge.*
—— [2] (1866). *Entom. Zeitschr.*
*Ludlow [1] (1902). *Jour. Amer. Med. Assoc.* p. 426.
* —— [2] (1902). *Jour. New York Entom. Soc.* X. p. 127.
* —— [3] (1903). *Ibid.* XI.
* —— [4] (1904). *Canad. Entom.* XXXVI. p. 297.
* —— [5] (1908). *Class. Geo. Dist. and Seas flight Mosq. (Philippine Islands).*
* —— [6] (1909). *Canad. Entom.* XLI.
*Lutz [1] (1904). In *Bourroul.*
McCracken [1] (1904). *Entom. Mus.* IX. Jan. 1904.
Macquart [1] (1825). *Mém. d. l. Soc. R. des Sciences de l'Agric. et des Arts de Lille.*
—— [2] (1834). *Histoire naturelle des Insectes Diptères.* Paris.
—— [3] (1854). *Mém. d. l. Soc. R. des Sciences de l'Agric. et des Arts de Lille.*
Meigen [1] (1804). *Klassifikation und Beschreibung der Europ. Zweif. Insekten*, Bd. 1.
—— [2] (1818). *Syst. Besch. der bekannt. Europ. Zweif. Insekten*, vol. I.
*Neiva (1908). In *Peryassu.*
Neveu-Lemaire [1] (1902). *Mém. d. l. Soc. Zool. de France*, XV.
—— [2] (1902). *C. R. Soc. Biol.* LIV.
* —— [3] (1905). *Archiv d. Parasit.* X. p. 238.
*Newstead and Carter [1] (1910). *Annals of Trop. Med. and Par.* IV. No. 3.
* —— [2] (1911). *Ibid.* V. No. 2.
*Newstead, Dutton and Todd (1907). *Ibid.* I. No. 1.
Patton (1905). *Jour. Bombay Nat. Hist. Soc.* p. 623.
Rothwell (1907). *The Entomologist*, XLV. p. 34.

*Skuse [1] (1889).  *Proc. Linnean Soc. N. S. Wales.*  2nd Ser. III.
—— [2].  *Indian Museum Notes;* III.  Calcutta.
Smith [1] (1901).  *Jour. Boston Soc. of Med. Sc.* v. p. 34.
—— [2] (1904).  *New Jersey Agric. Exp. Sta.* pp. 1–40.
Staeger [1] (1839).  *Syst. for. o. d. c. Denmark nid lil fundre Dipt.*
Stephens [2] (1828).  *Zoological Journal,* XII.
*Stephens and Christophers (1908).  *The Practical Study of Malaria,*
    3rd ed.
*Theobald [1] (1900).  *Reports to the Malaria Comm.·of Royal Society,* 1.
*  —— [2], [3] (1901).  *Monograph of the Culicidæ of the World,* vol. I
    and II.
*  —— [4] (1902).  *Proc. Roy. Soc.* LXIX. p. 367.
*  —— [5] (1902).  *Journ. Trop. Med.* v. p. 181.
*  —— [5a] (1903).  *Ann. d. l'Inst. Pasteur,* XVII. 2.
*  —— [6] (1903).  *Monograph of the Culicidæ,* vol. III.
*  —— [7] (1903).  *Reports of the Sleeping Sickness Commission.*
*  —— [8] (1903).  *The Entomologist,* XXXVI. p. 256.
*  —— [9] (1904).  *First Report Gordon College, Wellc. Labs.* I. p. 62.
*  —— [10] (1905).  *The Entomologist,* XXXVIII. p. 101.
*  —— [11] (1905).  *Jour. Econ. Biology,* I. No. 1, p. 17.
*  —— [12] (1905).  *Ann. Mus. Nat. Hung.* III. p. 65.
*  —— [13] (1905).  *Genera Insectorum Fam. Culicidæ.*  Brussels.
*  —— [14] (1907).  *Monograph of the Culicidæ,* vol. IV.
*  —— [15] (1909).  *Records of the Indian Museum,* III. No. 3.
*  —— [16] (1910).  *Ibid.* IV. No. 1.
*  —— [17] (1910).  *Monograph of the Culicidæ,* vol. V.
*  —— [18] (1901).  *Jour. of Trop. Med.* IV. p. 229.
*Theobald and Grantham (1905).  *Mosquitoes of Jamaica.*
Tsuzuki (1902).  *Cent. f. Bakt.* XXXI. pp. 15, 763.
Van der Wulp [1] (1839).  *Naturhist. Tijdschr.* II. p. 252.
—— [2] (1869).  *Tijds. voor Entom.*
—— [4] (1884).  *Leyden Museum Notes.*
Ventrillon [1] (1906).  *Bull. d. Mus. d'Hist. Nat.* XII. p. 100.
—— [2] (1906).  *Ibid.* XII. p. 198.
Walker [3] (1850).  *Insecta Saundersonii,* I.
Watson (1910).  *Annals of Trop. Med. and Par.* IV. No. 2.
Wiedemann [2] (1828).  *Ausser Europ. Zweif. Insekten,* I.

# CHAPTER IX

## ANOPHELINE-TRANSMITTED DISEASES

## MALARIA.

*Synonyms.* Ague, Paludism, Intermittent fever, Remittent fever ; Marsh, Climatic, Jungle, Hill, Mountain and Coast fever, Plasmodiose, Fièvre palustre, Wechselfieber, Kaltesfieber, Πυρετος, *Bimbi ou Moustique* (Galla), *Mbou ou Moustique,* and also many local names such as Roman fever, Sierra fever, etc., etc.

Definition. Under the term malaria is grouped together a number of intermittent fevers caused by plasmodial parasites living in the red blood corpuscles At the present time only three distinct species of these parasites are usually recognized, viz. *Plasmodium malariæ, P. vivax,* and *P. falciparum* ( = *Laverania malariæ*) ; each gives rise to a distinct type of fever and is transmitted by various Anopheline mosquitoes.

The common features of the disease, in addition to fever, are anæmia, hypertrophy of the spleen, and sometimes the liver, and the deposition of pigment (melanin) in the various organs and integument.

Historical. The periodicity of the febrile attacks of malaria had attracted attention long before the parasitic nature of this disease was known, or its transmission by mosquitoes suspected. Certain references have been taken as shewing that malaria was recognized even in the time of Homer (1100 B.C.) and in the Hippocratic Books (500 B.C.) fevers having quotidian, tertian and quartan periodicity are described. This characteristic periodicity, which finds expression in the term *intermittent fever,* even now sometimes used, represented, however, practically everything that was known about the disease in these early times.

A much more precise knowledge of malaria and a clear recognition of *remittent* and *pernicious* forms of the disease, where periodicity is not a feature, followed the introduction to Europe in the seventeenth century of *Cinchona* and its alkaloids, it being then possible to distinguish types of fever curable by quinine from those not affected by this drug.

A third feature of malaria, namely its frequent association with *paludic* conditions, although it seems to some extent to have been known to the ancients (*e.g.* Varro, 116 B.C.), was first fully realized as a result of the work of Doni, Morton, Lancisi and others, from the seventeenth century onwards. This association was explained as shewing that malaria was due to exhalations from decaying vegetable matter, or to minute forms of life present in such exhalations. Hence there resulted the *Miasm* theory of malaria, a theory universally held by mankind up to a few years ago and responsible for the name " Malaria " (= bad air).

In 1847 the occurrence of the characteristic *pigment* of malaria in the blood and organs was discovered by Meckel ; this pigment, it was thought, was the result of the chemical action of miasm on the blood.

In 1881 Laveran discovered the organism containing this pigment now known as the *malarial parasite*. Within a few years Laveran's organism, the first discovered protozoon parasitic in man, was universally recognized as the cause of malaria. Thus in modern usage it has followed that no diagnosis which has not been based upon the demonstration of this parasite, or its characteristic pigment in the blood, is accepted as of any value in a crucial case, malaria now being an example of a disease defined not on clinical but on parasitological grounds.

In 1886 Golgi demonstrated the nature of the life-cycle of the parasite in man, and shewed that the periodicity of the febrile attacks was dependent on the length of the cycle of development of successive broods of the parasite, and that the attack of fever occurred at the time when such broods simultaneously broke up into the spores which restarted the cycle. Golgi also differentiated two species of malarial parasite, the parasites of *quartan* and of *tertian* malaria, respectively.

In 1891 Marchiafava and Bignami, after studying certain irregular fevers prevalent in Rome in the summer and autumn, announced the existence of a third species of parasite, characterized by the occurrence of very minute forms, and now known as the *æstivo-autumnal, malignant tertian* or *tropical parasite*. It was shortly afterwards discovered that certain large and peculiar crescentic forms of the parasite, now very familiar as *crescents*, were a stage in the life-cycle of this third species. In addition these and other Italian workers by their collective researches made quite clear the real parasitic nature of Laveran's bodies and by elaborating methods by which they could be demonstrated, laid the foundation for the study of the malarial parasite by observers in other parts of the world.

In the decade or so following upon these early observations a great many important facts in regard to malaria were elicited. It was shewn that infection could be conveyed to healthy persons by the subcutaneous or intravenous inoculation of the blood of malarial subjects. It was also proved that in such cases only that form of parasite appeared which had been present in the original infection, thus greatly strengthening the view of a plurality of species. Other species more or less resembling the malarial parasite, but shewn to be distinct, were also found to occur in birds, bats and other animals, and were closely studied. Special methods of staining were elaborated and much work was done with regard to the peculiar crescent bodies and the process of exflagellation exhibited by these and by certain other forms of the parasite.

All efforts to discover how the parasites gained an entrance to the blood of man, however, failed. Experiments (Marchiafava ; Celli, 1885 ; Marino, 1890, and Zeri, 1890, etc.), undertaken with a view to producing malaria in healthy persons by causing them to drink water from notoriously malarious places, were without result. When marsh water was injected into animals a condition thought at first to be malaria was produced, associated with tumefaction of the spleen and the appearance of pigment in the organs. But it is now obvious that this condition was one of septicæmia, and with the discovery of the malarial parasite any significance attaching to these experiments had to be abandoned.

The possibility that mosquitoes might be concerned in the

transmission of malaria had been put forward already by King (1883). That mosquitoes·might convey malaria was also definitely suggested by Laveran on the analogy of the development of filarial embryos in the mosquito (1884). But it was Manson (1894) who more especially elaborated and emphasized the probability of mosquito transmission, and who by his remarkable deductions, based on the behaviour of the flagellate bodies, led directly to Ross's efforts to demonstrate this relation experimentally.

But none of these hypotheses, not even Manson's carefully thought out deductions, anticipated the mosquito cycle as we now know it, as a result of Ross's brilliant research, in all its beautiful simplicity. According to Manson it was the flagella breaking away from the parasite that underwent development in the mosquito, and it was by the medium of·water in which the mosquito eventually died that it was supposed re-infection of man took place. Ross's discovery of the cycle of development of *Proteosoma* shewed that it was the whole parasite which underwent development, and that re-infection did not take place through water, but that the parasites underwent growth and multiplication in the body of the mosquito, eventually finding their way to the salivary glands, to be injected with the salivary secretion when the mosquito next fed. The significance of flagellation was almost coincidently shewn by MacCallum, who observed in *Hæmoproteus* (= *Halteridium*), another parasite of birds, the fertilization of the female form, or macrogamete, by the flagella, or microgametes, liberated from the microgametocyte, or male form, of the parasite.

The discovery of the life-cycle of *Proteosoma*, and the fact that the protozoa, like the parasitic worms, might exhibit *melaxeny*, or the utilization of two or more hosts in their development, gave the clue to the method of transmission of human malaria, and the mosquito cycle of the malarial parasite, as worked out by Grassi and others, was found to follow almost exactly the development previously noted by Ross in the case of *Proteosoma*. But whereas the parasite of birds underwent development only in mosquitoes of the genus *Culex* (*C. fatigans*), that of man required those of the genus

*Anopheles.* (*A. maculipennis* and an *Anopheles* in which Ross had already seen zygote stages of the malarial parasite in India.)

Observations and experiments in Rome shewed that the occurrence of Anopheline mosquitoes was especially characteristic of malarious localities, and still more important that patients contracted the disease when exposed to the bites of *Anopheles* brought from notoriously malarious districts, or those which had been previously fed on malarious subjects. A final proof was the classical experiment of Manson, in which *Anopheles* infected in Italy were allowed to feed upon two volunteers in England, both of whom as a result contracted malaria.

This discovery, one of the most remarkable in the history of medicine, was so opposed to popular ideas of the way in which malaria was contracted, that for a time there were some who doubted whether the simple explanation given by Ross's experiments could explain all the facts regarding malaria transmission. Especially the idea that malaria was supposed to be contracted in remote and uninhabited swamps led to the frequently expressed suggestion that there might be channels of infection other than the mosquito, and a good deal was made of certain bodies found by Ross within the parasitic cysts, and called by him " black spores," as shewing that there might be a cycle of development over and above that already known. In order to explain the deadliness of tropical swamps and jungles, others suggested that *Anopheles* obtained infection by hereditary transmission from mosquito to mosquito, or from the blood of bats or other wild animals. " Black spores," however, are now known to be a species of *Nosema* attacking the mosquito independently of malarial infection, whilst it is now generally recognized that, contrary to current belief, remote jungles and swamps in themselves are harmless, in the absence of human inhabitants to yield infection. Neither hereditary infection of mosquitoes nor their infection from wild animals is now considered probable, and the view universally held at the present time is that malaria is an infectious disease passing from man to man, but requiring for this purpose the presence of an intermediary transmitting host, the mosquito.

This view, that malaria is a disease transmitted by *Anopheles*, but essentially of an infectious nature depending on pre-existing human infection for its origin, may be said to be that upon which all present day conceptions regarding the epidemiology and prevention of malaria are based. Such a conception of malaria is of course entirely opposed to the older notions of a "telluric" disease, and as a result the whole method of approaching malaria problems has so changed that writers sometimes refer to researches they may have conducted as being directed from the *New Ætiological Standpoint*.

But though all the more modern work upon malaria has been based upon the discovery of the mosquito cycle, yet it would be a mistake to suppose that no considerable advance in the knowledge of malaria has been made since this great discovery. Not only has there been a vast accumulation of knowledge regarding the circumstances connected with malaria in almost all parts of the world, but even in some cases a distinct modification, or rather expansion, of original conceptions of the disease has resulted. Thus the idea of malaria as an infectious disease requiring some previous *case of fever* from which infection was to be derived, has been modified, at least as far as tropical countries are concerned, and brought more into touch with the old telluric views by the discovery of the almost ubiquitous latent infection of native indigenous races and of the part played by native communities as "reservoirs of infection." Equally important have been the striking advances in the conception of the part played by economic influences in determining the degree of prevalence of malaria, for as stated by Celli it is not merely *malaria parasite + Anopheles + man* which determines the prevalence of malaria, especially the prevalence of this disease in epidemic form, but the formula *malaria parasite + Anopheles + man + X*. It is in fact the complicated factors involved in this unknown $X$ with which the most recent investigations on malaria have been mainly concerned, and the complete elucidation of Celli's formula will constitute still another step of no mean importance in the history of malarial research.

Again, with regard to advances in connection with

preventive measures directed against malaria, there has not only been a great increase of practical experience of such action under particular circumstances, but methods of combating the disease have sometimes become possible which at first sight were not self-evident. As examples may be mentioned the important method of dealing with malaria known as *Segregation*, now largely employed in Tropical Africa, and the no less remarkable development of prophylaxis as recently applied among British troops in India, where malaria has been combated not only by direct, but by a host of indirect and often extremely ingenious devices.

## *Life-cycle of the Malaria Parasite in Man and in the Mosquito.*

Like many other parasitic Protozoa, the malarial parasite has two periods of multiplication in its life-cycle, one in which it multiplies and over-runs its mammalian host, the other in which, to ensure its eventual translation to a fresh host, it multiplies in the body of the mosquito. The first period of multiplication in the blood of man, since it occurs independently of any fusion of male and female elements (*syngamy*), is known as the *asexual*, or, from the fact that multiplication goes on by a process of *schizogony*, the *schizogonous cycle*. The period of multiplication, which starts with the entry of blood containing suitable forms of the parasite into the stomach of the mosquito, is dependent on the fertilization of the female element (*macrogamete*) by a male element (*microgamete*) and is known as the *sexual* or *sporogonous cycle*, sporogony being the term applied to the analogous part of the life-cycle in other Sporozoa.

The schizogonous cycle can be repeated, as far as is known, an indefinite number of times, and apparently without the intervention of any sexual process may keep up a condition of infection of the host lasting for several years. Sporogony, on the other hand, occurs but once, with the formation of a vast number of the forms known as *sporozoites*, which, after accumulating in the salivary glands of the mosquito, remain without further development until introduced into the blood of man.

Schizogony occurs only in man, and the schizont forms, if ingested by the mosquito, are simply digested. But whilst the greater part of the sporogonous cycle takes place in the mosquito, the early stages, as far as the formation of the sexual forms is concerned, takes place in the blood of man. Thus in the blood of a malarious patient both asexual and sexual forms may be seen ; the former are those concerned in the production of fever and the clinical effects of malaria generally, the latter are of importance only if they are taken up by a suitable mosquito.

Although three species of *Plasmodium* occur in man and give rise each to a distinct type of fever, their methods of development and multiplication are essentially the same.

*Asexual cycle.—Schizogony.* We will commence with a description of the parasite as it is introduced into the blood by the bite of an infected mosquito. At this stage it consists of a small sickle-shaped body, about 10–20$\mu$ in length by 1–2$\mu$ in diameter. It is known as the sporozoite, and large numbers of these are extruded with the salivary secretion of an infected mosquito, as may be seen by allowing the insect to feed on a drop of glycerine on a slide. The sporozoite consists of a central nucleus surrounded by a uniformly staining elongate mass of cytoplasm. It is pointed at both ends, and by means of flexion is capable of progressive movements in the blood plasma. After being introduced into the blood of a human being three possibilities are open to these sporozoites. They may be killed in the body and thus produce no infection ; they may remain latent in the spleen or some other internal organ until a favourable opportunity to develop presents itself; and lastly, they may proceed at once to develop and give rise to the characteristic fever after a certain incubation period.

The sporozoite begins to develop by first boring into a red blood corpuscle and thus becoming an intracellular parasite. Once it has entered the red cell it assumes a rounded amoeboid form, which is known as the trophozoite.

The young trophozoite is actively amoeboid, giving off pseudopodia and absorbing nourishment from the contents of the red cell. At first it consists of a uniform mass of cytoplasm containing a single nucleus, but soon a "vacuole" appears in the parasite, causing it to assume a ring form (Fig. 40, 1).

As the parasite grows it feeds on the substance of the red corpuscle, and gradually destroys the whole cell, but during this process certain waste products are formed, one of which is deposited within the cytoplasm of the growing trophozoite in the form of pigment granules. These granules are composed of a brown or black substance allied to melanin, to which the name "hæmozoin" is sometimes applied. This substance is chiefly the result of the decomposition of the hæmoglobin, and has very pronounced physiological properties, being mainly responsible for the febrile attacks that occur in patients suffering from malaria.

The trophozoite grows until it reaches a certain size—about three-quarters the diameter of the red cell—when it becomes rounded off and withdraws all pseudopodia. The full grown trophozoite is then known as the schizont, and consists of a rounded mass of cytoplasm containing numerous pigment granules and a nucleus situated to one side of the centre. This nucleus now begins to divide, according to the species of *Plasmodium*, into 6 to 20 smaller nuclei (Fig. 40, 5), which become arranged around the periphery of the parasite. Each of the nuclei then becomes surrounded by a mass of cytoplasm which separates off from the remainder, and thus a number of small parasites are formed. These are known as the merozoites and are usually ovoid bodies, about $2\mu$ by $1\mu$, each containing a single nucleus. In the above-described process a certain amount of cytoplasm, containing all the pigment granules, is left unsegmented at the centre of the cell. After segmentation is complete the wall of the red cell bursts and the merozoites, together with the residual protoplasm and pigment granules, escape into the blood stream.

Many of the merozoites are now ingested by the leucocytes, but a certain number escape and at once proceed to attack other red cells. Unlike the sporozoite, the merozoite does not directly bore its way into the red cell, but usually becomes attached to the surface of the cell.

Very soon after the young parasite has attached itself, its

cytoplasm becomes spread out and exhibits a characteristic, comparatively large, clear, central vacuole, the effect of which is to give the parasite the appearance of a ring, such *ring forms* occurring in the early stages of development of all three forms of the parasite.    In fresh preparations these ring forms can be seen to possess on one part of their circumference a swelling like the stone of a signet ring which is the nucleus, and to extrude small pseudopodial processes, which in some forms are very long and slender, in others more lobose.    In specimens stained by the Romanowsky method the nuclear portion is conspicuous as a bright red mass, whilst lying around the vacuole is a thin crescentic portion of delicate blue-staining cytoplasm.

Many of the ring forms, especially in the case of the malignant tertian parasite, remain for some time attached to the surface of the red blood corpuscle, such forms being termed *accolé* or attached parasites.    Eventually in all species the parasite sinks into the substance of the cell.

The subsequent development is identical with that previously described, the termination of which is the formation of a schizont and the subsequent liberation of a number of merozoites into the blood stream.    This cycle may be repeated any number of times until a large proportion of the red cells is infected.

The asexual method of multiplication in the blood of the vertebrate host is characteristic of all species of *Plasmodium*. By this means the infection is carried from one cell to another within the vertebrate host, and very rapidly millions of the blood corpuscles become infected.    The destruction of the blood cells thus entailed rapidly produces anæmia in the affected patient, but much more harm is done by the waste products of the parasites.    These consist of the pigment granules and various other products of metabolism which are left behind in the residual protoplasm when schizogony occurs.    As they can only escape into the blood stream when the red cell bursts, these various toxic waste products are liberated together with the merozoites, and as most of the infected corpuscles rupture about the same time, the effect of the accumulated products is so considerable as to produce an attack of fever in the patient. The febrile attacks only occur when schizogony is taking place and the merozoites are being liberated into the blood stream. The interval between the attacks indicates, therefore, the time taken by the parasite to develop from the merozoite through the trophozoite stages up to the schizont, and to subdivide into a number of merozoites, or, in other words, to pass through the complete asexual cycle. It has been found that the time taken for the completion of this cycle varies in different species of *Plasmodium*, being 72 hours in the case of *P. malariæ*, 48 hours in *P. vivax*, and from 24 to 48 hours in *P. falciparum*. Hence the fevers caused by each of these parasites differ from one another by the intervals elapsing between the febrile attacks. The full description of these species, together with their distinguishing characteristics, is described below (*vide* p. 155).

In these few words we have briefly described the asexual cycle of development that takes place in the vertebrate host, but, as will be obvious, the only method by which the merozoites could infect another host would be by the inoculation of blood containing them. This method of transmission is successful, for if blood containing malarial parasites is inoculated into a normal human being, the latter becomes infected with malaria. However, such a mode of transmission probably never occurs in nature, for the merozoites are incapable of withstanding desiccation, or any other of the vicissitudes to which they would be exposed on the proboscis of a biting arthropod, the only conceivable agent for such direct transmission. Consequently, in addition to its asexual multiplication, which merely serves to increase its numbers in the infected individual, it is necessary for the parasite to possess some means of being carried from one host to another. We shall see that provision is made for this transmission, but first it is necessary to describe another development that the young trophozoite may undergo in the red cell.

*Development of the sexual forms in the blood.* About a week after a patient becomes infected with malaria certain large intracorpuscular forms may be observed that do not go through

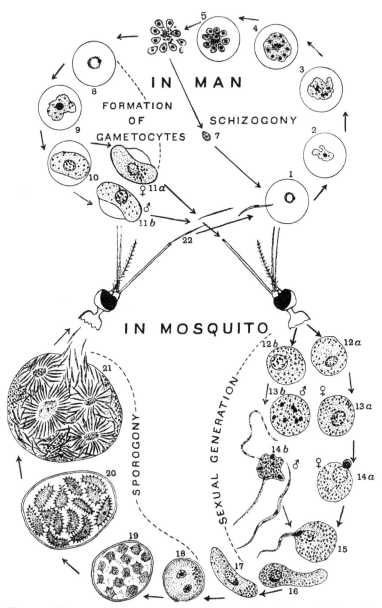

Fig. 40. Diagrammatic representation of the life-cycle of the malarial parasite of pernicious malaria. 1–6. The schizogonous cycle shewing successive stages in growth from the young ring form (1) up to the fully-grown parasite (4) in which the nucleus has divided. 5 and 6. Division of the body of the parasite to form the merozoites. 7. A single merozoite, which

is capable of entering another red cell and repeating the above-described cycle. 8–11. Formation of the gametocytes ; these arise by growth of merozoites and after reaching a certain size (10) develop into either male or female gametocytes (11a and 11b) ; in the male gametocyte (11b) the nucleus is larger and more scattered than in the female (11a). 12–16. Stages of the sexual generation in the stomach of the mosquito. 12a, 13a and 14a. The formation of the female gamete. 12b, 13b and 14b. Stages in the formation of the male gametes. 15. Fertilization, resulting in the formation of a zygote (16), which then becomes motile and is known as the oökinete (17). 18–22. Stages in the sporogonous cycle in the mosquito. The oökinete (17) bores into the stomach wall and forms a cyst (18) ; it increases in size, its nucleus multiplies and eventually each nucleus becomes surrounded by a mass of cytoplasm, forming a number of sporoblasts (19) ; each of these sporoblasts gives rise to numerous sporozoites (20–21). The ripe sporocyst is represented in 21, and the escaping sporozoites (22) enter the salivary gland of the mosquito and escaping with the salivary secretion, enter the blood and are capable of repeating the cycle.

the process of schizogony. These are the sexual forms, and are of two kinds, male and female. It is probable that the merozoites differentiate sexually at an early stage of the disease, but what determines the sex is unknown.

In its earliest stages the young sexual form is indistinguishable from an ordinary trophozoite, but it grows extremely slowly and never assumes the ring form.

As it grows its cytoplasm becomes filled with granules of pigment and soon certain differences can be noticed in the staining reactions of the protoplasm, resulting in the differentiation of what are known as the macrogametocytes and microgametocytes respectively. The former are destined to give rise to the female gametes, and are characterized by the possession of a small feebly-chromatic nucleus and a dense cytoplasm containing numerous granules and much pigment. The microgametocytes, which give rise to the male gametes, have each a large densely chromatic nucleus extending across the middle of the cell, and the cytoplasm is clearer and contains less pigment.

When full grown, the sexual forms are larger than the red cells which contain them ; consequently the latter are considerably distorted by the parasite and form conspicuous objects that were noticed long before their true nature was recognized.

At this stage there are now three types of parasites, viz. the schizonts, macrogametocytes and microgametocytes, the two latter belonging to the sexual and the former to the asexual cycle.

The sexual cycle cannot be completed in the blood but only in the internal organs of those species of mosquito which transmit the infection. In the absence of these the microgametocytes soon die off without any further development taking place.

The macrogametocytes, on the other hand, are much more resistant, and can remain in the body for very considerable periods. These are the forms that are supposed to be responsible for the cases of latent malaria, in which a patient may remain in good health for some years and then suddenly develop typical malaria without having been exposed to the possibility of re-infection. In these cases it is the macrogametocytes that have remained dormant in the body waiting for a convenient opportunity to develop, such as that afforded by a chill or any other diminution in the vitality of the patient. Under these circumstances the macrogametocyte develops parthenogenetically. Its nucleus divides into two parts, one densely chromatic and the other poor in chromatin. The pigment granules and other waste products gather round the latter, and the whole is divided off from the remaining protoplasm and constitutes a sort of residuum similar to that left behind by the merozoites. The remaining part of the macrogametocyte, now much clearer by the loss of its pigment granules, divides up into a number of merozoites in exactly the same way as an ordinary schizont, and the merozoites escaping into the blood plasma penetrate other red cells and thus start another cycle of schizogony.

*Sexual cycle.—Sporogony.* As mentioned above the macro- and microgametocytes only complete their development in the internal organs of the mosquito that is responsible for their transmission. When such a mosquito—in the case of malaria *only* Anophelines—feeds on the blood of a patient containing sexual forms, in addition to the latter, it ingests many parasites belonging to the schizogonous cycle. All these are digested, the macro- and microgametocytes being the only forms that are capable of resisting the secretions in the stomach of the mosquito. Here they undergo further development, the stimulus for which is probably the reduction in temperature, combined with the dilution of the blood that takes place in the gut of the insect.

The macrogametocyte escapes from its red cell and becomes spherical; then its nucleus divides and one of the daughter-nuclei, together with a small amount of cytoplasm, is extruded as a polar body (Fig. 40, 14 a). After this maturation process is complete the parasite is now ready for fertilization, and is known as the female or macrogamete.

The microgametocyte undergoes a different kind of development, for after becoming spherical and escaping from the red corpuscle, its nucleus breaks up into a number of fragments, sometimes known as chromidia, which travel outwards and become arranged round the periphery of the cell. Part of the nucleus remains behind at the centre as a residuum and is not used up in the subsequent development. The surface of the microgametocyte now grows out into a number of flagellum-like processes into each of which passes one of the nuclear fragments. These processes are highly motile, and by their lashing about cause the parasite to resemble a flagellate. In consequence the earlier observers referred these forms to the genus *Polymitus*, and they are still often referred to by this name. Each of the flagellum-like processes finally becomes free and swims away as an independent organism. These are the male or microgametes. The microgametocyte usually produces four to six of these microgametes which in their formation use up the protoplasm of the gametocyte, merely leaving a residuum composed of all the pigment granules, together with part of the original nucleus and a small amount of cytoplasm. The microgamete consists of an elongated filament with a slight thickening about the middle of its length, caused by the nuclear matter. It progresses by rapid wave-like movements and as it is only about 0·5 $\mu$ in diameter, is extremely difficult to observe in the living state.

Conjugation now takes place, one of the microgametes boring its way into a macrogamete. This is followed by union of the two nuclei, and the resulting structure is known as the zygote. At first the zygote is spherical, but it soon elongates into a small worm-like body which is actively motile, moving about in much the same way as a gregarine. The zygote is then known as the oökinete or, by some writers, the vermicule, because of the character of its movements.

The whole of this process, including the formation of the gametes and their union to form the oökinete, takes place in the stomach (= hinder part of the mid-gut) of the mosquito, and is completed within a comparatively short time. All the above stages may be observed by placing a drop of blood containing the gametocytes on a slide and slightly breathing on it. If the preparation be now covered with a cover-glass and examined under an oil-immersion lens, all the stages in the evolution of the micro- and macrogametes, and their subsequent union to form the oökinete, may be followed in the living state.

The subsequent development of the oökinete can take place only in the mosquito, and we shall proceed with the description of the changes which it undergoes in this site.

After moving about for some time, the oökinete bores through the epithelium of the gut-wall and comes to rest between this layer and the tissues immediately surrounding it. Here the parasite becomes rounded off and secretes a thin cyst-wall. This form is known as the oöcyst and is parasitic upon the mosquito, for it grows considerably in size, absorbing nourishment from the surrounding tissues. During its growth, the gut-wall is bulged out towards the body-cavity, and consequently at this stage the stomach of the infected mosquito has a very characteristic appearance (Fig. 53). As many as 500 oöcysts have been found in the stomach-wall of a single infected *Anopheles*.

As the oöcyst grows, its nucleus divides into a number of daughter-nuclei, each of which becomes surrounded by a mass of cytoplasm and gradually separated off from its neighbours. These are known as the sporoblasts ; they are irregular in form and remain slightly connected together by means of cytoplasmic processes.  After the formation of the sporoblasts a certain amount of protoplasm is left over, containing all the waste products and also some of the pigment granules originally present in the macrogamete.

The nucleus of each sporoblast now divides into a large number of smaller ones which become arranged around the periphery.  The surface of the sporoblast then exhibits a number of cytoplasmic projections, each of which increases in length and takes with it a daughter-nucleus.  Eventually the spindle-shaped process, with its contained nucleus, becomes free from

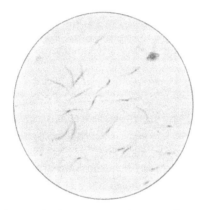

Fig. 41.  Photomicrograph of sporozoites of malaria from the salivary glands of *Anopheles (Pyretophorus) costalis.*  × about 1000.  After Hill and Haydon.

the mother sporoblast, and is then known as the sporozoite. Each sporoblast produces large numbers of these bodies, but a certain amount of protoplasm containing waste products is always left unused in their formation.  The oöcyst, which contains the whole of the sporozoites derived from the many sporoblasts, and by this time has increased enormously in size, eventually bursts, and the sporozoites are set free in the body-cavity of the mosquito.  As the cœlomic fluid bathes all the organs of the mosquito, the sporozoites are brought in contact with all parts of the body.  They appear to have a predilection for the salivary glands and the majority bore their way into these organs and may be seen filling the secretory cells and also becoming free in the lumen. The sporozoites are now incapable of further development in the mosquito, but if the latter feeds on a human being, large numbers of them are introduced into the wound together with the salivary secretion. They thus enter the blood and there penetrate into the red blood corpuscles and start the schizogonous cycle with which we commenced.

The whole of this process, from the differentiation of the macro- and microgametocytes to the formation of the sporozoites, is known as the sexual or sporogonous cycle, and is completed in from ten to twelve days. Thus a mosquito that has ingested blood containing the gametocytes does not become infective until this incubation period has elapsed. Then its salivary glands contain the sporozoites, and the insect probably remains infective during the remainder of its life.

### *Bionomics of Mosquitoes in Relation to Malaria.*

The habits of the particular species of mosquito concerned in the transmission of malaria in any particular locality are of the highest importance, and therefore, at the risk of repetition, some of the more important features may be briefly mentioned.

The majority of Anophelines are more commonly associated with village life, and are especially prevalent in more or less uncultivated districts, and, unlike the Culicines, their breeding habits are usually unsuitable for their persistence in towns.

With respect to this point, however, there are exceptions, and it will be necessary to refer to the connection between the habits of various species in relation to the spread of malaria.

At the time of the discovery of the mosquito cycle, only some half-dozen species of *Anopheles* were known, most of which are European species. There are now more than 100 well defined and accurately described species, as well as many named varieties, and these taken collectively have a distribution which extends almost all over the globe. These species differ not only in morphological details, but what is more important from our present point of view, they vary greatly in their habits and in their relation to malaria.

Among habits affecting the conditions of malarial dissemination may be mentioned the predilection of particular species for particular kinds of breeding place. Some species are essentially stream breeders and are even adapted by their habits, and probably to some extent by structure, to prevent themselves being carried away by flood conditions. An example of a species

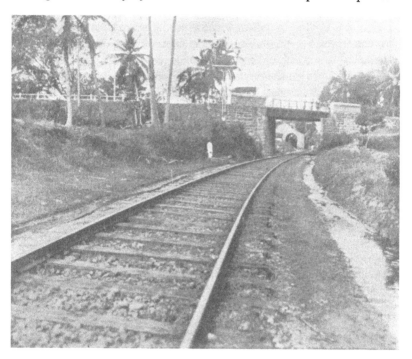

Fig. 42. Breeding places of Anophelines. Railway cutting at Kurunegala. The water course flowing on each side of the permanent way supplying the engines with water. These channels are blocked with weeds, from amongst which larvæ of *A. culicifacies* and *A. rossii* have been taken. After Bahr (from the *Tropical Diseases Bulletin*).

having this habit is *A.* (*Myzomyia*) *listoni* (*M. christophersi* Theobald), which swarms in the streams of the sub-Himalayan terai, and is largely responsible for the high prevalence of malaria in these regions. Another example is *A.* (*Nyssorhynchus*) *willmori*, a species which is very difficult to eradicate, because of its power of breeding freely in the small streams of Malay

Other species are pool-breeders, and some may even restrict themselves, or be able to flourish only in some particular kind of pool. Thus the numerical prevalence of the common Indian species *A. (Myzomyia) rossii* is dependent usually on the occurrence of small freshly-filled shallow muddy rain-pools, such as are formed in countless thousands during the Indian monsoon. In the forests of South America a malaria-transmitting species, *A. (Myzomyia) lutzi*, breeds in various pitcher-plants, and especially in the cups of various epiphytic tree pines. An even more remarkable choice of breeding place is seen in the Malayan species *A. (Lophoscelomyia) asiatica*, which is found breeding only in bamboos that have been perforated by a borer.

Over a large tract of the earth's surface, where mangrove swamps and salt marshes are a feature of the sea coasts, the species *A. (Myzomyia) ludlowi* breeds in brackish water, in pools that are entered by the sea at spring tides. In the case of the Andaman Islands, Christophers has recently shewn that this species is the chief carrier of malaria, and as it is not found at a greater distance than half-a-mile from the coast, is the cause of a *littoral* distribution of malaria in these islands.

Another good example of the extent to which habits of particular species in regard to the choice of breeding place may affect the dissemination of malaria is seen in the case of the very interesting *Anopheles, A. (Nyssorhynchus) stephensi*. This species ordinarily is found in pools in large sandy river beds, and has a predilection for quite small collections of water, such as the hoof-marks made by cattle coming to drink, or shallow surface wells made in the sand at the river margin. It was found, however, by the Royal Societies Commission, to possess, like Culicines, the power of breeding in water pots and other domestic utensils, when these were filled with comparatively clean water. More recently this species has been shewn by Liston and by Bentley to be the species concerned in the spread of malaria in Bombay City, where the population is as dense as in the heart of London, and under conditions where no other species of this genus has been able to survive. It is entirely due to the power of *N. stephensi* to breed in wells, covered cisterns, and such like places, that it has been able to establish itself in these novel and, to the genus as a whole, quite unsuitable surroundings.

Apart from the differences in regard to the ability to flourish in particular kinds of breeding places, are other habits which sometimes influence very considerably the epidemiological conditions under which malaria is spread. Thus many species of

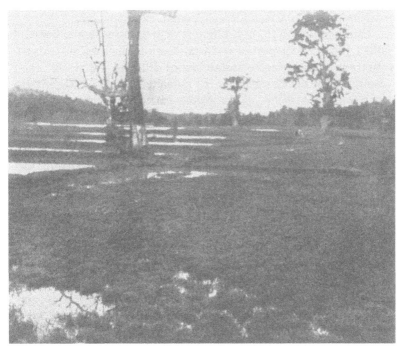

Fig. 43. Flooded Paddy Fields in Ceylon. The picture shews in the foreground the pools formed by the hoof-marks of cattle ; in these Anophelines breed. After Bahr (from the *Tropical Diseases Bulletin*).

*Anopheles* are naturally little addicted to entering or remaining in human habitations, and in nature are not found particularly associated with man. Other species readily take up a life of dependence on man and utilize his dwellings as shelter. It is to this latter class that the more important malaria carriers belong. Again, under ordinary circumstances, some species are entirely nocturnal in their habits, whilst others bite freely on cloudy moist days, and others again may have actively diurnal habits and feed by day like *Stegomyia*. An example of the latter habit is seen in the species *A. (Myzorhynchus) barbirostris*, which swarms in the forests of Malay and is most bloodthirsty throughout the daytime. Another diurnal species is *Anopheles aitkeni*. Even the boldness and persistence, or even the small size of particular species, may add greatly to their effect in transmitting malaria under particular circumstances.

But in addition to these differences in habits which indirectly affect the transmission of malaria, there is the very important question of the relative suitability of different species of *Anopheles* for the development of the parasite. When it was shewn that certain species of *Anopheles* carried malaria and that *Culex* and other biting insects did not, it was assumed that the power to act as a suitable host to the malaria parasite was common to all Anophelines. The first instance of an *Anopheles* being shewn not to transmit malaria was in the case of the common Indian species *A. (Myzomyia) rossii*. This species is found quite commonly in very large numbers associated with every degree of prevalence of malaria, but it has not yet been shewn to act as a transmitting agent under natural conditions, though it can be infected experimentally. Not infrequently this species occurs along with others which are actively concerned in the spread of malaria, but though under these circumstances a considerable percentage of both *A. (Myzomyia) culicifacies* and *A. (Nyssorhynchus) stephensi* have been found with sporozoites in the salivary glands, *A. (Myzomyia) rossii* has never been found infected. This peculiar fact, regarding which the following independent figures have been given, is not easy to explain, but there seems little doubt that

|  | M. culicifacies | N. stephensi | Myzomyia rossii |
|---|---|---|---|
| Stephens and Christophers Lahore (Punjab) | 4·6 °/₀ | — | o |
| Ennur (Madras) | 8·6 °/₀ | — | o |
| Bentley Bombay | — | 3·5 °/₀ | — |

for some reason, *A. rossii* is not an active transmitter of malaria, if it transmits at all, under natural conditions.

Another species not suitable as a carrier, and which in this case was refractory even to experimental infection, is the North American species *Anopheles punctipennis*. In this case *A. maculipennis* and *A. punctipennis* were fed together on an infected patient; the former became infected whilst the latter remained free from infection.

The development of the three species of malarial parasites does not take place with the same facility in any given species of mosquito. Thus Kinoshita found that in Formosa, *Plasmodium falciparum* was incapable of development within *A. (Myzorhynchus) sinensis*, whilst this species of mosquito could easily be infected with *Plasmodium vivax* (seven times out of eleven) and less easily with *Plasmodium malariæ* (one in seven). In the same region *A. (Myzomyia) christophersi* almost invariably became infected when fed on a patient containing the gametes of *P. falciparum* in his blood.

Other species have also been noted as probably not taking an active part in malaria transmission or to be actually refractory to experimental infection with the malaria parasite.

But though some species are possibly incapable of acting as hosts, and whilst some are more suitable hosts than others, there is reason to believe that very many of the species are at least potential transmitters. Thus in India, Stephens and Christophers succeeded in experimentally infecting all but one species out of a considerable variety of Anophelines. Similarly, Darling at Panama has produced infection in many of the Anophelines of that region.

The most important point in regard to the transmitting power of a species is the extent to which it is found actively concerned in transmission under natural conditions. In this respect there are certain species which must be looked upon as the chief carriers in particular parts of the world.

In Europe the common carrier is *Anopheles maculipennis*, but the common species, *Anopheles bifurcatus*, is also capable of transmitting malaria. *A. maculipennis* is the common carrier in the Mediterranean islands and is largely concerned in the spread of malaria in Algeria and Palestine. It is also the chief agent in North America.

In Algeria, besides *A. maculipennis*, the species incriminated are : *Anopheles algeriensis* (Ed. and Et. Sergent, 1905), especially occurring in the coast regions ; *A. hispaniola* (Sergents, 1905), found chiefly in the hilly broken country ; *A. (Pyretophorus) myzomyfacies* (Ed. Sergent) ; *A. (P.) superpictus* and *A. (P.) chaudoyei*. *A. chaudoyei* is capable of breeding freely in saline waters and is the species chiefly concerned in malarial transmission in the Saharan oases.

In Egypt, *A. (Cellia) pharoënsis* is a proved and important carrier.

*Anopheles funesta* and *A. costalis* have both been shewn by Ross to transmit the infection, and are the most important and widely distributed carriers of malaria in Tropical Africa.

In India, Stephens and Christophers shewed that *A. (Myzomyia) listoni* is a very actively transmitting agent in the Duars or terai country at the foot of the Eastern Himalayas. A more general, and perhaps the commonest Indian transmitter is *A. (Myzomyia) culicifacies*. *A. fuliginosus* Giles has also been shewn to transmit the disease, but apparently is not a very important carrier. *A. maculipalpis* has been found infected in nature in various parts of India. Amongst the most important and active Indian carriers are *A. (Nyssorhynchus) stephensi* and *A. (N.) willmori*.

In Malay, in addition to *M. listoni*, the proved carriers in nature are *A. (Myzomyia) albirostris*, *A. (Myzomyia) ludlowi*, and *A. (Nyssorhynchus) willmori*.

In Central America a number of species are active carriers, the most important being *A. (Cellia) argyrotarsis* and *A. (C.) albimana*.

In addition there are numbers of species very probably concerned in malaria transmission, perhaps even important carriers in particular parts of the world, *e.g. A. formosaënsis* in the island of Formosa ; *A. arabiensis* in the Aden hinterland; *A. (Myzomyia) lutzi* in the forests of Brazil ; and *A. (Nyssorhynchus) annulipes* in Formosa, Australia, etc.

*Influences affecting Malaria through the Transmitting Host.*

The most powerful influences affecting *Anopheles* are temperature, rainfall and humidity. Added to these must be considered the physical characters of the country under consideration, the nature of the soil, the prevalence of natural enemies, and even the races of mankind inhabiting the countries.

With regard to physical conditions, generally hot moist climates are suitable, cold and also excessively dry climates unsuitable, to the development of *Anopheles*. In this respect, however, the question of species and even of special adaptive habits becomes important.

*Temperature* plays a double *rôle*. If low it not only delays or prevents the propagation of *Anopheles*, but it even more actively interferes with the development of the parasite within the mosquito. A perennial low temperature may altogether prevent the propagation of the parasites, for it is found that the gametocytes cannot develop below a temperature of about 15° C. As a result, one can trace northern and southern limits to the occurrence of malaria, corresponding to the mean summer isotherm of 15° to 16° C. Moreover, the different species of malaria require different degrees of warmth in order to ensure their development. Thus *Plasmodium malariæ* develops best at comparatively low temperatures, and consequently is found in much colder regions than the other two species. On the other hand *P. falciparum* will only develop at comparatively high temperatures, and therefore in temperate regions it only occurs during the summer and autumn months, whilst throughout the tropics it is prevalent the whole year round. *Plasmodium vivax* occupies a somewhat intermediate position, for it is capable of development throughout a wide range of temperature and, as one would expect, this species is the most widely distributed, occurring in both tropical and temperate regions. A perennial low temperature within limits, however, does not prevent the propagation of certain species of *Anopheles*, e.g. *A. bifurcatus* reaches a particularly large size in the north of Scotland. Still less does a temporary or seasonal period of low temperature destroy or permanently affect the prevalence of *Anopheles*, such periods being tided over by "hibernation." It is thus easy to see how, as regards the northern and southern limits of malaria, we may have these fairly corresponding with the limits of the distribution of *Anopheles*, and to understand how, even apart from any other reason, a considerable altitude may be associated with a freedom from malaria, even though *Anopheles* are still found.

*Rainfall*, up to a certain point, is very favourable to *Anopheles*, but if excessive it may have an adverse effect by washing away the larvæ and destroying them. *Humidity* would seem to be entirely a favourable circumstance, and has been shewn to affect favourably the development of the malarial parasite within the mosquito.

The nature of the soil may affect conditions as regards *Anopheles*, not only by its power to retain surface water or to allow of the formation of springs, but often by reason of its chemical nature ; surface waters in some soils readily develop a ferruginous scum or other conditions, unsuitable to the development of mosquitoes.

The occurrence of natural enemies, especially circumstances which favour the general presence in surface waters of small fish, is a most powerful influence checking the multiplication of *Anopheles*. Under conditions of alternate rainfall and drought many pools utilized by *Anopheles* are of too temporary a nature for the presence of fish, or even of other natural enemies, such as various predaceous insect larvæ. On the contrary, in very moist countries, even the smaller pools are usually stocked with fish and other predaceous animals. There may thus often be a very fortunate regulating mechanism which may completely reverse the normal order of affairs and make *Anopheles* comparatively scarce under conditions that at first sight might appear wholly favourable.

Besides being open to attack by fish and various predaceous aquatic insects, *Anopheles* are frequently the victims of parasites. Among such may be mentioned acarid ectoparasites, an encysted trematode, nematodes, gregarines, flagellates of the genus *Leptomonas*, and at least one species of *Nosema*. They are also liable to invasion by certain fungi.

The part played by *Anopheles* in the transmission of malaria is often distinctly modified by the method of life and customs of man. Thus the type of dwelling may be such as to minimize the chances of *Anopheles* obtaining human blood or, on the other hand, to greatly favour such a chance. Thus, the introduction of glass windows into English houses may well have hastened the disappearance of malaria from this country. Again, communities, by housing cattle or other domestic animals, often favour the occurrence of *Anopheles*, whilst the amount of clothing worn and special modes of livelihood, may similarly affect the prevalence of malaria.

*Malaria in Relation to Man.*

So long as man was supposed to be the victim of animal-culæ, that before entering his body lived a free life in marsh water, etc., the part man himself played in the continuance and preservation of the parasite was not considered. But as we now understand the rationale of malaria transmission, it is evident that man, no less than the mosquito, is essential to the continued life of the parasite, and the nature of man's influence as a host is at least equal in importance to those circumstances we have discussed in the previous section.

It will be evident from what has already been said that it is man and not the mosquito which forms the chief reservoir of infection. A man once infected, even though no longer exposed to re-infection, may harbour the parasite for years. So long as he does so, and is liable to relapses with the formation of gametes, such a man is capable of infecting mosquitoes and of restarting active transmission of the disease. The ability to maintain a prolonged state of infection in man is therefore a very valuable asset to the parasite, and all conditions which favour or are adverse to a maintenance of the parasite in the blood of man are of epidemiological importance. Similarly, the *amount* of infection passed on to the mosquito has been shewn to be an important matter, a mosquito which has taken in blood containing many gametes being capable of giving rise to a much more severe infection than one which

has taken in but a few parasites.   Thus questions of susceptibility and immunity, whether natural or acquired, or due to
the use of drugs, have to be considered.   Also the condition
of nutrition of the members of a community, and its effect
on the natural resistance of the human organism against the
parasite, and the extent to which influences favourable to
relapses prevail, are all factors in the epidemiology of malaria.

Susceptibility to malaria may be evidenced either by increased liability to infection, or by the degree to which *toleration*
of the presence of the parasite exists.   In the case of primitive
and aboriginal races there is evidence to shew that apart from
any possible lessened liability to infection, there is often a greater
degree of toleration than is exhibited, for example, in Europeans.
A real *immunity* with a lessened liability to infection is also
undoubtedly developed in those persons long exposed to
malarial infection.   When in any race toleration and immunity
are well marked, a considerable degree of malaria may occur
in a latent form.   In such cases susceptible strangers suffer
far more than the native residents.

The importance of the part played by susceptibility and
immunity in malaria was demonstrated by Koch at Stephansort
in New Guinea, where, at the time his observations were made,
malaria was very prevalent.   Koch was able to shew that after
a batch of Chinese immigrant coolies, who formed a large portion
of the population, had been resident for some years in the
colony they suffered distinctly less from malaria than they did
on their first arrival, and that in the absence of fresh immigration,
malaria amongst the community, as a whole, shewed a steady
decline, but with each successive large immigration of new
coolies there was a marked recrudescence of the disease.   These
observations of Koch establish a principle in malarial epidemiology which may be termed the law of *non-immune immigration* (Christophers and Bentley), and which applies to all
immigration of susceptible individuals into a malarial focus.

Where the number of strangers is small, the effect is chiefly
exhibited upon them, as in the case of Europeans residing in
Africa.   Here, as shewn by Stephens and Christophers, the
whole epidemiological outlook as regards the European is

dominated by the presence of a more or less latent native malaria.

Where the influx of strangers is comparatively very large, the whole community is adversely affected, and under certain circumstances the prevalence of malaria through a whole tract of country may be greatly increased.

Since the new-born child is, in a sense, an immigrant, in any community the young children are especially affected. Where malarial infection is intense, but the population is stable and possibly possesses a certain degree of racial tolerance, the amount of infection is highest in the young children and at a minimum in the adults. In this case the children go through life more or less permanently infected and with a certain amount of splenic enlargement. At about the age of puberty, they cease to shew parasites in their blood, or to exhibit enlargement of the spleen.

Where malaria is more or less seasonal in its occurrence, or where there is any serious degree of immigration or shifting of populations, the restriction of infection to children is less marked. All grades of difference in this respect may be encountered, the usual rule being that strictly indigenous and primitive tribes shew the greatest amount of tolerance, and along with a high proportion of infection amongst children, exhibit the greatest adult immunity from infection.

Recently much stress has been laid upon the influence of economic factors in determining a high or a low degree of malaria prevalence. Poverty stricken and squalidly living communities in malarious countries usually exhibit a far greater degree of malarial infection than do communities in a condition of prosperity. Besides the " social " distribution of malaria, very grave manifestations may be brought about at least partly by conditions of general stress, such as the occurrence of famines or scarcity following failure of rainfall, especially when this is followed by floods still further adding to the distress and supplying all the requisites for an active transmission of the disease by Anopheline mosquitoes. Thus, in Denmark, epidemics of great severity have frequently followed great storms, which had led to extensive inundations associated with much hardship, and a similar condition has been described in India, where, during exceptional monsoons, many large rivers overflow their banks, causing extensive inundations. Under such conditions malaria may prevail with such intensity as to cause a mortality with which it is not usually associated, and may equal or exceed the ravages of even bubonic plague.

Besides purely economic influences, the prevalence of malaria is often greatly enhanced in a community, or even in a population, by circumstances leading to unusual conditions of labour, increased physical fatigue, exposure to the sun and to rain. In such cases the mere production of relapses alone may lead to a greatly increased prevalence of malaria, but where *Anopheles* are present there is naturally associated with an increased output of parasites an increased transmission of the disease. Malaria may from such reasons be greatly increased during certain seasons, *e.g.* the rainy season in the Canal Zone, even though the number of *Anopheles* has not been increased. An increase of malaria during the harvests is another familiar example.

Where unusual exposure and hardship are associated with inadequate food and general distress, the result is usually for malaria to assert itself in a very grave form, even though the conditions as regards *Anopheles* are not especially favourable.

## *The Prevention of Malaria.*

Under present-day conceptions there can be no transmission of malaria under any of the following conditions :

1. Absence of Anophelines, by which infection would be conveyed.

2. Absence of infected persons in the community, from whom infection could be obtained by the mosquitoes, even if these were present.

3. The existence of adequate " protection " by means of which either

    (a) The healthy cannot be bitten.

    (b) The infected cannot be bitten.

Preventive action therefore aims at bringing about more or less perfectly one or more of these conditions. Theoretically any one of the three, if completely realized, would suffice to prevent any fresh transmission of malaria, and finally to exterminate the disease. Unfortunately in practice it is usually possible only very imperfectly to achieve the desired end in any of these directions, and it becomes necessary to combine the effects of as many methods as possible. Circumstances alone can determine in any given case which line of action is most called for, or what combination of methods is likely to be most effective.

Under the first head come all measures which have as their object the reduction in the number of Anophelines present. Such action may be direct, as in the case of anti-mosquito campaigns, or indirect as by the extension of agriculture, or large drainage measures. Under the second head come various methods of quinine prophylaxis, all agreeing in the use of quinine as a destroyer of the parasite in the human host, but differing a good deal in the immediate object arrived at. Under this head also come certain measures applicable to mixed communities as the " Removal or prophylactic treatment of the reservoir of infection," " Segregation of the healthy," and the avoidance by the individual of sources of infection generally. Under the head of protection are included such measures as the screening of dwellings and barracks, the use of suitable protective clothing, and the use of the mosquito net.

1. Many methods of attacking *Anopheles* are now known, the more important being :

*The obliteration of breeding places.* By minor drainage measures, filling up pools or depressions with earth and, in some cases, subsoil drainage, pools utilized by *Anopheles* for breeding may be completely done away with. In cases where it is difficult or impossible to carry out such action, breeding places may be made less suitable by clearing out weeds, deepening, and perhaps even lining with masonry, the edges of large sheets of water. Not infrequently the chief sources of *Anopheles* are to be found in connection with small streams, in which case training in some form or another should be performed. Where

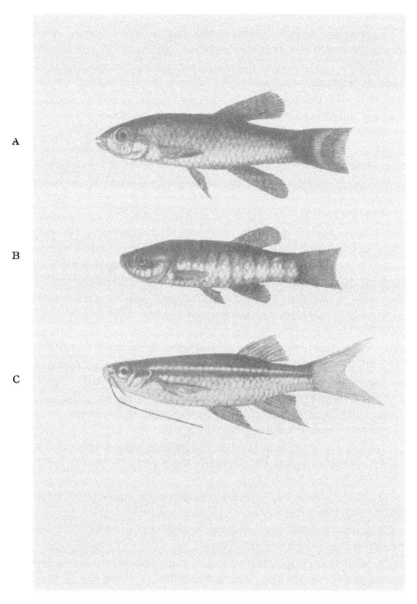

Fig. 44. Indian fish of utility as mosquito-destroyers. After Sewell and Chaudhuri (from the *Tropical Diseases Bulletin*).
A ( ♂ ) and B ( ♀ ). *Lebias dispar* (nat. size).
C. *Nuria danrica* (nat. size).

wells are an important source of *Anopheles* they often require special devices to prevent them being a source of danger whilst allowing water to be obtained from them, and other breeding places of a special nature may require special measures to deal with them. On the whole the most important consideration in such measures is that the action taken should be of as permanent a nature as possible.

*The use of larvicides.* Many substances have been experimented with in respect to their lethal effect upon the larvæ of mosquitoes. The larvicide in most general use is some form of kerosene or mixture containing this substance. The oil floats on the surface of the water and thus interferes with the respiration of the larvæ and pupæ. Certain aniline dyes, and other chemical bodies which dissolve in the water, have very powerful larvicidal properties, and their use has been suggested. The chief difficulty with regard to all larvicides is the temporary nature of the effect they produce, and the necessity for regular and periodical treatment of the breeding places attacked in this way. Ordinarily such substances are now used only where more permanent measures are not possible.

*The introduction of natural enemies.* So far the hope that by the introduction of some natural enemy, the number of *Anopheles* in a country could be at all affected, has not met with much encouragement. Nevertheless, under certain circumstances, the use of suitable small fish has an application. The most effective larvæ-eating fish for the most part belong to the family *Cypriondontidæ*, but species of *Anabas*, *Ophiocephalus* and others are also of practical use in this respect.

*Measures directed against the adult mosquito.* The fumigation of houses with burning sulphur, pyrethrum and other substances, has been found of use. In Panama the catching of adult mosquitoes by children for a small reward is said to be very effective. Whitewashing and improvement in lighting during the daytime may be called for sometimes.

The various measures briefly outlined above are but some of the tools in the hand of the sanitarian, to be used as circumstances require them. Before they can be applied with success it is almost always necessary for the conditions relating to

A

B

C

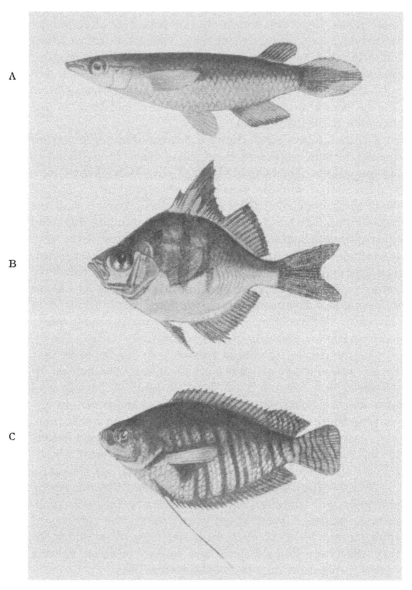

Fig. 45. Indian fish of utility as mosquito-destroyers.   After Sewell and Chaudhuri (from the *Tropical Diseases Bulletin*).
  A.   *Haplochilus panchax* (nat. size).
  B.   *Ambassis ranga* (nat. size).
  C.   *Trichogaster fasciatus* (nat. size).

transmission to have been very thoroughly studied and the whole area accurately and thoroughly surveyed.

Of measures indirectly affecting the prevalence of *Anopheles*, the most important are " drainage " and " agriculture." The drainage of marshes, lakes, etc. has long been known to have a favourable effect upon malaria. Agricultural operation, by which waste lands are reduced to the condition of tilled fields, is another general measure having a very definite influence upon malaria. Both these measures, though they do not aim directly at mosquito reduction, bring about this result indirectly by lowering the level of the subsoil water, lessening humidity and so forth. A measure of this general kind, which may assume importance under certain circumstances, is protection against flooding. It has recently been shewn that some of the worst manifestations of epidemic malaria follow in the wake of floods, arising from the overflowing of rivers and swollen mountain torrents. In such cases various engineering devices may be important anti-malarial measures of this general kind.

2. Where preventive action against malaria takes the form of attacking the parasite in the human host it usually consists of some method of quinine prophylaxis. In the method advocated by Koch an attempt is made to sterilize, as far as the malarial parasite is concerned, the blood of every member of the community by systematically searching out and treating every infected person. The method to which the term *quinine prophylaxis* is generally applied, is one in which as many of the community as possible are persuaded to take quinine regularly and systematically. Where large and at the same time poor and ignorant populations are concerned, it has generally been found impossible to apply either of the above measures sufficiently thoroughly to be effective, and it is now recognized that under these circumstances the greatest benefits are obtained by treating the sick and encouraging in every way the use of quinine in its curative rather than its prophylactic capacity. This method is usually designated as *quinine treatment of the sick*. Though directed especially to the saving of life, it has been found also to have a general influence upon malaria.

In addition to this direct action of quinine upon the source of infection in man, there are a number of indirect methods of reducing the sources of infection.

3. (a) Very often where mixed communities are concerned, it may be desirable to protect especially the more susceptible class of individuals. When possible this is brought about by some form of segregation. Where the reservoir of virus is small in comparison with the community of susceptibles, as frequently happens in Algerian stations, segregation takes the form of removal of the indigenous community to a short distance from the station. Where the number of the susceptible persons is small in comparison with the reservoir, as is usual in the case of Europeans in Africa, it is advisable to build quarters for this community at some distance from the native settlement. In some cases it may be desirable to undertake measures against malaria in a small community acting as a "reservoir," not so much for the direct effect upon this community, as for the indirect effect upon the larger susceptible community surrounding it. In this way, the actual application of segregation may vary, though the principle remains the same.

Still another indirect method of diminishing the amount of human infection, and thus reducing the activity of malaria transmission, is the protection of a community from influences likely to bring about repeated relapses. For example, among labourers or convicts, or even among agricultural people, any amelioration of the conditions under which they are living may be looked upon as an anti-malarial measure coming under this head.

(b) Protection against the bites of *Anopheles* by the screening of dwellings with wire gauze, etc. is a measure which has been found especially valuable in Panama and elsewhere. The protection brought about by the habitual and careful use of a mosquito net is perhaps the most effective measure of private prophylaxis known against malaria, and with some other minor precautions is quite sufficient to enable the educated individual to enter the most malarious tracts unharmed. The use of mosquito nets by the sick is a valuable prophylactic measure in hospitals, where in the absence of any such precaution the dissemination of malaria may result from the bringing together of many cases of the disease.

## DESCRIPTIONS OF THE THREE PLASMODIA CAUSING MALARIA.

### I. *Plasmodium vivax* (Grassi and Feletti, 1890) and Tertian Malaria.

SYNONYMS : *Oscillaria malariæ* Laveran, 1881, *pro parte*. *Hæmosporidium tertianum* Lewkowicz, 1887. *Plasmodium* var. *tertiana* Golgi, 1889. *Hæmamœba vivax* Grassi and Feletti, 1890. *Plasmodium malariæ* var. *tertianæ* Celli and San Felice, 1891. *Hæmamœba laverani* var. *tertiana* Labbé, 1894. *Plasmodium malariæ tertianum* Labbé, 1899. *Hæmamœba malariæ* var. *magna* Laveran, 1900. *Hæmamœba malariæ* var. *tertianæ* Laveran, 1901. *Plasmodium tertianæ* Billet, 1904, *pro parte*.

*Description.* The young trophozoite appears in the red blood corpuscles as a very actively amœboid body about $1-2\mu$ in diameter. It is much more active than the other two species of malarial parasites and it was because of this feature that the specific name *vivax* was applied to it. The young trophozoite very soon assumes the ring form, and by means of its pseudopodia and the large amount of exposed surface, it grows rapidly at the expense of the contents of the red cell. The latter becomes pale and swollen, and on staining with Giemsa its protoplasm presents certain degeneration phenomena, taking the form of scattered red granules, known as Schüffner's dots. The presence of these dots in the protoplasm of the infected red cells generally serves to distinguish *P. vivax* from the other malarial parasites, but similar appearances occur in the red cells of dogs infected with *Babesia (Piroplasma) canis*.

As the trophozoite grows, melanin is formed and deposited in the form of fine rods scattered throughout the cytoplasm of the parasite. The period of growth occupies about 30 hours, by which time the trophozoite almost fills the corpuscle, the fully formed schizont being $8\cdot5-10\mu$ in diameter.

From the thirtieth to the forty-eighth hour the schizont divides up into from 15 to 20 merozoites, or rarely as many as 24. The stages in this process have been described above, but it may be well to repeat that all the melanin, together with a certain amount of waste protoplasm is left unused. The melanin granules are packed together in the form of one or two conspicuous brown masses, usually situated at the middle of the parasite.

The merozoites are somewhat irregularly arranged, often in two concentric circles ; rosette forms, such as occur in *P. malariæ* and *P. falciparum*, are absent.

About the forty-eighth hour the wall of the red cell bursts open and the contained merozoites together with the melanin and other waste products are liberated in the serum. The cycle of schizogony therefore occupies 48 hours, and in consequence the febrile attacks recur after this interval.

In *P. vivax* the gametocytes are common in the peripheral circulation as well as in the internal organs, and consequently their development can be followed without much difficulty. The macrogametocytes are large spherical bodies about 12–16$\mu$ in diameter, and in addition to their size may be distinguished from the schizonts by their denser protoplasm and larger and more numerous melanin granules. The nucleus is usually situated at the periphery and is an oval structure containing numerous chromatinic granules. The microgametocytes are similar in shape to the macrogametocytes, but are much smaller (9–11 $\mu$), and in addition may be distinguished from the latter by their large densely staining nucleus. In addition, the cytoplasm is very much lighter and less granular.

Both the kinds of gametocytes originate from ordinary merozoites, but during their development can be distinguished from the schizonts by their much slower growth and absence of active amœboid and ring forms.

The development of *P. vivax* in the mosquito was first worked out in *Anopheles maculipennis*, one of the common mosquitoes of Europe, but many other species are known to transmit the infection equally well. When ingested by the mosquito, the development of the gametes will not take place below 16° C., but the most favourable temperature is much higher (24–30° C.).

The microgametocyte gives rise to 4 to 8 microgametes, and the macrogametocyte undergoes division of the nucleus and extrusion of a polar body before becoming a macrogamete ready for fertilization. After this process has taken place, the male and female pro-nuclei are said to remain apart for some time before uniting to form the single nucleus of the oökinete. At a temperature of 28° C. the latter has penetrated the gut-wall and become an oöcyst by the end of about 40 hours after the mosquito's feed. At this stage the oöcyst is an almost transparent spherical body containing thin brown strands of melanin, and is surrounded by a well-defined wall. The nucleus has already commenced to divide and several daughter-nuclei are scattered through the cytoplasm.

The following day the oöcyst increases in size and the sporoblasts begin to separate off from each other. The melanin is aggregated together into clumps lying between the sporoblasts. On the fourth day the oöcyst is now seen to contain well-defined sporoblasts, each of which is covered by the growing sporozoites. During the fourth and fifth days the oöcyst still continues to grow, attaining a diameter of about 50 $\mu$ and projects outwards into the cœlom of the insect. The sporozoites become completely formed and thus the oöcyst is transformed into a hollow sphere containing innumerable sporozoites each about 14 $\mu$ in diameter. About the seventh or eighth day the cyst ruptures and the numerous sporozoites are liberated into the cœlomic fluid. From ·here large numbers find their way to the salivary glands, but some of them bore into the developing eggs in the ovary. The fate of these latter is unknown, for up to the present, beyond this fact, there is nothing to support the view that the infection is transmitted to the offspring of an infected mosquito.

The above cycle of sporogony is thus complete in about eight days, under these favourable conditions of temperature, and after the sporozoites have entered the salivary glands the mosquito becomes infective. At lower temperatures the development is very much prolonged and consequently the mosquito does not become infective until after a much longer incubation period.

The length of time that a mosquito remains infected has never yet been proved, but it is probably for the remainder of its life.

*Distribution.* This species is widely distributed throughout the world, occurring in most tropical and subtropical regions. It also occurs somewhat scantily in Northern Europe below 60° north latitude.

As a result of successful mosquito campaigns and other prophylactic measures the distribution of the disease is being restricted, and it has been eradicated from some parts of the world. Tertian fever or ague was formerly prevalent in Britain and it is interesting to note that one or two isolated cases of malaria in patients that had never left England have been recorded within the present century. Consequently the conditions for the transmission of the disease have not yet entirely disappeared from this country.

II. *Plasmodium malariæ* (Laveran, 1881) and Quartan Fever.

SYNONYMS : *Oscillaria malariæ* Laveran, 1883. *Plasmodium* var. *quartana* Golgi, 1890. *Plasmodium malariæ* var. *quartanæ* Celli and San Felice, 1891. *Hæmamœba malariæ* Grassi and Feletti, 1892. *Hæmamœba laverani* var. *quartana* Labbé, 1894. *Hæmosporidium quartanæ* Lewkowicz, 1897. *Plasmodium malariæ quartanum* Labbé, 1899. *Hæmomonas malariæ* Ross, 1900. *Hæmamœba malariæ* var. *magna* Laveran, 1900. *H. malariæ* var. *quartanæ* Laveran, 1901. *Plasmodium golgii* Sambon, 1902. *Plasmodium quartanæ* Billet, 1904. *Laverania malariæ* Jancsó, 1905.

*Description.* The young trophozoite is somewhat smaller than that of *P. vivax*, and also much less active. The pseudopodia are usually blunt, so that the parasite is rather compact in appearance. The pigment is deposited in the form of very coarse darkly-coloured granules, or rodlets, which are commonly gathered at the periphery of the parasite. In contra-distinction to the granules of the other species of malarial parasites, those of *P. malariæ* are non-motile. A vacuole is formed, but is comparatively small and disappears during the growth of the trophozoite. The presence of the parasite in the red cell does not produce any evident changes in the corpuscle beyond a slight decrease in size and a darker colour. The trophozoite takes about 60 hours to grow up into the mature schizont, which is a somewhat angular body 6–7 $\mu$ in diameter.

During the next 12 hours the nucleus of the schizont divides up into 6–12 smaller ones, which become arranged in a single circle at the periphery. Each becomes surrounded by a mass of cytoplasm which separates off from its neighbours and thus a regular circle of 6–12 merozoites is formed. The pigment granules form a dark clump at the centre and as the merozoites radiate from it, a very typical rosette appearance is produced.

The merozoites (about 1·75 $\mu$ in diameter) are now set free by the rupture of the corpuscle and may enter another red cell and repeat the cycle. More often, however, they seem to be killed off by the phagocytes, and thus it is only rarely that this parasite produces fatal effects in its host.

The whole of the above cycle takes place in the peripheral blood, and occupies 72 hours.

Accordingly the fever which is caused by this parasite occurs every fourth day (hence the name Quartan Fever) after the schizogony takes place.

In addition to the simple quartan fever in which the attacks recur every fourth day, cases of double and triple quartan are also met with. In double quartan fever the attacks recur on the first, second, fourth, fifth, seventh, eighth days, etc. This is merely a case of a double infection, and the parasites being the descendants of two separate lots of sporozoites, are at different stages of development. The first infection will undergo schizogony on the fourth, seventh, tenth days, etc. after the entry of the sporozoites, whilst if the second infection occurs on the day following any of these attacks the latter

parasites will complete their cycle of schizogony every 72 hours
from this date onwards, *i.e.* on the fifth, eighth, eleventh days, etc.
The result of such a double infection will be the occurrence of
febrile attacks on two successive days followed by an interval
of one day, and to this type of fever the term Double Quartan
is applied.

In the same way a patient may again become infected on
the only day on which schizogony is not taking place, and after
this last infection has developed will shew a rise in temperature
every day. This type of fever is known as Triple Quartan
Fever ; it may be distinguished from the other kinds of malaria
by the shape of the parasites.

III.   *Plasmodium falciparum* (Welch, 1897) and Quotidian,
        Malignant Tertian, or Æstivo-Autumnal Malaria.

SYNONYMS : *Oscillaria malariæ* Laveran, 1881, *pro parte.*
*Hæmamœba præcox* Grassi and Feletti, 1890. *Hæmamœba
malariæ præcox + H. malariæ immaculatum* Grassi and Feletti,
1890. *Laverania malariæ* Grassi and Feletti, 1890. *Plasmodium malariæ* var. *quotidianæ* Celli and San Felice, 1890.
*Hæmosporidium undecimanæ* Lewkowicz, 1892. *H. sedeci-
manæ* Lewkowicz, 1892.   *H. vigesimotertianæ* Lewkowicz,
1892. *Hæmamœba laverani* Labbé, 1894. *Hæmatozoon falciparum* Welch, 1897. *Hæmamonas præcox* Ross, 1899. *Plasmodium malariæ præcox* Labbé, 1899. *Plasmodium præcox*
R. Blanchard, 1900. *Hæmamœba malariæ* var. *parva* Laveran,
1900. *Plasmodium immaculatum* Schaudinn, 1902. *Laverania
præcox* Nocard and Leclainche, 1903.

*Description.* This is the smallest of the three species of
*Plasmodium* affecting man, the fully developed schizont being
not more than about 5μ in diameter. The young sporozoite
is very small and, after penetrating a red cell, as a rule at once
assumes the ring form. The latter is characteristic in appearance as the nucleus is always peripheral and the contours of
the ring are very dark and clear. The trophozoites have the
peculiarity of frequently appearing at the surface of the red cell.
They are distinguished from those of the other two species of

malaria by their active amœboid movements. The trophozoites grow rapidly and assume an oval form; they contain a few
pigment granules which are small, irregular and only feebly
motile. During its growth the parasite causes an alteration
in the substance of the red cell, which in stained preparations
is seen to contain a number of granules known as Maurer's
dots. Otherwise the erythrocyte remains unaltered in appearance until the formation of the merozoites results in its
destruction.

The fully developed schizont is 4·5 to 5μ in diameter, and is
very rarely present in the peripheral circulation. It segments
into 8–10 or sometimes 15 merozoites, which may either be
arranged in the form of a rosette, or irregularly. The segmentation almost invariably takes place in the capillaries of the
internal organs, and when it is in process there is a tendency
for the red cells to cling together and also adhere to the wall of
the blood-vessel, thus causing obstruction of the circulation.

The whole cycle of schizogony takes from 24 to 48 hours
to be completed, and thus the febrile attacks are more or less
irregular, but often occur each day.

The gametocytes develop from the trophozoites in the usual
manner, but are distinguished from those of the other two
human species of *Plasmodium* by their crescentic form. The
macrogametocyte may be distinguished by the arrangement
of the pigment, which is usually concentrated in the neighbourhood of the compact nucleus, leaving the remainder of the
cytoplasm clear. In the microgametocyte the pigment is
irregularly scattered through the cytoplasm and the nucleus
is somewhat diffuse. Moreover the shape of the two kinds of
gametocytes is different, being long and thin in the case of the
former, and broad and somewhat rounded in the latter. The
remains of the distorted red cell may be seen surrounding the
" crescents," the hæmoglobin often being concentrated in the
form of a small clump attached to the side of the parasite. The
dimensions of a fully grown macrogametocyte are about
12 μ × 4 μ.

These gametocytes are very conspicuous in the circulation
of patients suffering from *P. falciparum*, and under the name of

"crescents" were known for many years before their true nature was discovered. On being taken into the gut of a susceptible species of mosquito, the gametocytes escape from the red cells and give rise to the gametes. The macrogamete is vermiform, whilst the microgametocyte becomes spherical before giving rise to the microgametes. The cycle of development in the mosquito at the most favourable temperature, 28-30° C., is complete within eight days. In this species development cannot take place below 18° C., and consequently it is only found in warm countries, the disease to which it gives rise being often known as "Malaria Tropica." The development of *P. falciparum* in the mosquito is more easily followed than that of the other species of malarial parasites, for when a mosquito is susceptible to this species, as in the case of *A. (Myzomyia) christophersi*, practically all the insects become infected when fed on a patient suffering from this infection.

In consequence of the comparatively high temperature required for the development of *P. falciparum* within the mosquito, the disease does not occur in temperate regions except during the summer. Usually associated with *P. vivax*, it is found throughout the whole of the tropics, except in regions like the Sahara, where mosquitoes are absent owing to the lack of water.

## LITERATURE.

The more important and accessible general treatises upon malaria, and papers dealing with recent work upon epidemiology and preventive measures against malaria.

†Bahr, P. H. (1913). Malaria in Kurunegala. *Report Colonial Office.* April, 1913.

†Bentley (1910). *Malaria in Bombay* (Report). Govern. Central Press, Bombay.

†Celli (1901). *Malaria according to the New Researches.* Longmans, Green & Co. London, 1901.

†Christophers. Malaria in the Punjab. *Scientific Memoirs by Officers of the San. and Med. Depart. of the Gov. of India*, No. 46.

† —— Malaria in the Andamans. *Ibid.* No. 56.

Christy. *Mosquitoes and Malaria.* Good elementary account.

Craig (1909). *The Malarial Fevers, Hæmoglobinuric Fever and the Blood Protozoa of Man.*

† Works representative of the more recent lines of investigation on malaria.

TABLE III.

METHODS OF DISTINGUISHING THE THREE SPECIES OF *PLASMODIUM* OCCURRING IN MAN[1].

| | P. malariæ | P. vivax | P. falciparum |
|---|---|---|---|
| Young trophozoites | Contours very sharp; amœboid movements very slow | Contours indistinct; amœboid movements active | Contours distinct; amœboid movements active |
| *Schizonts* Shape and size | Quadrilateral—smaller than a normal red cell | Round; larger than a normal red cell | Round; diameter equal to the radius of a red cell |
| Pigment | Grains large and irregular; feebly or non-motile | Grains in the form of short rods, actively motile | Grains few, small and irregular, feebly motile |
| Appearance of infected blood corpuscle | Contracted, and more pitted than the normal cells. By staining one cannot distinguish any protoplasmic granulation | Hypertrophied, soft and pale. By staining one can distinguish Schüffner's granules | Normal |
| Schizogony | Distinct rosette forms; present in the peripheral circulation | Segmentation forms somewhat hat-shaped; frequently present in peripheral circulation | Segmentation forms either rosette-shaped or irregular. Confined to the capillaries of the internal organs |
| Number of merozoites | 6 to 12 | 15 to 20 | 8 to 10, sometimes more |
| Gametes | Spherical | Spherical | Crescentic, rarely becoming spherical in blood |
| Time occupied by evolution of asexual cycle | 72 hours | 48 hours | From 24 to 48 hours |
| Clinical form of Fever | Quartan; simple, double or triple | Tertian, simple or double | Subtertian; quotidian; malignant tertian; (æstivo-autumnal malaria) |

[1] From Brumpt, *Précis de Parasitologie.*

Darling (1910). Factors in the Transmission and Prevention of Malaria in the Canal Zone. *Annals Trop. Med. and Parasitology*, IV. part 2.

Droderick (1909). *A Practical Study of Malaria*. Saunders & Co. Philadelphia.

Grall and Marchoux (1910). *Traité de Pathologie Exotique*. Baillière et fils. Paris.

Hirsh (1883). *Handbook of Geographical and Historical Pathology*. New Sydenham Society. Vol. I.

*Laveran (1907). *Traité du Paludisme*. Masson & Co. Paris.

Lühe (1906). Article on Blood Protozoa in Mense's *Handbuch der Tropenkrankheiten*.

Mannaberg (1905). Malaria, in Nothnagel's *Encyclopedia*. English edition.

†Mathis and Leger (1911). *Recherches de Parasitologie et de Pathologie humaines et animales au Tonkin*. Masson & Co. Paris.

†Ross, R. (1909). *Report on the Prevention of Malaria in Mauritius*. Waterlow and Sons. London.

† —— (1911). *The Prevention of Malaria*. John Murray. London.

Ruge, R. (1903). *Introduction to the Study of Malarial Diseases*. Rebman, London.

† —— (1912). *Malariaparasiten*. In Kolle and Wassermann's *Handbuch* (a comparatively short but very complete account).

†Sergent, Ed. and Et. Campagne antipaludique en Algérie, etc. *Annals de l'Instit. Pasteur*. Jan. 1903, Feb. and Mar. 1904, April and May 1906, Jan. 1907, May 1908, and *Campagne antipaludique* (Gov. gén. de l'Algérie), 1908–10.

Stephens and Christophers (1907). *The Practical Study of Malaria* (deals with technique, Malaria Survey, etc.).

†Watson (1910). *Prevention of Malaria in the Federated Malay States*. University Press, Liverpool.

*Ziemann. In Mense's *Handbuch*, 1906.

*Vide* also :

†*Atti della Soc. per gli studi della Malaria*. Annual volume. 1899–1908.

†*Malaria*. Vols. I and II, now discontinued.

†*Paludism*. Nos. 1–5.

†Various articles in Ross's *Prevention of Malaria*.

The more important publications dealing with the question of transmission of malarial parasites by particular species of *Anopheles*.

Adie (1903). A note on *Anopheles fuliginosus* and Sporozoites. *Indian Med. Gazette*, XXXVIII. p. 246.

Adie, Mrs (1911). *Ne. Willmori*, a proved carrier in nature. *Paludism*, No. 3.

Banks (1907). Experiments in Malarial Transmission by means of *M. ludlowi*. *Philippine Journal of Science*, B. vol. II. No. 6, p. 513.

---

* Complete treatises dealing minutely with every side of the subject.

† Works representative of the more recent lines of investigation on malaria.

Bastianelli and Bignami (1899). *Atti d. Soc. per gli studi d. Malaria*, I. p. 28.

Bastianelli, Bignami and Grassi (1898). *Atti d. R. Accad. dei Lincei*, VII. p. 313.

Bentley (1911). *Myzomyia rossi* and Malaria. *Paludism*, No. 2.

—— (1911). The Seasonal Malarial Infection of *M. stephensi* in Bombay. *Paludism*, No. 2.

—— (1912). *Malaria in Bombay*. Gov. Central Press, Bombay.

Billet (1903). Sur un Espèce nouvelle d'*Anopheles* (*A. chaudoyei*) et sa relation avec le paludisme à Touggart. *C. R. Soc. Biol.* LV. p. 565.

Christophers (1912). Malaria in the Andamans. *Sci. Memoirs by Officers of the San. and Med. Departs. of Gov. of India*, No. 56.

Cruz (1910). Prophylaxis of Malaria in Central and Southern Brazil. In Ross's *Prevention of Malaria*.

Daniels (1900). Development of Crescents in the small dark *Anopheles* prevalent in British Central Africa. *Reports to Mal. Com. of R. S.* Ser. v.

—— (1909). Mosquitoes in the Federated Malay States. *Studies from the Institute for Med. Research* (*Fed. Malay States*), vol. III.

Darling (1909). Transmission of Malarial Fever in the Canal Zone by *Anopheles* Mosquitoes. *Jour. Amer. Med. Assoc.* LIII. p. 2051.

—— (1910). Factors in the Transmission and Prevention of Malaria in the Canal Zone. *Annals of Trop. Med. and Par.* IV. part 2.

Grassi (1902). *Die Malaria, Studien eines Zoologen*. 2. Aufl. Jena.

Hill and Haydon. *Annals of the Natal Government Museum*.

Hirshberg (1904). An *Anopheles* mosquito which does not transmit malaria. *The Johns Hopkins Hosp. Bull.* Feb. 1904.

James (1902). Malaria in India. *Sci. Memoirs by Officers of the San. and Med. Departs. of the Gov. of India*, No. 2.

James and Liston (1911). *The Anopheline Mosquitoes of India*. Calcutta.

Jancsó (1904). Zur Frage der Infektion der *Anopheles claviger* mit Malariaparasiten bei neiderer Temperatur. *Cent. f. Bakt.* XXXVI. p. 624.

—— (1905). Der Einfluss der Temperatur auf die geschlechtliche Generationsentwicklung der Malariaparasiten, etc. *Cent. f. Bakt.* XXXVIII. p. 650.

Kinoshita (1906). Über die Verbreitung der Anophelen auf Formosa und deren Beziehung zu der Malariakrankheiten. *Arch. f. Schiffs- u. Tropen-Hyg.* X. p. 708.

Koch (1899). Über die Entwicklung der Malariaparasiten. *Zeit. f. Hygiene*, XXXII.

Liston (1908). The present Epidemic of Malaria in the Port of Bombay. *Jour. Bombay Nat. Hist. Soc.* 15 Nov.

Lutz (1903). Waldmosquitos und Waldmalaria. *Cent. f. Bakt.* XXXIII. p. 282.

Macdonald (1910). Malaria in Spain. In Ross's *Prevention of Malaria*.

Newstead, Dutton and Todd (1907). Insects and other Arthropoda collected in the Congo Free State. *Annals of Trop. Med. and Par.* I. p. 10.

Patton (1905). The Culicid Fauna of the Aden Hinterland. *Jour. Bombay Nat. Hist. Soc.* p. 623.

Ross (1908). *Report on the Prevention of Malaria in Mauritius.* London.

—— (1910). *The Prevention of Malaria.* London: John Murray.

Ross, Annett and Austen (1900). *Report of the Malaria Expedition of the Liverpool School of Tropical Medicine.* Memoir II.

Schaudinn (1904). Die Malaria in dem Dorfe " St Michele di Lerne " in Istria, etc. *Arb. a. d. Kaiserl. Gesundh.* XXI. p. 403.

Schüffner (1902). Die Beziehungen der Malariaparasiten zu Mensch und Mücke an der Ostküste Sumatras. *Zeits. f. Hygiene,* XLI. p. 89.

Sergent, Ed. and Et. (1905). *Anopheles algeriensis* et *Myzomyia hispaniola* convoient le Paludisme. *C. R. Soc. Biol.* LIX. p. 499.

—— (1908–10). Campagne antipaludique en Algérie. *Ann. Inst. Pasteur,* vols. XXII. and XXIV.

Staunton (1913). The Anopheles Mosquitoes of Malaya and their Larvæ, with some notes on Malaria-carrying Species. *Jour. of the London School of Trop. Medicine,* vol. II.

Stephens and Christophers (1899–1902). *Reports to the Malaria Committee of the Royal Society,* I–VIII.

—— (1907) *The Practical Study of Malaria.* University Press, Liverpool.

Tsuzuki (1902). Malaria und ihre Vermittler in Japan. *Arch. f. Schiffs-u. Trop.-Hyg.* VI. pp. 9, 285.

Van der Scheer and V. Berlekom (1900). Malaria and Mosquitos in Zealand. *Brit. Med. Jour.* I. p. 202. 26 Jan. 1901.

Vogel (1910). *Myzomyia rossi* as a Malaria Carrier. *Philippine Jour. of Science,* vol. v. No. 3, p. 277.

Watson (1910). *The Prevention of Malaria in the Fed. Malay States.* University Press, Liverpool.

# CHAPTER X

## CULICINÆ

The main characters of the Culicinæ have already been described in Chapter VIII and therefore we shall at once proceed to a description of by far the most important member of the group, namely, *Stegomyia fasciata,* notorious as one of the commonest domestic mosquitoes and also for the part it plays in the transmission of Yellow Fever.

## Stegomyia fasciata (Fabricius, 1805)[1].   The Tiger Mosquito.

*Synonyms: Culex fasciatus* Fabricius, 1805. *C. calopus* Meigen, 1818. *C. frater* Desvoidy, 1827. *C. tæniatus* Wiedemann, 1828. *C. konoupi* Brullé (?), 1832. *C. viridifrons* Walker, 1848. *C. annulitarsis* Macquart, 1848. *C. excitans* Walker, 1848. *C. inexorabilis* Walker, 1848. *C. formosus* Walker 1848. *C. exagitans* Walker, 1856. *C. impatibilis* Walker, 1860. *C. bancroftii* Skuse, 1886. *C. mosquito* Arribalzaga, 1891. *C. elegans* Ficalbi, 1896. *C. rossii* Giles, 1899. *Stegomyia fasciata* Theobald, 1901.

*Description.* In addition to possessing the characters of the genus (p. 109), according to Theobald this species may be distinguished by the following features :

" Thorax dark-brown to reddish-brown, with two median parallel pale lines and a curved silvery one on each side, a small line in front between the two median ones. Abdomen black, with two white basal bands and lateral spots. Legs black, with basal white bands, last joint of hind-legs pure white." (Theobald.)

The **female** has a head densely covered with broad flat scales, which are black and grey on each side. There is a white patch on each side and another

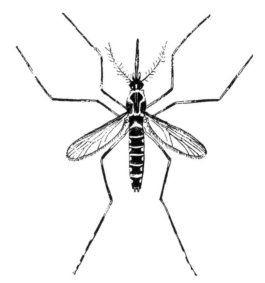

Fig. 46. *Stegomyia fasciata*, adult female ; enlarged. (After Howard.)

[1] According to Howard, Dyar and Knab (1913) the correct name of this species is *Aëdes calopus.*

in the median line extending from in front back to the neck. The scales at the back of the head are in the form of long black bristles and project forward. The eyes are black surrounded by a white border and sometimes contain white patches.

The antennæ are brown, excepting the basal segment, which is black with a patch of white scales on its inner side. They are longer than the proboscis and have a banded appearance. The proboscis is brown, almost black towards the extremity, but lighter about the middle. The palps are black, and only about one-third the length of the proboscis ; each is composed of three segments covered with large flat scales, those of the first two being brown, and silvery-white on the last segment.

The dark-brown thorax is covered with reddish-brown, pale-golden and cream-coloured scales and is ornamented with various white spots and lines. In front, near the neck, there is a white spot on each side. The dorsal surface has a white, broad curved band on each side extending from the anterior edge of the thorax and curving inwards about the middle of the mesonotum, from which it is continued backwards as a thinner pale line to the scutellum. Between them are two parallel pale lines extending about half way across the mesonotum and on to the scutellum, and anteriorly is a short white line between these two. The scutellum has a thick row of white scales and also three tufts of bristles. The metanotum is brown. The pleuræ are dark-brown with several patches of white scales.

There is much variation in both the size and colour of the thoracic scales and many of the varieties have been described as distinct species. The arrangement of the ornamentation is however very constant and will serve to distinguish *fasciata* from any other species of the genus *Stegomyia*.

The abdomen is brownish-black, circled with a white band at the base of each segment ; the posterior four bands before the last one are more or less tinged with yellow. There is a triangular white spot on the sides of each segment, and in addition the first segment is almost covered with cream-coloured scales and edged with pale hairs.

The legs are brown, circled with white. The coxæ are yellowish. The femurs are yellowish towards the base, brown towards the apex, but with white scales on the ventral surface, and finally the extreme tip is pure white. Those of the third pair are swollen at the extremity. The tibiæ are black. The metatarsi have basal white bands. The fore tarsi have the first joint basally white and the rest black ; the mid tarsi are the same. The hind tarsi are all basally white except the last joint, which is white, and the penultimate segment, which is white with the exception of a black apex. The claws of the first two pairs of legs are toothed and those of the hinder pair without teeth.

The wings are clear, unspotted, a little longer than the abdomen, with brown scales, those of the lateral nervures being very long and narrow, and of the median, short and broad. The first sub-marginal cell is longer and only slightly narrower than the second posterior cell, and the base of the former is a little nearer the base of the wing than the latter. The posterior cross-vein is about one and a half to twice its length distant from the mid cross-vein. The latter unites with the supernumerary forming a very obtuse angle, almost straight. The balancers are ochraceous and sometimes the knob is slightly fuscous.

The length is 3·5 to 5·0 mm.

The **male** is darker than the female.  The head is black with white scales in front and in the middle.  The antennæ are brown, marked with paler bands, sometimes almost white.  The proboscis and palps are black, the latter possessing four white basal bands.  The thorax is marked in the same way as the female, but the scales are more silvery and the markings more distinct.

The first segment of the abdomen is covered with cream-coloured scales, the bases of the second to the fifth with white, and the fifth to the eighth have clear white lateral spots.  The latter also occur on the sides of the anterior segments.

The claws of the fore-legs are unequal, the larger one being toothed and the smaller, simple ; those of the mid-legs are simple, and unequal ; the hind claws are equal and simple.

The genital armature is of the usual form.

The length is 3·0 mm. to 4·5 mm.

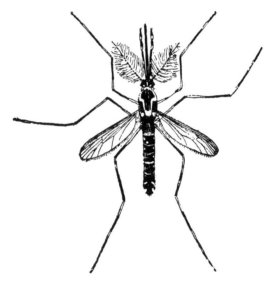

Fig. 47.  *Stegomyia fasciata,* adult male ;  enlarged.  (After Howard.)

*Habitat.*  This is one of the commonest species of mosquitoes and is widely distributed throughout almost all tropical and subtropical regions.  Although sometimes occurring in temperate countries it is essentially a tropical species, for below a temperature of 23° C. the female refuses to feed and at 20° C. loses all activity and will not oviposit.  The most favourable climatic condition for its development is a humid atmosphere, at a temperature of 25–30° C. all the year round.

In the laboratory *S. fasciata* may be kept alive for some time at 7–8° C., if kept in a refrigerator and thereby protected from currents of air. When exposed to a similar temperature in the open air it soon dies. At 0° C. the insect succumbs in a few seconds and, on the other hand, a temperature of 37° C. is also rapidly fatal.

This susceptibility to variations in temperature causes this mosquito to be confined to certain degrees of latitude, from 40° N. to 40° S., or more exactly between the two isothermal lines of 20° C. Owing to the ease with which it may be carried from one country to another by means of ships, the species is now found in most of the regions between these limits. The accompanying map (Fig. 48) represents the distribution of

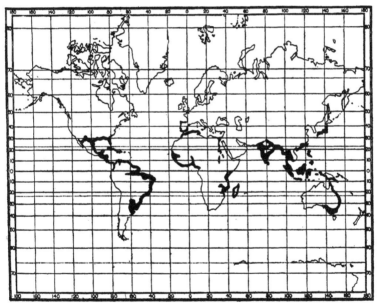

Fig. 48. The distribution of *Stegomyia fasciata*.

*S. fasciata*, and it will be noticed that the insect especially occurs along the coast lines and the banks of large rivers, where the requisite conditions of humidity are fulfilled. It is absent from those regions in which the temperature during the night falls so low as to be harmful to reproduction.

In addition to its susceptibility to cold *Stegomyia* is even more affected by dryness, especially when accompanied by heat. The insect is somewhat protected from the vicissitudes of the climate by its domestic habits, as it is generally found inside houses. In fact its fondness for houses is so great that, according to Boyce, it is never found breeding at distances of more than 50 to 100 yards from buildings.

On emerging from the pupa, the imago at once flies into a house or other shelter, and generally settles down in some dark corner and, like most other blood-sucking flies, it has a great preference for dark-coloured objects.

If the mosquitoes are breeding close to ships they often enter them, and in consequence *Stegomyia* is the commonest species found on board ship. In the old sailing ships, not only could these insects live for weeks in the cabins, store-rooms, holds, etc., but actually breed in the water that was often left exposed in various receptacles. Although modern steamers do not afford such facilities for the persistence of this insect on board, yet recently there have been cases in which live *Stegomyia fasciata* were found on ships that had been at sea 13 to 20 days.

*Feeding habits.* As in the majority of mosquitoes the female *Stegomyia* is the only one which feeds on blood and this food is necessary before the insect is able to lay its eggs. The male, which is fully developed on emergence, does not bite, in spite of statements to the contrary. It feeds on fruit juices and also settles on the skin, to which it is attracted by the secretions of the body. Although the male does not actually bite, the singing noise produced by its wings is very annoying; its note is much higher than that of the female.

The female does not feed on all persons indiscriminately, but seems to exercise some choice in the selection of its victims. Thus it prefers white people to black, in spite of its fondness for dark objects. Similarly blondes are preferred to brunettes, children to adults, and fresh arrivals from temperate regions suffer more than acclimatized persons. The factors which guide the insect in the selection of its host are not known, but scent is probably the most important, after the effect of the body-heat.

According to Marchoux, who has given one of the most complete accounts of *S. fasciata*, the female is entirely nocturnal in its blood-sucking habits, except for a short time after it emerges from the pupal case. Under these latter conditions the insect is so hungry that as soon as it is able to fly it sets off to find a host. Once having succeeded in obtaining a meal, the female comes to rest in some dark corner, and in future only attempts to feed towards the evening, or at night. This statement, however, as to the nocturnal feeding habits of *S. fasciata* has been denied by many subsequent investigators, who agree in the view that this mosquito is mainly diurnal in its feeding habits. Although in nature blood appears to be the only food of the females, Goeldi succeeded in keeping them alive for more than three months on a diet of honey. These insects, however, were unable to lay any eggs.

*Length of life.* In a state of captivity, female *S. fasciata* have been kept alive for a period of more than four months, so that their duration of life is comparatively long, but in nature, it is doubtful whether an insect would often be able to live such a long time. The occurrence of isolated cases of yellow fever long after an epidemic has ceased may be due to the persistence of infected mosquitoes or, on the other hand, to the presence of mild and unrecognized cases of the disease.

The male has a much shorter life than the female, for as it feeds on the nectar of flowers, and moreover is very active, it requires to feed much oftener. As a result of its continual search for nourishment, and also for females, the male is continually exposed to accidents and soon loses his protective scales. From this moment the slightest drop of moisture is sufficient to cause the suffocation of the insect.

The maximum period that female *S. fasciata* have been kept alive when nourished on honey is 102 days, whilst under similar circumstances males only lived for periods varying from 28 to 72 days.

*Fertilization and egg-laying.* Copulation is usually accomplished in the open air, especially during the warm hours of the day. The union is made when the insects are flying, only rarely when at rest, as the two ventral surfaces are brought in apposition.

The spermatozoa are stored in the spermathecæ, but although a fertilized female may thus remain fertile for a long time, eventually the sperm becomes used up and another copulation is necessary before more fertile eggs can be produced.

The female lays the first batch of eggs a few days after taking its first meal of blood, the exact period varying according to the conditions of temperature and humidity. When these are very favourable the period may be as short as two days, but at temperatures below 20° C. the interval may be prolonged indefinitely and two or three feeds may elapse before egg-laying commences. The average number of batches of eggs laid is usually two or three, but in individual cases as many as nine batches have been observed.

The eggs are extruded singly and the number laid on the first occasion is generally 60 to 90. The number of eggs comprising the subsequent batches is always less than that of the first one, this being the most important. Goeldi has found that the females usually die immediately after the final act of parturition, though in two instances individuals survived 12 and 14 days respectively.

The same author also states that fertilized eggs may remain latent in the body of the female for from 23 to 102 days. A meal of blood was capable of causing the female to lay her eggs after these two periods respectively.

The eggs are generally laid at night, on the surface of almost any stagnant water. They may be found in the water collected in old tins, saucepans, rain-tubs, broken bottles, holes in trees, and practically in every accumulation of water, however slight, occurring in the vicinity of the houses the mosquito inhabits. The nature of the water seems to be indifferent, for the eggs hatch out in the most stagnant and evil-smelling water, almost as readily as in pure water.

*The egg.* The egg consists of an ovoid body, rather more pointed at one end than the other, and is blackish in colour, dotted over with small white hemispherical particles of excretory matter. In addition the egg is surrounded by a series of small air-chambers which help to keep it afloat.

As each egg is laid by the female a small drop of liquid is also extruded on the surface of the water and may help to keep the egg floating, as this secretion is of somewhat oily consistency. Certainly a slight agitation of the water is sufficient to cause the eggs to sink, but development proceeds almost as well beneath the water as at the surface. In the former case, however, the eggs are more liable to the attacks of bacteria, etc. Under favourable conditions the eggs hatch out in about two or three days. In the Amazons the normal incubation period is said to be from three to eight days, but its duration depends almost entirely on the temperature. If this falls below 20° C. the eggs are unable to develop, and if the thermometer falls to this temperature for a few hours each day the development is greatly prolonged.

The eggs are very resistant and can withstand long exposures to cold and dryness. They may be exposed to a temperature of 37° C. for one hour, or kept at 0° C. for many days, without their vitality being affected. Eggs have been maintained for several months between 10° C. and 20° C. and when the temperature was raised, about one-twentieth of them hatched out.

The most striking results, however, are those obtained with eggs that have been dried. These may be kept for three months without more than 40 per cent. of them dying. Francis has also shewn that they may remain alive for six and a half months if kept dry. Newstead describes an experiment with eggs of *S. fasciata* that had been sent from Manaos on the Amazon. The eggs had been laid on moist white filter paper ; they were then dried in air and subsequently for 24 hours over calcium chloride. They were then packed in tubes and sent across to England. Forty-five to 47 days later, on their arrival at Liverpool, they were placed in water at 23° C. and several larvæ hatched out within 12 hours. Moreover, these larvæ developed very rapidly and the adult insects emerged within 12 days. From these results it is evident that the eggs of *S. fasciata* under certain conditions may remain alive for considerable periods without developing.

*The larva.* The egg gives birth to a small, colourless, and very active larva, which occasionally swims and wriggles along the surface of the water in the same manner as certain Anophelines. This larva under favourable conditions grows rapidly, and after a succession of moults attains the pupal stage.

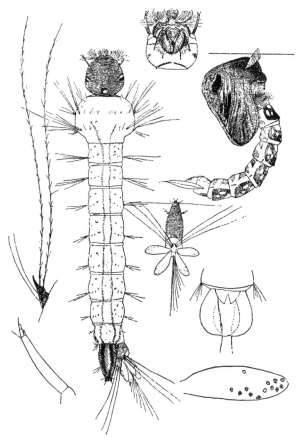

Fig. 49.　Larva and Pupa of *Stegomyia fasciata*, with enlarged parts.　(After Howard.)

The larva of *Stegomyia* may generally be distinguished by two characters, viz. its comparatively colourless appearance and the short black respiratory syphon, one-quarter the total length of the abdomen. The larvæ of *Culex* are darker coloured

and generally possess long respiratory syphons. In addition
the larvæ of *S. fasciata* possess the following characters :

The antennæ are smooth, the tuft being represented by a
single short hair. At the apex there is a minute but distinct
second joint and a few delicate hairs. The labial plate possesses one large terminal tooth and 11 or 12 smaller ones on
each side of it. The thorax is rather hairy and bears four
large chitinous hooks, two on each side. Each of these hooks
gives off one or two hairs. The abdomen is very broad, and
is almost the same width all the way down.

The two lateral combs, situated on the eighth segment,
each consist of eight to ten serrated spines, varying in size
and the number of serrations. The syphon is comparatively
short and stumpy, being only one-quarter the total length
of the abdomen, and about two and a half times as long as its
width at the base. The syphon spines vary both in number
and arrangement ; they are succeeded by a triple hair. The
terminal segment of the abdomen is very short and almost
rectangular and bears a number of blunt bifurcate hairs.
The papillæ are broad and rounded ; their length is about
one and a half times that of the last segment.

The larvæ feed on decaying organic matter, especially on
nitrogenous substances. They thrive best in neutral or slightly
alkaline water, and soon die if free acids are present. Although
still capable of development in very brackish water, *S. fasciata*
cannot live in sea-water, as at least one other species of the
genus (*S. pseudoscutellaris*) has been shewn capable of doing.

After a number of moults the larva gives rise to the pupa.
The duration of the larval stage at fairly warm temperatures
varies from seven to fifteen days, but a temperature of below
20° C. will prolong development almost indefinitely. The young
larvæ are remarkably tenacious of life under water and will
stand submersion for three to five hours. The fully grown
larvæ can still endure a submergence of at least one and a
half to two hours, a property which enables them to feed at
the bottom of comparatively deep water.

There is no record of the live larvæ of *Stegomyia* ever
having been found in ice, as in the case of those of the allied

genus *Culex*. Miss Mitchell has found them in water at 1° C. and states that some pupated at 12° C., but in the laboratory the larvæ generally die if the temperature falls to 10° C. It is noteworthy that these low temperatures are more fatal to the fully grown larvæ than to the earlier stages.

If the temperature of the water in which the mosquitoes are developing falls daily below 20° C., the duration of the larval stage may exceed a month. The adults which eventually emerge, moreover, are generally so weak and unhealthy that they are unable to feed and soon die.

*The pupa.* The duration of the pupal stage varies from one to five days, after which the adult insect emerges. The pupæ are very sensitive to cold and a fall of temperature is almost invariably fatal to them, as their organization is not adapted to withstand the vicissitudes of climate. The pupæ resemble those of *Culex* in their general appearance.

The duration of the complete life-cycle from the new laid egg to the emergence of the imago may be as short as 11 days, but is usually from 15 to 20 days. A prolonged exposure to cold, on the other hand, may increase this period to as much as five months, and as mentioned above, the dried eggs are capable of living for long periods without developing.

*Stegomyia fasciata and disease.* In addition to being one of the commonest species of mosquito occurring in the tropics, *Stegomyia fasciata* is entirely responsible for the transmission of " Yellow Fever." It also has been shewn capable of transmitting *Filaria bancrofti* to man, but as this parasite is more commonly carried by members of the genus *Culex*, the infection will be described later.

Ed. Sergent and Neumann have shewn that *Plasmodium* (*Proteosoma*) *præcox* or *relicta*, parasitic in birds, will develop in *S. fasciata*. Finally, Fülleborn and Mayer, by feeding this mosquito on the blood of animals swarming with trypanosomes and subsequently, after short intervals, on normal animals, have succeeded in the mechanical transmission of *Trypanosoma gambiense*. It is very doubtful, however, whether in nature *S. fasciata* ever carries sleeping sickness, and in any case such transmission can only be very exceptional.

REFERENCES.

Boyce, R. (1911). *Yellow Fever and its prevention.* John Murray. London.

Francis, S. W. (1907). Observations on the life-cycle of *Stegomyia calopus. Publ. Health Reports,* vol. xxii. pp. 381–3.

Goeldi, E. A. (1904). Os Mosquitos no Pará. *Bol. Mus. Goeldi (Pará),* vol. iv. fasc. 2, pp. 129–197.

Howard, L. O. (1901). *Mosquitoes.* McClure, Phillips and Co. New York.

—— Dyar and Knab (1912). *The Mosquitoes of North and Central America and the West Indies.* Publ. 159. Carnegie Inst. Washington.

Marchoux, E. (1910). *Fièvre Jaune,* in Chantemesse and Mosny's *Traité d'Hygiène.* Baillière et fils. Paris.

Theobald, F. V. (1901–10). *A Monograph of the Culicidæ or Mosquitoes.* Vols. i to v. Brit. Museum, London.

# CHAPTER XI

## DISEASES TRANSMITTED BY CULICINÆ. YELLOW FEVER, DENGUE, BIRD MALARIA, ETC.

### I. Yellow Fever.

*Synonyms.* Bilious remittent fever. Tropical toxæmic jaundice. Typhus Icteroides. Pestis Americana. Febris Flava. Yellow Jack. Magdalena fever. Fièvre Jaune. Gelbfieber. Febbre Gialla. Fiebre Amarilla. Typhus Amaril. Matlazahuatl. Coup de Barre.

*General account and history.* Yellow fever is an acute non-contagious fever, usually characterized by the occurrence of two paroxysms of fever separated by an intermission, and accompanied by albuminuria, hæmorrhages and jaundice. The presence of the latter symptom has given rise to the name by which the disease is usually known, but it should be emphasized that this feature is often absent in mild cases. The disease is widely distributed in tropical and subtropical America, and also, according to most authorities, on the West Coast of Africa. It is endemic only in those regions where *Stegomyia fasciata* can exist all the year round, and in consequence only appears sporadically in subtropical and temperate regions. It is mainly a disease of seaport towns and practically all the great epidemics have occurred in such localities.

About the early history of yellow fever very little is certain. It is said to have been known by the Aztecs under the title of "Matlazahuatl." Other authorities believe that the disease originally occurred in the Antilles and was carried by the Spaniards to the mainland of America. There is little doubt that the disease originated in America and was fully established by the time that the early explorers arrived from Europe.

On the other hand certain authors have thought that it might have been introduced from West Africa by the slave-boats, but such a view is not in accordance with the fact that the disease seems to have been already known in America when Columbus discovered the continent. From Central America yellow fever has been carried by ships to various parts of the world, in some of which it has become endemic, and in others only occurred in epidemic form.

Its distribution is shewn in Fig. 50, which represents the extreme range of all places in which yellow fever has been known to occur within recent times. At present many of these localities are quite free from the disease and, as a result of anti-mosquito campaigns, many more are likely to become so in the near future.

At present the chief endemic foci of the disease are the States of Central and South America, with the exception of Panama, and the West Coast of Africa. In the United States, the Gulf States have frequently been the site of great epidemics, but the climatic conditions prevent the disease from becoming endemic. In West Africa yellow fever seems to have been known since 1778, when it was recorded from St Louis. The fact that the disease has existed in an unbroken line for more than a century, is strong evidence of its endemic character in West Africa, and although there have been no outstanding epidemics, yet the number of patients who annually succumb to " Bilious Remittent Fever " is considerable. One of the greatest difficulties in the way of studying the disease is the fact that mild cases of yellow fever cannot be diagnosed with any certainty. As a result, although the natives of endemic regions must frequently harbour the virus in their blood, up to the present it has been impossible to discover any direct proofs of it.

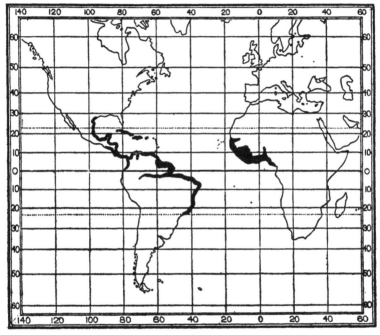

Fig. 50. The approximate distribution of Yellow Fever at the present time. Infected regions are coloured black.

The cause and method of infection of yellow fever have been a puzzle ever since the disease became known, and although the latter of these two points has now been settled the causal agent is still a matter of discussion.

In early times it was believed that the virus was in some way transmitted through the air, and the fact that it usually occurred in the vicinity of water led to the belief that it was produced by bacterial fermentation. Subsequently a number of bacteria were described as the cause of the disease, but all of them have been shewn to be merely secondary invasions.

In addition to being regarded as a highly infectious disease, yellow fever was always considered to be contagious, and patients suffering from it were strictly isolated and their clothing, etc. thoroughly sterilized. In spite of this isolation of patients, however, epidemics were not checked, and it was noticed that many persons became infected without ever having come in contact with infected cases, whilst frequently doctors and nurses, who worked in the same rooms as the patients, did not suffer from it.

It was also observed that ships coming from infected ports frequently carried the infection and consequently quarantine ordinances were brought into force, which to some extent reduced the spread of the disease, but the wars at the end of the eighteenth century caused these measures to be relaxed, with the result that some very serious epidemics occurred about this time. These afforded some opportunities for the study of the disease and several American observers called attention to the large numbers of mosquitoes and other insects that occurred during yellow fever epidemics. In 1848, Nott, of Mobile, accused some insect or mosquito of being the possible carrier. It was not, however, till 1881 that Charles Finlay of Havana definitely attributed the transmission of the disease to a mosquito. He had noticed in Cuba the connection that seemed to exist between the prevalence of yellow fever and the presence of large numbers of the tiger mosquito, *S. fasciata.* Accordingly, he attempted to transmit the infection experimentally by feeding mosquitoes on patients suffering from the disease and subsequently on normal persons. Although his experiments were open to many objections, there is no doubt that Finlay did succeed in transmitting the disease by means of the bites of mosquitoes and he energetically advanced his theory in a number of articles. Eventually his views began to attract the attention they deserved and finally, in 1899, an American Commission was sent to Cuba to study the disease.

This commission was composed of four members, Reed, Carroll, Lazear, and Agramonte, and the way in which they investigated the problem of the transmission of yellow fever will always remain famous. During their investigations Dr Lazear succumbed to the disease, but the research was carried on by his fellow workers, who succeeded in proving beyond all doubt that yellow fever is carried by the tiger mosquito, *Stegomyia fasciata*.

The earlier work of the commission was devoted to an examination of the various bacteria that had been described as the cause of the disease. Of these the most notorious were Sanarelli's *Bacillus icteroides*, and Sternberg's *Bacillus* X, which had been found in a certain number of cases. Reed and Carroll found that both these bacteria played no part in the ætiology of the malady, but were merely the result of a secondary infection. Subsequently, in 1900, Reed, Carroll, Agramonte and Lazear shewed that the disease could be produced in non-immune persons by the subcutaneous inoculation of blood from an infected patient. They also proved that the disease was not contagious but could only be spread by the bites of infected *S. fasciata*. These results have been thoroughly confirmed by subsequent investigators.

The work of the French Commission, composed of Marchoux, Salimbeni and Simond, is the most important of all subsequent researches on the disease, for these authors were able to elucidate some of the necessary conditions for the transmission of the malady. They also found that the first generation of the offspring from an infected mosquito is capable of infecting persons. Their results will be considered in detail in the section devoted to a description of the mode of transmission of yellow fever.

The practical benefits that have resulted from the application of the discovery of the mode of transmission of yellow fever are only paralleled by those following Ross's work on the development of *Plasmodium* in the mosquito.

In the Panama Canal zone, which used to be one of the worst endemic regions in Central America, as a result of anti-mosquito campaigns the number of cases of yellow fever was reduced so rapidly that within five years the disease had completely disappeared from this region.

*Geographical distribution.* In considering the distribution of yellow fever it is necessary to emphasize the fact that the disease is being rapidly eradicated from the more civilized regions of the world, and comparatively few endemic centres exist at the present time.

The most important of these are the following :

Guatemala, Nicaragua, Costa Rica, Ecuador, Spanish Honduras, Venezuela, French Guiana, certain parts of Mexico and the West Indies, and along the banks of the Amazon, Orinoco, and Magdalena Rivers. It will thus be seen that the States of Central and South America are the great centres of the disease, and from these regions it has spread into many other countries. It is probably endemic in West Africa for the continual recurrence of small epidemics cannot be explained on the supposition that these represent infections introduced by ships.

The endemic centres of yellow fever do not extend beyond latitudes 40° N. and 40° S., where the mean isotherm is not below 26° C. The malady, however, often extends into colder regions during the summer months, and may produce great epidemics, which, however, always disappear on the return of cold weather.

Great epidemics of yellow fever have occurred in many of the seaport towns of the Southern United States, especially in New Orleans where, in 1878, there was a record of 4046 deaths as the result of one epidemic. The Gulf ports were probably endemic centres during the eighteenth century and first half of the nineteenth, but as the result of improved hygienic conditions and better drainage the breeding places of the mosquitoes have been reduced until now the disease is almost extinct.

The Atlantic ports, as far north as New York, were also frequently visited by more or less severe epidemics, as the disease was continually being introduced by ships coming from Cuba and other endemic centres. The infected *Stegomyia* carried from these places would be able to live on board for some weeks and thus be capable of spreading the infection at the ports at which the ship called.

On the West Coast of America the general conditions are so unfavourable to the breeding of the mosquito, that the disease has not been able to establish itself and has only appeared sporadically in one or two localities, with the exception of the Isthmus of Panama, which until recently was one of the noted endemic centres. With this exception, therefore, the West Coast has never been the scene of any severe epidemics, for comparatively few ships sail up the coast and consequently there has been little chance of their spreading infected mosquitoes. Colon is practically the only port that has hitherto been liable to infection, but with the opening of the Panama Canal and the increase in trade which this is sure to effect, the question of the possibility of thus extending the range of yellow fever will have to be carefully considered. The recent outbreak at St Nazaire in 1908 has shewn clearly that even modern ships are capable of carrying infected *Stegomyia* for considerable distances.

In Europe the appearances of the disease have been very similar to those in North America, and many epidemics occurred during the eighteenth and nineteenth centuries, when the growth of commercial intercourse resulted in an increase in the number of ships coming from endemic centres.

In Southern Europe numerous epidemics of considerable severity have occurred, and the ports of France, and even Swansea and Southampton in England, have been the scenes of small outbreaks. In the south of Europe *Stegomyia fasciata* is capable of breeding, and therefore epidemics could easily become established during the summer months, but in the more northerly regions this is out of the question. In these cases the infection is strictly limited to persons who have been near a ship carrying infected mosquitoes on board.

Thus in the case of the outbreak at St Nazaire in 1908, infected *Stegomyia* were taken on board a ship at Martinique. These were carried across the Atlantic and on arrival at St Nazaire, several of the mosquitoes escaped and fed on persons either on board or in the vicinity of the ship. Eleven individuals were known to be infected in this way, of whom seven died.

Unless greater care is taken to screen ships during their stay in infected ports, there is little doubt that occasional epidemics of this nature now and then will appear. In North Europe, where the absence of *Stegomyia* prevents any further spread of the infection, these slight outbreaks are of comparatively slight danger, but in regions where the mosquito is abundant, *e.g.* Malay and India, the introduction of a few infected *Stegomyia* might lead to the production of terrible epidemics, such as those which raged in Barcelona during the eighteenth century.

*Mode of infection.* The various theories as to the nature of this disease have been sufficiently discussed in the previous chapter, and we shall at once proceed to a description of the work of the American Commission of 1899, on the transmission of yellow fever.

The first attempts of this commission to transmit the disease by mosquitoes were made with some *Stegomyia fasciata* that hatched in the laboratory from eggs supplied by Finlay. These insects were fed several times on patients suffering from yellow fever at various stages of the illness. Eleven persons having offered themselves for experiment, each day these infected mosquitoes were fed on a fresh human subject. Only two of these persons became infected, and both of them had been bitten by mosquitoes that had fed 12 days previously on the blood of a yellow fever patient in the first stage of the disease.

In this preliminary experiment the possibility of these two patients having become infected by other means had not been definitely excluded. It was decided, therefore, to continue these experiments, after taking more rigorous precautions against any external contamination. A camp was established in the neighbourhood of Tuemados, on a plateau that was well drained, and absolutely free from yellow fever. Twenty-eight non-immune subjects, mostly Americans and Spaniards, were shut up in this camp and carefully examined for several days in order to make sure that none of them were infected. If any of the patients shewed the slightest febrile symptoms they were at once removed from the camp, but none of the others were allowed to go out of it. After these preliminary precautions, some *Stegomyia* that had fed 12 days previously on a yellow fever patient in the first stages of the disease, were allowed to bite twelve persons. Ten of them became infected after incubation periods varying from 41 hours to five days. Twelve other persons who remained in the camp never shewed the slightest signs of infection, although living in close proximity with these yellow fever patients.

This experiment proved that not only is this mosquito the carrier of the infection, but that contact with patients is harmless. The latter is most important from an economic point of view, and therefore the commission carefully investigated the question.

A mosquito-proof house was constructed so as to present the worst possible hygienic conditions. It was badly ventilated, and badly lighted, and the windows were kept shut all day. The air inside the house was very humid and the temperature often rose to 35° C. Into this house was introduced the soiled linen from beds that had been occupied by yellow fever patients. A certain number of persons occupied this house for 20 days, sleeping between bed-clothes that had been soiled by the excrement and black vomit of yellow fever patients. In spite of these conditions none of the persons occupying the house became infected and the experiment has been repeated several times with similar results. No matter under what conditions of sanitation, etc., in the absence of *Stegomyia*, nobody became infected with the disease.

Finally, a house was constructed of the same dimensions as the preceding, but well lighted and ventilated, so as to present the best hygienic conditions. This house was rendered mosquito-proof by wire gauze, and also was divided into two halves by means of a partition of the same material. On one side the persons occupying the room were exposed to the same conditions as in the preceding experiment, namely, sleeping between the soiled bed linen from yellow fever patients, etc. In the other half only carefully sterilized material was allowed to enter but, in addition, there were introduced 15 mosquitoes that had fed, at least 12 days previously, on patients at the commencement of their infection. A young American doctor, Dr Moran, entered this half of the house and was bitten by a number of the mosquitoes. After a short incubation period, he developed a typical attack of yellow fever, whilst persons who occupied the other half of the house for at least 20 days remained healthy.

In this manner was established the important truth that yellow fever is only carried by means of the mosquito, and the above-mentioned results have been repeatedly confirmed by subsequent investigators.

*The causal agent.* In spite of numerous researches the causal agent is still under discussion, for most of the organisms that have been described from yellow fever patients may be explained as the result of secondary infection, or in other cases, as artefacts. Because of the many points of resemblance between relapsing fever and yellow fever, it has been suggested that the latter is also due to a spirochæte. Recently Seidelin has described the occurrence of a parasite, belonging to the Babesiidæ, in the blood and organs of yellow fever patients. To this parasite Seidelin has given the name of *Paraplasma flavigenum*, and he considers it to be the causal agent of yellow fever.

Whatever the causal agent may be, it is present in the circulation in large numbers, for the subcutaneous injection of minute quantities of infected blood into a non-immune person is followed by an attack of yellow fever. It is said to be present in the circulation only during the first three days of an attack, for blood taken from a patient on the fourth day, when his temperature was still high (40° C.) was found to be non-infective. However, as there has only been one attempt made to infect persons with the blood taken from patients after the third day, this statement is still open to question. On the whole it seems probable that yellow fever patients may remain infective even after all signs of the disease have disappeared, for it is difficult to explain its prevalence in certain cases except on the theory of latent infections. The organism must be excessively minute for it can easily pass through a Chamberland Filter F. When the infected serum is diluted with an equal quantity of water the virus is even capable of passing through a Chamberland Filter B, 0·033 c.c. of the filtrate producing a typical attack when injected into a non-immune person.

The virus is extremely fragile, for a drop of infected blood may be placed on an excoriated part of the skin with impunity, as the slightest desiccation destroys the disease agent. Moreover, it is very susceptible to heat, for at a temperature of 55° C. it loses its virulence within five minutes.

*Development within the mosquito.* Under ordinary circumstances when a *Stegomyia* has fed on the blood of a yellow fever patient during the first three days of an attack, it becomes infective after an incubation period of about 12 days. The conditions of development within the mosquito are very uncertain, however, for it often happens that mosquitoes remain uninfective, even though fed on infected blood.

The effect of temperature is very important and probably accounts to some extent for the restricted range of the disease. If a mosquito is kept at a temperature of about 22° C., instead of becoming infective 12 days after an infected feed, the incubation period is prolonged to three or four weeks. At 20° C. the virus is incapable of developing within the mosquito and thus the latter does not become infected.

If an infected mosquito, capable of transmitting the disease, is exposed to a low temperature, it ceases to be infective, but recovers this power on again being warmed. It is possible that changes in temperature alter the virulence of the disease, for during the cool season the cases of yellow fever are often benign, the most severe ones occurring during the hot weather.

Under certain conditions it seems that the infection may be transmitted to the offspring of an infected mosquito.

Marchoux and Simond kept a female *Stegomyia*, which laid its eggs 16 days after an infective feed. These eggs were kept at a temperature of about 28° C. and developed in a comparatively short length of time into the adult insects. The latter were found to be infected and produced a typical attack of yellow fever when fed on a non-immune subject. Although no one else has succeeded in repeating this experiment, the

French investigators were so careful to exclude all chance of error, that there is little doubt that under certain conditions, a *Stegomyia* infected with yellow fever is able to transmit the infection to its offspring. The reappearance of yellow fever in places where it had apparently become extinct may possibly be explained by this factor.

Once a mosquito has become infected, it probably continues so for the remainder of its life, but there are not sufficient observations on this question. In nature the insects are certainly still infective after being nourished on sugar for two or three weeks, as shewn in the case of the St Nazaire epidemic.

It is possible for the virus of yellow fever to be preserved indefinitely in the mosquito and thus the cycle of development must be quite different from that of *Plasmodium*. This was clearly shewn by an interesting experiment performed by Marchoux and Simond. Mosquitoes, that had fed on an infected patient more than 12 days previously, were ground up in thick syrup and some freshly hatched *Stegomyia* fed on this mixture. Fifteen days later these insects were found to be infected, although they had never fed on a yellow fever patient.

*Vaccination.* Although no successful means of preventing infection by this means have yet been discovered, the results obtained by the use of various sera are of some interest.

We have previously referred to the extreme susceptibility to temperature of the virus of yellow fever. Warming for five minutes at 55° C. destroys all its activity. If preserved at a temperature of 29° to 30° C. in an ordinary tube plugged with cotton, the serum loses its virulence within 48 hours. The same temperature acts much more slowly if the infected serum is covered with a layer of oil in order to protect it from the air. At the end of five days some serum kept in this manner was still infective, and produced an attack of yellow fever when injected into a non-immune person. It should be added that it only produced a very mild attack. After being thus preserved for eight days the serum lost its virulence entirely and could be injected into non-immunes without producing any infection.

The inoculation of serum that had either been warmed, or kept for eight days at 25° C., was found to confer a partial immunity against yellow fever. All the subjects that had received such injections, were subsequently inoculated with a virulent strain of yellow fever, and in every case the resulting attack was found to be extremely mild in character, shewing that the serum had had an immunizing effect.

During the course of an attack of yellow fever the presence of antibodies in the blood of the patient may easily be demonstrated. The serum of a patient taken on the eighth day of an attack and injected into a non-immune person, completely protected the latter against infection when subsequently inoculated with virulent blood. The serum of a convalescent patient is even more effective, and if injected into non-immune persons will protect them against all attempts at infection for a period of about 20 days. By the twenty-sixth day the immunity begins to disappear but is still present, for the inoculation of virulent blood only produces a slight attack of fever.

Such immune serum may also be applied therapeutically, and when injected into infected patients is said to diminish the severity of the symptoms and hasten the recovery. Unfortunately, all these methods are of little use, because they require the presence of infected patients and convalescents to furnish the necessary materials.

REFERENCES.

Boyce, R. (1911). *Yellow Fever and its prevention.* London : John Murray.

Clarac, A. and Simond, P. L. (1912). *Fièvre Jaune,* in Grall and Clarac's *Traité Pratique de Pathologie Exotique.* Paris. Vol. III. pp. 21–176.

Finlay, C. (1883). Sur une nouvelle théorie de la fièvre jaune. *Ref. Arch. de méd. nav.* January, 1883.

Marchoux, E. (1910). *Fièvre Jaune,* in Chantemesse and Mosny's *Traité d'Hygiène.* Paris : Baillière et fils.

Marchoux, Salimbeni and Simond (1903). La fièvre jaune. *Ann. Inst. Pasteur,* vol. XVII. pp. 665–731.

Marchoux and Simond (1906). Études sur la fièvre jaune. *Ibid.* vol. XX. pp. 16, 104 and 161.

Reed, Carroll, Agramonte and Lazear (1900). Preliminary note on the Etiology of Yellow Fever. *Phil. Med. Journ.* Oct. 27.

Reed and Carroll (1902). Recent researches concerning the etiology, propagation, and prevention of Yellow Fever, by the U.S. Army Commission. *Journ. of Hygiene*, vol. II, pp. 101–119.

Sanarelli, G. (1897). Etiologie et pathogénie de la fièvre jaune. *Ann. Inst. Pasteur*, XI. p. 433.

Seidelin, H. (1911). The Etiology of Yellow Fever. *Yellow Fever Bulletin*, vol. I. pp. 229–258.

For a complete bibliography see the *Yellow Fever Bulletin*, and also Scheube's *Die Krankheiten der warmen Länder*. (Jena : G. Fischer.)

## II. DENGUE.

*Synonyms.* The synonymy of this disease is very extensive, upwards of 100 names having been applied to it. The most important of these are as follows : Dandy Fever ; Breakbone Fever ; Febris Endemica cum Roseola ; Exanthesis Arthrosia ; Arthrodynie ; Knokkelkoorts ; Eruptive Rheumatic Fever ; Fièvre rouge, etc.

*History.* The first records of dengue do not appear before the end of the eighteenth century, though there is some possibility that an epidemic noted by Pazzio as occurring in Seville from 1764 to 1768 was caused by this disease.

In 1779 dengue was noted in Cairo and Arabia, by Gaberti ; in India, by Persin ; and also in Batavia, by David Bylon. The following year Rush described an epidemic occurring in Philadelphia, and in 1784 the disease was introduced from the West Indies into Spain, where it caused severe epidemics in Cadiz and Seville, which were well described by Cristobal Cubillas.

During the nineteenth century epidemics have been recorded from most tropical and subtropical regions. According to Manson there is a tendency for these epidemics to occur at intervals of about 20 years. The last epidemic to occur in Europe was in 1889, when the disease was especially prevalent in Turkey, Greece, and the Eastern Mediterranean region generally.

*Distribution and epidemiology.* Dengue is essentially a tropical disease, but occasionally it extends into subtropical regions. It has occurred in practically every country between

32° 47′ N. and 23° 23′ S., and during the summer months it may extend up to as much as 42° N. The disease is usually more prevalent in low-lying lands well supplied with water, probably because such sites provide better opportunities for the breeding of *Culex*. There are exceptions to this rule, however, for during the epidemic in Syria in 1888–9 the disease extended to villages having an altitude of nearly 4000 feet.

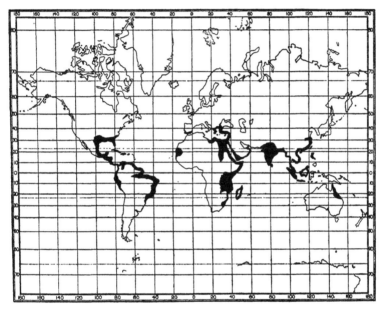

Fig. 51. The distribution of Dengue. The countries from which cases have been recorded are coloured black. (Compare this chart with that on page 193, shewing the distribution of *Culex fatigans*.)

The distribution of dengue, past and present, is represented in the accompanying map (Fig. 51). At the present time the chief endemic centres of the infection are India and the East Indies, and, in the New World, the West Indies and Central America. From these centres the disease, in warm summers, may even extend into temperate regions, but on the approach of winter it gradually disappears, as a certain amount of heat seems to be necessary for its transmission.

Neither age, sex, race, nor social conditions, seem to have any effect on this disease, which attacks rich and poor, old and young, black and white, with the utmost impartiality. The rapid spread of epidemics of dengue is another feature which was noticed even by the earliest observers. The rapidity with which it extends is probably unequalled by any other malady, and usually within a few days of its appearance in any particular locality a considerable proportion of the population will be found suffering from the disease. In 1884 an epidemic in Nouméa broke out so suddenly that the majority of the public services were disorganized ; a regiment of marines was reduced to less than one section, and so many of the sailors were affected that the ships were temporarily put out of action.

The disease is usually conveyed from one place to another by means of ships carrying infected passengers. Thus dengue was introduced into Tahiti by a steamer that carried a single infected passenger, who had contracted the disease in Nouméa. This case was sufficient to start an epidemic in the island.

When any particular maritime locality becomes the centre of an epidemic, all ships visiting the place are liable to become infected. Occasionally the disease is spread by means of trains as, for example, in India, where it was carried from Calcutta across Bengal by these means. Such a method of expansion, however, is somewhat unusual and seaports continue to be the localities most visited by epidemics, the infection being introduced by ships. An epidemic generally lasts for about five or six months, gradually diminishing in the number of cases until it finally disappears.

It is interesting to note that the distribution of dengue shews a remarkable coincidence with that of *Culex fatigans.* (Figs. 51 and 52.)

*Causal agent.* Our knowledge of dengue is still very imperfect and in spite of numerous researches the cause of the disease remains unknown. McLaughlin, in 1886, found a micrococcus in the blood of infected patients and supposed that this was the causative agent, but his results have been disproved by subsequent investigators. In 1903, Graham believed that he had discovered the cause of the disease, in the form of small hyaline bodies occurring in the red cells, which he considered to be related to *Babesia*. In addition, he fed *Culex fatigans* on infected patients and claimed to have found his parasites in the insects up to the fifth day after feeding, without, however, observing any signs of their development. Nevertheless the salivary glands were said to contain spores from two days up to a month after the mosquito had

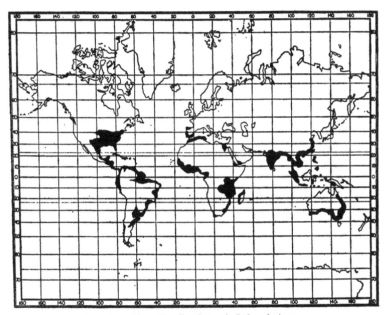

Fig. 52. The distribution of *Culex fatigans*.

fed on infected blood. A typical attack of dengue was produced in a healthy person by the injection of the salivary glands of a mosquito, that had fed on an infected patient 24 hours previously.

Although Graham's work on the transmission of dengue by *Culex fatigans* has been confirmed, the organism which he described has never been observed by any subsequent investigators, but from the nature of the disease there seems little doubt that it is caused by some protozoal parasite living in the blood. Ashburn and Craig have studied the ætiology and transmission of dengue in the Philippines, and were able to produce the disease in normal persons by the intravenous injection of 20 c.cs. of blood from an infected patient. The incubation period was two to three days, and was followed by typical attacks of dengue. These authors also found that the pathogenic agent was so small that it would pass through the pores of a filter which retained organisms 0·4 $\mu$ in diameter, filtered serum being equally as infective as non-filtered blood.

The blood shews little alteration except in the leucocyte count, a slight or well-marked leucopenia being a fairly constant character. The number of polymorphonuclear leucocytes may be reduced to forty or fifty per cent., but at the same time there is an increase of the large mononuclears and lymphocytes, the latter predominating. Some authors maintain that the leucocyte formula remains essentially the same throughout the disease, whilst others are of the opinion that considerable variations occur. Dengue is not accompanied by any anæmia, the red cells remaining normal both in number and appearance.

*Mode of infection.* The *transmission* of this disease is still somewhat obscure in spite of the work of Graham, and Ashburn and Craig. For a long time it was considered to be a highly contagious infection and Düring recorded a case in which five families that received their washing from the same laundress all became infected about the same time and before the other inhabitants.

Arnold, in 1846, was the first to support the idea that the disease is not contagious and based his theory on two facts noticed in Havana, namely, that the epidemic was localized in the town and did not spread into the surrounding country, and that among the first cases, not any of the patients had been in contact with one another, either directly or indirectly.

The belief in the contagious nature of dengue has now been abandoned by the majority of investigators, but, in addition to the idea that it is carried by *Culex*, various other theories of animal transmission have been advanced. In America it is a common idea that the spread of the disease depends in some way on the cattle. In India, Martialis has noticed that the cows and horses are sometimes attacked by dengue, often presenting a temporary paralysis of one or more legs, but usually recovering after three or four days. Also, Duchateau, during an epidemic in the Senegal, noticed that it coincided with a high mortality amongst the wild birds and fowls.

None of these theories has received any support from experiments, for up to the present all attempts to infect animals have remained negative.

Finally, in 1903, Graham propounded the theory that *Culex fatigans* is responsible for the transmission of this disease and supported his theory by experiments. Ashburn and Craig, however, are the only investigators who have actually succeeded in transmitting the disease by the bites of infected *Culex fatigans*. It should be noted, however, that they only succeeded on one occasion and their results have not been confirmed.

The details of Ashburn and Craig's experiments are as follows :

On September 12th, a non-immune soldier was placed under a mosquito net with about 20 *Culex fatigans* that had fed on a dengue patient the previous night. The man was bitten on the night of the 12th, approximately one day after the mosquitoes had fed. About three and a half days later he shewed a distinct rise of temperature and a day later developed a typical attack of dengue.

It is evident that in this experiment the parasite causing the disease had no time to undergo any cycle of development in the mosquito, except a very short one. As all attempts to infect persons by the bites of mosquitoes after an interval of more than one day gave negative results, Ashburn and Craig are of the opinion that the parasite of dengue is merely capable of living in the stomach of the mosquito and does not need to undergo any cycle of development before becoming infective.

It must be admitted that the experimental evidence in support of the mosquito transmission theory is very incomplete, but a consideration of its epidemiology leaves no doubt as to the usual mode of infection.

In the first place the disease has been definitely proved to be non-contagious, but is infectious in the same way as yellow fever and malaria. Secondly, the distribution of dengue more or less coincides with that of *Culex fatigans*. Additional support, however, is that brought forward by E. H. Ross, who shewed that in Port Said, Egypt, dengue entirely disappeared after the destruction of mosquitoes. Previously the town had been subject to severe epidemics, but since the extermination of the mosquitoes, not a single case of dengue has been recorded, although the disease has been rife in other parts of Egypt.

Of course, it is possible that other Culicines may be capable of transmitting the infection, and the observations of Legendre in Hanoi suggest that *Stegomyia* is probably a carrier of the virus.

### REFERENCES.

Ashburn and Craig (1907). Experimental investigations regarding the etiology of Dengue Fever. *Philippine Jour. Sci.* Sect. B, *Med. Sci.* vol. II. No. 2.

Graham (1903). The Dengue ; a study of the pathology and mode of propagation. *Journ. Trop. Med.* 1903, p. 209.

Legendre (1911). *Bull. Soc. Path. Exot.* vol. IV. p. 26.

Seidelin, H. (1913). Dengue. A summary. *Yellow Fever Bulletin,* vol. II. pp. 335–358. (Contains a very good general account of the disease.)

III. BIRD MALARIA (*Plasmodium præcox* [Grassi and Feletti]).

*General account.* A great variety of birds, such as finches, sparrows, crows, etc., have been found infected with a parasite closely resembling the *Plasmodia* of man. By some authors this bird parasite has been separated off into a distinct genus, *Proteosoma*, but the differences between it and *Plasmodium* are so slight that now the two are generally united. There is also some doubt as to whether all the *Plasmodia* occurring in birds should be regarded as one species, and some observers have preferred to give specific names to the *Plasmodia* from different species of birds, but there is no justification for this course, as hitherto all attempts to find any specific differences, apart from the kind of host, have failed. Therefore, for the present, all the plasmodial parasites occurring in birds may be regarded as belonging to one species, *Plasmodium præcox* (Grassi and Feletti, 1890).

The parasites have a decidedly pathogenic action upon the birds they infest. They grow at the expense of the red corpuscles, which lose their hæmoglobin, and gradually degenerate. As a result infected birds become anæmic and, in addition, the substances produced by the parasites seem to have a general toxic effect upon the organs of the body. As in the case of human malaria, the body temperature rises, but rarely more than 1–1·5° C. Birds not infrequently succumb to the infection, especially during the early part of the year, when climatic conditions are somewhat severe.

*Causal agent.* *Plasmodium præcox* in its general form somewhat resembles *P. vivax*. The small amœboid sporozoites penetrate into the red cells and there generally assume a somewhat triangular form, with a round vesicular nucleus containing a karyosome. This young trophozoite grows at the expense of the contents of the red cell and deposits waste materials in the form of pigment granules, which are scattered through its protoplasm. Danilewsky refers to these young forms as "pseudo-vacuolæ." The protoplasm is finely granular and contains numerous vacuoles.

According to Labbé there are two kinds of schizogony in the circulating blood. Sometimes the parasite divides up into six or seven merozoites arranged in the form of a rosette, whilst at other times the parasite divides up into very numerous merozoites scattered irregularly throughout the infected blood corpuscle. In both cases the pigment and waste materials are left behind in the form of a residual body. The merozoites escape and penetrate other blood corpuscles, where they either develop and repeat the schizogonic cycle, or give rise to the gametocytes. The development of the latter closely resembles that of the corresponding forms in other species of *Plasmodia* (*e.g. P. vivax*).

## The Morphological Changes.

*Development in the mosquito.* The experiments of Ross, Sergent, Ruge and Neumann have shewn that at least four species of Culicinæ are capable of transmitting *P. præcox*, viz. *Culex pipiens, C. fatigans, C. nemorosus* and *Stegomyia fasciata.* In all these species the development of the parasite is practically identical with that of *P. vivax* in *Anopheles*, and therefore it is unnecessary to describe it in detail.

The development, however, does not take place with equal facility in all these species, even under the same conditions of temperature and humidity.

Thus Neumann found that out of 501 *Stegomyia fasciata* which fed on an infected canary, only 57 (= 11·4 per cent.) subsequently shewed the development of ripe cysts and the sporozoites of the parasite. On the other hand out of 104 *Culex pipiens* fed under similar conditions, 85 (= 81·7 per cent.) became infected. Moreover the time occupied in the development of the parasite, from the ingestion of the gametocytes to the appearance of sporozoites in the salivary gland of the mosquito, was longer in the case of *Stegomyia* than in *Culex.*

At a temperature of 27° C., with a relatively high humidity of about 75 to 80 per cent., the times occupied by the various stages of development were as follows :

|  | In *Culex* | In *Stegomyia* |
| --- | --- | --- |
| Formation of microgametes    .. | 30 to 45 mins. | 30 to 60 mins. |
| Copulation ..    ..    ..    .. | 30 to 60 mins. | 39 to 90 mins. |
| Formation of oökinete, | | |
|     commencement of    .. | About 10 to 12 hours | About 16 hours |
|     majority formed  .. | 20 hours | 26 hours |
| Disappearance of oökinetes from | | |
|     the stomach ..    ..    .. | After 48 hours | After 72 hours |
| Formation of sporocyst ..    .. | About 30 hours | Not before the 3rd or 4th day |
| Development of sporozoites in the | | |
|     cyst  ..    ..    ..    .. | 6 to 7 days | 8 to 10 days |
| Total developmental period, from the ingestion of the infected blood to the appearance of sporozoites in the salivary glands of the infected mosquito | 9 to 11 days | 13 to 15 days |

At a temperature of 20° to 22° C. the formation of the oökinete and its subsequent development is very greatly prolonged, but the liberation of the microgametes and the process of copulation does not seem to be delayed. If the humidity is lowered to about 40 per cent. the development of the cysts is prolonged for at least two days, so it seems that a dry atmosphere is relatively unfavourable to the infection of mosquitoes.

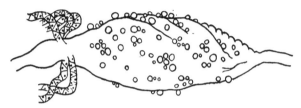

Fig. 53. View of the stomach of a *Culex* shewing large numbers of the sporocysts of *Plasmodium præcox* on its walls. (After Ross.)

Neumann kept very large numbers of *Culex* and fed them entirely on the blood of an infected canary. Although the majority of these mosquitoes were heavily infected with the *Plasmodium*, none of them seemed to shew any ill-effects from the presence of these parasites. On the other hand Koch, who similarly fed a number of *Culex nemorosus* on birds infected with *P. præcox*, found that many of the insects succumbed to the infection.

REFERENCES.

Grassi, B. (1901). *Die Malaria-Studien eines Zoologen.* Jena: Fischer.
Koch, R. Ueber die Entwicklung der Malariaparasiten. *Zeitschr. f. Hyg. u. Infektionskrankh.* vol. xxxii.
Neumann, R. O. (1909). Die Übertragung von *Plasmodium præcox* auf Kanarienvögel. *Arch. f. Protistenkunde,* vol. xiii. pp. 23–69.
Ross, R. (1905). Nobel Prize Essay, 1905.
Ruge, R. (1901). Untersuchungen über das deutsche *Proteosoma. Centralbl. f. Bakt.* i. vol. xxix. pp. 187–191.
Sergent, Ed. and Et. (1907). Études sur les Hématozoaires d'Oiseaux. *Ann. Inst. Pasteur,* vol. xxi. pp. 251–280.

IV. APPENDIX. *The Blood Parasites of* Athene noctua.

In addition to the above-mentioned infections, it is probable that most of the blood parasites of birds are transmitted by the agency of some species of mosquito. Schaudinn, in his famous memoir on the life-cycles of the parasites of the Little Owl (*Athene noctua*), described the development of these organisms in the alimentary canal of the common gnat, *Culex pipiens*.

The Little Owl harbours in its blood at least six forms of avian parasites, namely, (1) a proteosoma ; (2) a halteridium ; (3) a small form of trypanosome ; (4) a large form of trypanosome ; (5) a leucocytozoon ; and (6) a spirochæte.

According to Schaudinn all these forms belong to the life-cycle of only three species of parasites. The proteosoma is certainly a distinct form unrelated to any of the others. On the other hand the halteridium and the small trypanosome were said to be phases of the same parasite, whilst the large trypanosome, leucocytozoon and spirochæte were considered as stages in the development of another parasite.

The halteridium was supposed to be the resting intracorpuscular stage of the small trypanosome, which at night developed a locomotor apparatus, became free from the red cell and swam about as an ordinary trypanosome ; in the morning it penetrated another red cell, its locomotor apparatus disappeared, and it again became a halteridium. Three forms of the parasite were distinguished, known respectively as male, female and indifferent forms. The latter were the forms which multiplied in the blood, and from these small trypanosomes either indifferent, male, or female forms, might develop.

The two latter developed slower than the indifferent forms, and as they grew larger were unable to change from the halteridium to the trypanosome form, but became exclusively intracorpuscular or halteridium forms. The further development of these sexual forms could only take place if they were ingested by a gnat, *Culex pipiens*. In the alimentary canal of this insect the male and female forms became free and copulated, forming typical oökinetes. The latter developed into trypanosomes which again might be either female or indifferent, or divide up into a large number of male forms. Ultimately the indifferent and male trypanosomes were inoculated back again into an owl; the female trypanosomes being too bulky could not pass through the proboscis of the gnat, and as the male forms soon died out in the blood the new infection was started by the indifferent trypanosomes.

This extraordinary account of the life-cycle of the parasite of the Little Owl has been the subject of much discussion during the past few years.

Mayer has brought forward evidence in support of one of Schaudinn's statements, for he found that when owl's blood containing only halteridia was kept in hanging drops under the microscope, eventually trypanosomes made their appearance and these could only have come there by the transformation of the halteridia.

On the other hand no other confirmation of the life-cycle has hitherto been published, whilst there are many serious objections to it. In the first place the careful researches of Minchin and Woodcock, who worked at Rovigno, the place where Schaudinn made his observations, have shewn that in the blood of *Athene noctua* there is every stage between the small trypanosomes and the large ones, and there is every reason to suppose that in this case, as in many other vertebrates, these are all merely forms of one polymorphic trypanosome.

Further the development of *Hæmoproteus columbæ*, the halteridium of the pigeon (*v.* Chapter XXIII), is of a totally different kind, as the transmitting host is not a mosquito and moreover the development does not include any trypanosome phases.

Minchin suggests a solution of the difficulty by supposing that the trypanosome of the Little Owl, like other known species of trypanosomes, has intracorpuscular forms which have been confused with true halteridia.

With regard to Schaudinn's account of the life-cycle of the *Leucocytozoon* there is not the slightest doubt that no relation exists between this parasite and the spirochætes and trypanosomes, which are supposed to be stages in its development.

The bacterial nature of the spirochætes is now generally admitted, and the life-cycles of those species that have been investigated have been found to be of the simplest nature, not involving any sexual phenomena, or anything in the slightest degree comparable with Schaudinn's account. Up to the present, no observer has succeeded in working out the life-cycle of any *Leucocytozoon*, but it is unlikely that a gnat is responsible for its transmission.

On the whole, therefore, it seems better to disregard Schaudinn's statements concerning this parasite, and to consider its life-cycle as still an open question.

REFERENCES.

Dobell, C. C. (1912). Researches on the Spirochæts and related organisms. *Arch. f. Protistenkunde*, vol. XXVI. pp. 117–240.

Mayer, M. (1911). Über ein Halteridium und Leucocytozoon des Waldkauzes und deren Weiterentwicklung in Stechmücken. *Ibid.* vol. XXI. pp. 232–254.

Minchin, E. A. (1912). *An Introduction to the Study of the Protozoa*, pp. 389–394. London : Edward Arnold.

Minchin and Woodcock, H. M. (1911). Observations on the Trypanosome of the Little Owl (*Athene noctua*). *Quart. Journ. Micr. Sci.* vol. LVII. pp. 141–185.

Schaudinn, F. (1904). Generations- und Wirtswechsel bei Trypanosoma und Spirochæte. *Arb. a. d. kais. Gesundheitsamt.* vol. XX. p. 387.

# CHAPTER XII

## DISEASES TRANSMITTED BY ANOPHELINÆ AND CULICINÆ. FILARIASIS

### I. *Filaria bancrofti* Cobbold, 1877.

*Synonyms.* *Trichina cystica* Salisbury, 1868. *F. sanguinis hominis* Lewis, 1872. *F. sanguinis hominis ægyptiaca* Sonsino, 1874. *F. dermathemica* da Silva Aranjo, 1855. *F. wücheresi* da Silva Lima, 1877. *F. sanguinis hominum* Hall, 1885. *F. sanguinis hominum nocturna* Manson, 1891. *F. nocturna*

Manson, 1891. *Microfilaria nocturna* Manson, 1891. *F. philippinensis* Ashburn and Craig, 1906.

*History.* The embryo of this species was discovered by
Demarquay in 1863, in the chylous fluid from a case of dropsy
of the tunica vaginalis, occurring in the West Indies. Wücherer
in 1866 noticed the parasites in the urine of several cases of
tropical chyluria, and in the next few years these embryos
were found in similar cases from various parts of the world.
In 1872 Lewis found that the parasites occurred in the blood
of man, and Manson, da Silva Lima and Crevaux established
the identity of these blood filariæ with those occurring in cases
of chyluria and lymph scrotum. In 1876 the adult filaria
was discovered by Bancroft in an abscess of a lymphatic gland
of the arm and also in a hydrocele of the spermatic cord.
Manson studied the disease in China, and was the first to notice
the periodic increase and decrease in the number of parasites
in the peripheral circulation. From these observations he
deduced that some blood-sucking insect was responsible for
the spread of the infection, and his discovery in 1878 that
mosquitoes were the agents in the transmission of the disease
constitutes one of the landmarks in the history of tropical
medicine. In 1879 he described the changes undergone by
the filaria in the body of the mosquito, *Culex pipiens*, but the
method in which the parasite again reached man remained
undiscovered till 1900, when Low observed the worms in the
proboscides of mosquitoes infected with *Filaria bancrofti*.

*Distribution.* This species has been recorded from tropical
and subtropical countries in most parts of the world. In
Europe one case has been observed in Spain and another in
Italy ; it is also probable that it occasionally occurs in Greece
and Turkey. In Asia this filaria is widely spread throughout
China, Japan, the Philippines, and India. It is rare in Indo-
China. In Oceania it is extremely common in the majority
of the islands, and in Samoa at least one half the inhabitants
are said to be infected. In Australia it occurs as far south as
Brisbane. In Africa it has been recorded from many localities
in the north, east and west, and probably occurs throughout the
whole continent north of latitude 20° S. It is also common

in Mauritius, Reunion and Madagascar. In America, it is common in many parts of the West Indies and Brazil, and cases occur in the southern United States up to latitude 40° N.

*Description.* The adult filariæ do not occur in the peripheral blood circulation, but are found in various parts of the lymphatics. The males and females generally occur together, often coiled about each other. Sometimes several occur together in small cyst-like dilatations of the distal lymphatics ; they are also found in the larger lymphatic vessels and in the glands themselves, and, probably not infrequently, in the thoracic duct.

The female is a long, hair-like, transparent, motile worm, 50–155 mm. in length, and 0·15–0·715 mm. in breadth. The two uterine tubes, easily seen through the transparent integument, occupy the greater length of the body, and are filled with ova and embryos at various stages of development. The body is plain, tapering rather abruptly towards the anterior end to form a distinct neck, beyond which is the slightly enlarged rounded oral extremity. The tail is also tapered, but ends rather abruptly. The cuticle is finely striated. At a short distance behind the head a luminous V-shaped spot is visible, that may represent the water-vascular system. The vulva is situated on the ventral surface at a distance of about 2·56 mm. from the anterior extremity. The anus opens immediately in front of the tail, 0·13–0·28 mm. from the posterior extremity. The worm is ovo-viviparous. The ova measure 25–38 µ in length by 15 µ in breadth.

The male resembles the female in its general appearance but is somewhat smaller, usually about 70–80 mm. in length by 0·40 mm. in breadth. When living it may further be distinguished from the female by its marked tendency to curl, and also by the shape of the tail, the extremity of which is sharply incurvated, often making one or two spirals. The anus is situated 0·11 mm. from the posterior extremity and from its aperture emerge two slender, unequal spicules, respectively 0·2 and 0·6 mm. in length. According to Looss there are three pairs of post-anal papillæ ; pre-anal papillæ seem to be absent. The anterior end is rounded and not marked off from the rest of the body by a distinct neck as in the case of the female.

The embryos, or microfilariæ as they are frequently termed, occur in the peripheral blood. Manson describes the movements of the living parasite in the following words : " In fresh blood, *F. nocturna* (= *bancrofti*) is seen to be a minute, transparent, colourless, snake-like organism which, without materially changing its position on the slide, wriggles about in a state of great activity, constantly agitating and displacing the corpuscles in its neighbourhood. At first the movements are so active that the anatomical features of the filaria cannot be made out. In the course of a few hours the movements slow down, and then one can see that the little worm is shaped like a snake or an eel—that is to say, it is a long, slender, cylindrical organism, having one extremity abruptly rounded off, the other for about one-fifth of its entire length gradually tapering to a fine point. When examined with a low power, it appears to be structureless ; with a high power, a certain amount of structure can, on close scrutiny, be made out. In the first place, it can be seen that the entire animal is enclosed in an exceedingly delicate, limp, structureless sack, in which it moves backwards and forwards. This sack or " sheath " as it is generally called, although closely applied to the body, is considerably longer than the worm it encloses, so that that part of the sack which for the time being is not occupied is collapsed, and trails after the head or tail or both, as the case may be. It can be seen also that about the posterior part of the middle third of the parasite there is what appears to be an irregular aggregation of granular matter which, by suitable staining, can be shown to be viscous of some sort. This organ runs for some distance along the axis of the worm. Further, if high power be used, a closely set, very delicate transverse striation can be detected in the musculo-cutaneous layer throughout the entire length of the animal. Besides this if carefully looked for at a point about one-fifth of the entire length of the organism backwards from the head end, a shining triangular V-shaped patch is always visible. This

V-spot is brought out by very light staining with dilute logwood. The dye brings out yet another spot, similar to the preceding, though very much smaller ; this second spot is situated a short distance from the end of the tail. The former I have designated the V-spot ; the latter the " tail spot." Staining with logwood also shows the body of the little animal is principally composed of a column of closely packed, exceedingly minute cells enclosed in the transversely striated musculo-cutaneous cylinder ; at all events, many nuclei are thereby rendered visible. Dr Low has recently pointed out to me that the break seen in all stained specimens in the central column of nuclei occurs at a point slightly posterior to the anterior V-spot. This break can only be recognized in stained specimens."

According to Annett, Dutton and Elliott, if preparations of the living filaria are examined directly after being made from the patient, the embryos are seen to exhibit, for a short period, a rapidly progressive movement across the field of the microscope—at first so rapid that the parasites can only be traced with difficulty. This movement quickly ceases, as the sheath of the embryo soon becomes attached to the slide, as described above.

The embryos vary from 270 to 340 $\mu$ in length, by 7 to 11 $\mu$ in breadth.

*Life-cycle in the vertebrate host.* We shall commence with the adult female in the lymphatics of the infected patient. The fertilization is internal and the fertilized female usually contains large numbers of embryos at various stages of development. As this animal is ovi-viviparous, the eggs are not liberated from the body of the parent until the embryonic filariæ (= microfilariæ) are well formed and capable of independent motion. The egg is surrounded by a transparent sheath, within which the embryos are enclosed the whole time they remain in the vertebrate host. The young filariæ, each enclosed in its sheath, on being liberated make their way into the blood-vessels of the host and may be found in the peripheral circulation. Whilst remaining in the blood they are incapable of further development, but are enclosed within their sheaths, presenting an appearance similar to that shewn in Fig. 54.

These are the filariæ that one encounters on examining the blood of a filarious patient, and as will be seen they are merely immature forms and, consequently, it is very difficult to classify them, as the various species are distinguished mainly by the characters of the adults. These embryos are often termed " microfilariæ " in order to distinguish them from the mature " filariæ," but it should be remembered that such a term cannot be used in a generic sense.

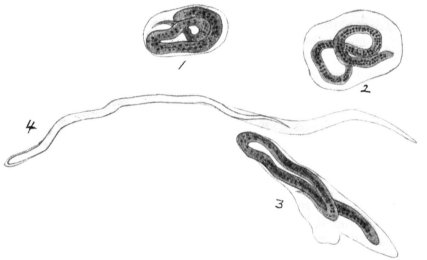

Fig. 54. Microfilariæ of *F. bancrofti* emerging from the uterus of the parent filaria, uncoiling in their chorionic envelopes. (After Bahr, from *Filariasis and Elephantiasis in Fiji.*)

*Periodicity.* The number of filariæ in the peripheral circulation presents remarkable periodic variations, a phenomenon which was first noticed by Manson. In the case of *Filaria bancrofti*, this author found that, in China, the parasites were present in the peripheral circulation during the night, but disappeared during the day ; and he proposed the specific name *nocturna* in order to express this habit. Under normal conditions of health and habit, during the day the parasite is rarely seen in the blood of a patient, or, if present, only in very small numbers, but as evening ·approaches about five or six o'clock the filariæ begin to enter the peripheral circulation in gradually increasing numbers. The maximum is usually attained about midnight, when it is no uncommon thing to find 300, or even 600, in every drop of blood. The numbers then begin to diminish, and by eight or nine o'clock in the morning the filariæ have disappeared again for the day. This diurnal periodicity may be maintained with regularity for years. Manson was able to shew that during the daytime the parasites retire to the lungs, heart and larger arteries, where they may be found in enormous numbers. In the case of a filarious patient who had committed suicide during the daytime, the parasites were found to occur in the various organs in the following numbers, which indicate the average per slide : liver, $\frac{2}{3}$ ; spleen, 1 ; brachial venæ comites, 28 ; bone marrow, 0 ; muscle of heart, 122 ; carotid artery, 612 ; lung, 675. In the lungs the filariæ were found lying outstretched or coiled in the blood-vessels, both small and large. In the carotid they occurred in enormous numbers on its inner surface, though how they managed to maintain their position in the blood current remains unexplained.

Many authors have attempted to explain this remarkable periodicity in the occurrence of the parasites in the peripheral circulation. Mackenzie shewed that it was in some way connected with sleep, for by reversing the usual habits, and making a patient sleep during the day and work at night, it was found that, after a few days of hesitation, the filariæ became diurnal instead of nocturnal. These results have also been confirmed by Annett, Dutton and Elliott working in Nigeria. Carter supposed that the embryos were carried into the circulation at the end of each day by the overflowing of chyle that follows alimentation. Myers suggested that the embryos are only laid at night and all die before the morning. Scheube supposed that the passage of the embryos from the lymphatics into the blood was prevented during the day by muscular work and digestion, and facilitated at night by the relaxation of the muscles. Von Linstow explained it on the supposition that during the night the dilatation of the cutaneous capillaries facilitated the entrance of the filariæ into the circulation.

Against all these theories can be brought the objection that a closely related species, *Filaria diurna*, is normally diurnal, and yet presents a somewhat similar life-cycle to that of *F. bancrofti*. A still more serious difficulty in the way of any mechanical explanation is the occurrence, in some parts of the world, of varieties of *F. bancrofti* that are diurnal in habit, and yet others which exhibit no periodicity. The researches of Bahr have shewn that in Fiji and Oceania generally, the filariæ occur in the blood of patients in no regular manner, and yet the parasites are morphologically identical with *F. bancrofti*. Similarly, Ashburn and Craig, because it exhibited no periodicity, considered the human filaria of the Philippines to be a distinct species, and gave it the name of *F. philippinensis*, but Low has shewn that it is identical with *F. bancrofti*.

Bahr's observations are of great interest, for they suggest that in Fiji the absence of periodicity in the filaria is a partial adaptation to the habits of its usual invertebrate host in this locality, *Stegomyia pseudoscutellaris*, a mosquito which only feeds during the day.

At present, however, there is no hypothesis that will satisfactorily account for the phenomenon of filarial periodicity.

*Life-cycle in the mosquito—the intermediate host.* As mentioned above, the filarial embryos are incapable of further development within the body of their host, but require to be ingested by a mosquito belonging to one of the species that serve as the invertebrate hosts for *F. bancrofti*. Then the parasites undergo further evolution in the body of the mosquito. The various stages in the metamorphosis of this species in the body of *Culex pipiens* have been worked out by Manson. The development may be conveniently divided into seven stages.

*First Stage.* Shortly after being ingested by the mosquito the transverse striation of the embryo becomes well marked, as if from longitudinal shrinking. Within about one hour the embryo breaks out of its sheath and then shews active movements. The parasite bores its way through the walls of the stomach and eventually comes to rest in the thoracic muscles of the mosquito. This process is usually complete in about 12 to 18 hours, but some of the worms die in the stomach. In the thorax all movement ceases, the striation disappears and various changes take place in the interior of the filaria.

*Second Stage.* This generally occupies about two to three days, during which the body thickens, and a mouth begins to appear. The posterior V-spot appears as a large vacuole and the anterior V-spot becomes very distinct.

*Third Stage.* The mouth becomes open and four large fleshy lips are formed. The posterior V-spot enlarges and definitely becomes the anus, appearing in front of the tail as a break in the cuticle, from which granular matter exudes. A row of cells appears in the previously apparently homogeneous body and terminates in front of the anus in some large cells. This row of cells later gives rise to the alimentary canal and a tegumentary layer with a cavity between. The larva is now 0·03–0·3 mm. in length by 0·029–0·05 mm. in diameter. At this stage the tail becomes large and sickle-shaped and the cells of the body usually dip into it. The alimentary canal extends from the mouth to the anus. Motion is entirely suspended.

*Fourth Stage.* Rapid growth takes place and the body retracts from the tail, which becomes a mere appendage. The length of the worm varies from 0·35–0·5 mm.

*Fifth Stage.* When the body has attained its maximum thickness the anterior end commences to elongate and become thinner, and the mouth begins to close. The anterior and posterior ends may elongate simultaneously, but more often this process occurs along the whole length of the larva. The mouth eventually closes and all, or nearly all, traces of the viscera disappear. About the seventh day of development the body of the worm assumes a fibrous and very transparent appearance, but before this stage is reached a well developed alimentary canal with pharynx and œsophagus may be distinguished. Slight movements now commence at the neck of the animal and extend downwards, and about this stage a general ecdysis takes place and the sickle-shaped tail is cast off, a new skin being developed within the old one. Large cells appear at the end of the tail and form three or four papillæ which characterise the larva at the end of this and during the next stage.

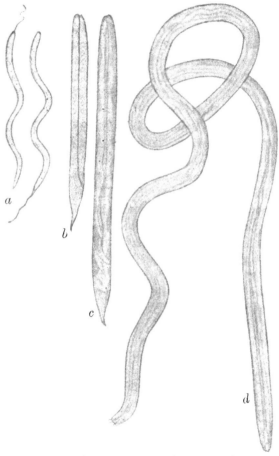

Fig. 55. *Filaria bancrofti* × 200. Stages in the development within the mosquito. (After Nuttall.) *a*, young filaria immediately after escaping from the sheath; *b*, 5 days, *c*, 10 days, and *d*, 16 days after ingestion by the mosquito.

The worm is now about 1·5 mm. in length, and its breadth has diminished to about one-half. The anterior end tapers but is abruptly rounded off; the posterior end also tapers slightly from the anus backwards, and bears the above-mentioned papillæ.

*Sixth Stage.* The movements now become more active. The lips of the mouth are closely pressed together in the form of a cone and minute horny papillæ are present. The worm now measures about 1·5 mm. by 0·03 mm.

Until 1900 it was supposed that this was the final stage in the development, and that the worm now required to escape into some water, in which it swam about until it was taken up by man in drinking water. In that year Low shewed that there was yet another stage.

*Seventh Stage.* When the filariæ have reached their highest development in the thoracic muscles they leave that tissue and begin to travel forwards, probably as a result of some chemiotactic attraction. They pass into the loose cellular tissue in the prothorax near the salivary glands, then force their way through the neck and coil themselves up in the loose connective tissue just below the cephalic ganglion and salivary sac. Finally, they pass into the proboscis of the mosquito by making an independent passage through Dutton's membrane at the base of the labrum, and pushing forward between the labrum and hypopharynx amongst the stylets. Here the worms are found stretched along the length of the proboscis, head foremost Two worms, probably male and female, are nearly always found together.

In this stage the worm is usually about 1 mm. in length and 0·025 mm. in breadth. It tapers slightly towards each extremity, and at the anterior end the cuticle is thickened in places to form a few small papillæ arranged round the terminal mouth. The posterior end, which is rounded off, is provided with three papillæ almost at right angles to the axis of the body of the worm. The alimentary canal is straight and shews no marked differentiation into œsophagus and intestine. Towards the anterior end, 0·14 mm. from the extremity, there is an indication of the presence of an orifice, towards which the genital duct is seen to bend.

These young filariæ remain in the proboscis of the mosquito until it feeds on some host. The worms then escape and may be

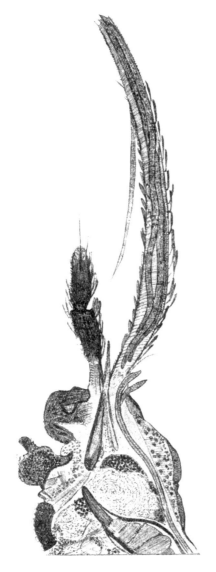

Fig. 56. Head and proboscis of *Stegomyia pseudoscutellaris*, 15 days after feeding, shewing two filariæ lying in the head and three in the proboscis. After Bahr from *Filariasis and Elephantiasis in Fiji*. (N.B. The cephalic ends of two filariæ are protruding from the under-surface of the head. This is not their natural situation but they have been forced into this position in cutting the section.)

found on the skin in the neighbourhood of the wound caused
by the bite of the insect. If the skin is sufficiently moist
the filariæ then bore their way through the epidermis into
the subcutaneous tissues. In some cases they may select the
wound caused by the mosquito as the point of entrance into
the body of their vertebrate host, but in most cases it is probable that they make an independent entrance through the
undamaged skin, as Looss has shewn to be the case for the larvæ
of *Agchylostoma duodenale.* Moreover, Bahr has actually
observed the larvæ of *Filaria bancrofti* bore into the pores of
the skin. The filariæ were dissected out of infected mosquitoes
and placed in a drop of saline on the back of a man's hand.
The larvæ could easily be seen wriggling about in the water,
but when placed on the skin, after a few convulsive movements, they suddenly disappeared, apparently through the
orifices of the gland ducts. Six filariæ were observed to
disappear in this manner, "with almost lightning-like rapidity."

When the skin is very dry the young filariæ often die before
they are able to effect an entrance, and therefore a person may
be bitten by an infected mosquito without developing filariasis.
If, however, the young worms effect an entrance, they make
their way to the lymphatics of their host and there develop
into the adult filariæ. After fertilization the females then
develop embryos, which, on being liberated, make their way to
the blood circulation, and thus the life-cycle may be repeated.

*Conditions affecting the development of the filaria within the
body of the mosquito.* One of the most important factors influencing development is the species of mosquito in which this
process takes place. In some species development occurs much
more readily and occupies a shorter period than in others.
For example, in Fiji, Bahr found that *F. bancrofti* developed
very readily in *Stegomyia pseudoscutellaris*, under favourable
conditions, the young worms appearing in the proboscis within
ten days. On the other hand, in *Culex fatigans* the development proceeded much less regularly and occupied a longer
period, whilst in *C. jepsoni* and *S. fasciata* the worms developed
very slowly, and eventually degenerated in the thoracic muscles
without arriving at maturity. The effect of different species

on the development is well shewn by the number of filariæ that developed in each species. *Stegomyia pseudoscutellaris* and *Culex fatigans* are both efficient intermediate hosts for *F. bancrofti*; but in the former practically all the embryos develop in the insect and come to maturity, whereas in the latter only two or three ever complete their development. The effect of temperature on the rate of development is very marked; at a high temperature the worms may be found in the proboscis after six days, but during cold weather the same evolution is not complete for at least 20 days, or may even be totally arrested.

The following species of mosquitoes are capable of acting as the intermediate hosts for *F. bancrofti*, and with further researches there is little doubt that the list will have to be considerably extended. In many cases the development in the mosquito has not been followed completely:

| Species | Locality | Observer |
|---|---|---|
| ANOPHELINES : | | |
| A. (*Myzomyia*) *rossii*[1] .. .. | India .. | .. James |
| ,, (*Pyretophorus*) *costalis*[1] .. | West Africa | .. Annett, Dutton and Elliott |
| ,, (*Myzorhynchus*) *sinensis*[2] .. | Malay .. | .. Leicester |
| ,, ,, *barbirostris*[2] | ,, .. | .. ,, |
| ,, ,, *peditæniatus*[2] | ,, .. | .. ,, |
| ,, (*Cellia*) *argyrotarsis*[2] .. | West Indies | .. Low |
| ,, ,, *albipes*[2] .. .. | ,, | .. Vincent |
| CULICINES : | | |
| *Culex pipiens*[1] .. .. .. | China .. | .. Manson |
| ,, *fatigans*[1] .. .. | Australia .. <br> St Lucia .. <br> West Indies .. <br> Philippines | .. Bancroft <br> .. Low <br> .. <br> .. Ashburn and Craig |
| ,, *gelidus*[2] <br> ,, *sitiens*[2] .. .. | Malay, Sumatra, the <br> Celebes and Malacca | Leicester |
| *Stegomyia fasciata*[3] .. | St Lucia, W. Indies, | Low etc. |
| ,, *gracilis*[2] <br> ,, *perplexa*[2] <br> ,, *scutellaris*[2] | Malay .. | .. Leicester |
| ,, *pseudoscutellaris*[1] .. | Fiji .. | .. Bahr |
| *Mansonia uniformis* (? *africana*)[2] | Central Africa | .. Daniels |
| ,, *annulipes*[2] <br> *Scutomyia albolineata*[2] <br> *Tæniorhynchus domesticus*[2] | Malay .. | .. Leicester |

[1] Species in which complete development has been observed.
[2] Species in which in all probability complete development takes place, but forms have not been actually seen in proboscis.
[3] Species in which an incomplete partial development occurs. Forms never reach stage suitable for proboscis.

*Effect of filariæ on the mosquito.* The developing filariæ have a very deleterious effect on the health of the mosquito, and heavily infected individuals can easily be recognized by their sluggish appearance. When a very large number of embryos are ingested by a favourable intermediate host, the resulting development usually causes the death of the mosquito. In the case of *S. pseudoscutellaris*, Bahr noticed that when mosquitoes were fed on a slightly infected patient nearly all of them were alive 21 days later, but out of a batch of 200 insects that fed on a patient shewing very numerous filariæ in his blood, only 17 managed to survive an equal length of time. The period at which the infected mosquitoes died was dependent apparently upon the degree of development of the filariæ. Thus, in warm weather most of the insects died on the sixth day after feeding, and in the cooler season on the tenth. The last stages of development, when the filaria is entering the proboscis, seem to be the most critical time for the mosquito, as in one batch 23 *Stegomyia* were alive on the 15th day after infection, but only three of them lived four days longer.

*Possibility of another "indirect" mode of transmission by the mosquito.* The pathogenic effect of *F. bancrofti* upon its intermediate host is of considerable interest, for it suggests that the worm has only recently become adapted to its present mode of transmission. Moreover, it seems possible that Manson's theory that the filariæ first escape into water and subsequently enter man, has been discarded rather too hastily. When the mature larvæ migrate from the thoracic muscles, although most of them come to rest in the proboscis, it is no uncommon occurrence to find them in the legs and other regions of the mosquito. These " mistakes " on the part of the larvæ also afford support to the theory that this filaria has only recently adopted its present mode of entry into the body. When the young filaria escapes from the proboscis of the mosquito on to the skin, it is only capable of penetrating the surface in the presence of moisture. On the other hand the young filariæ will live in water for several hours, and if a drop of water containing them is placed on the skin the parasites at once disappear down the openings of the gland-ducts.

It is evident, therefore, that if this filaria escapes into water, either by the death of its insect host, or some other cause, it is perfectly adapted for the penetration of any skin with which it may come in contact. This was probably the original manner in which the parasite was carried by mosquitoes, and the possibility of the occurrence of such an "indirect" mode of transmission, concurrently with the more recently acquired "direct" method, should not be ignored.

*Pathological effects.* In most cases *F. bancrofti* does not seem to exercise any marked injurious effect on its host; patients often shew filariæ in their blood for many years and all the time appear in perfect health. Under certain conditions, however, the adult filaria may give rise to various pathological symptoms, mainly as a result of obstructing lymphatics. Amongst these affections may be mentioned chyluria, lymph scrotum, varicose groin glands, etc. In some instances a living worm, or a bundle of worms, may plug the thoracic duct and act as an embolus, or originate a thrombus; in others, they give rise to inflammatory thickening of the walls, as a result of irritation, and thus lead to obstruction from the consequent stenosis. In such cases the embryos may disappear from the blood, usually as a result of the death of the adults.

Sometimes adult filariæ occur in large numbers in the lymphatic glands and also in the epididymis, testis and tunica vaginalis. In these situations the worms may die and become cretified, and whether alive or dead they cause fibrosis and blocking of the glands.

*Elephantiasis.* Of all the affections that are supposed to be due to filariasis, elephantiasis is the most important, as it occurs in most tropical countries. The disease may be defined as a chronic inflammatory hypertrophy of the fibrous connective tissue in some region of the body, induced by lymph stasis and resulting in a considerable hypertrophy of the skin and subcutaneous tissues. It most commonly affects the legs, scrotum, vulva, arms and breast. The resulting growths may become of enormous size, especially in cases of elephantiasis of the scrotum, in which this organ may attain the weight of over 230 pounds. According to Manson the condition of lymph stasis, necessary for the production of elephantiasis, may be due to the blocking of the lymphatic ganglia by the unripe eggs of filariæ, expelled from the parent before the embryos are able to uncoil. These eggs are five times as wide as the embryo, and being more or less rigid would be incapable of passing through any lymph glands. This theory accounts for the fact that the filaria embryos are rarely found in the circulation of patients affected with elephantiasis.

The reasons for regarding elephantiasis as a filarial disease are given by Manson as follows :

" (1) The geographical distribution of *Filaria bancrofti* and of elephantiasis correspond ; where elephantiasis is common there the filaria abounds and *vice versa*. (2) Filarial lymphatic varix and elephantiasis occur in the same district and frequently concur in the same individual. (3) Lymph scrotum, an unquestionably filarial disease, often terminates in elephantiasis of the scrotum. (4) Elephantiasis of the leg sometimes supervenes on the surgical removal of a lymph scrotum. (5) Elephantiasis and lymphatic varix are essentially diseases of the lymphatics. (6) Filarial lymphatic varix and true elephantiasis are both accompanied by the same type of recurring lymphangitis. (7) As filarial lymphatic varix is practically proved to be caused by the filaria, the inference that true elephantiasis—the disease with which the former is so often associated and has so many affinities—is attributable to the same cause, appears to be warranted."

On the other hand the filarial nature of elephantiasis is strongly opposed by certain authors, who bring forward arguments in support of the view that the disease is caused by bacteria. Le Dantec considers it due to a symbiotic infection with a *Streptococcus* and a *Dermococcus*. Dubruel obtained *Streptococci* in pure culture from cases of elephantiasis, and lately favourable results in the treatment of the disease seem to have been obtained by employing a vaccine prepared from this streptococcus. This author remarks that in the Island of Mooréa (Tahiti), where about one-twelfth of the inhabitants shew elephantiasis, he examined the blood of 200 persons without finding a single filaria. Moreover, he cites examples in which the contagious nature of the disease seems to be admissible.

REFERENCES.

Annett, Dutton and Elliott (1901). *Report on the Malaria Expedition to Nigeria.* Part II, Filariasis. *Liv. Sch. of Trop. Med.* Liverpool.
Ashburn and Craig (1907). Observations upon *Filaria philippinensis* and its development in the mosquito. *Phil. Journ. Sci.,* Sect. B, vol. II. pp. 1–14.
Bahr, P. H. (1912). Filariasis and Elephantiasis in Fiji. *Journ. of the School of Trop. Med.,* Supplement No. 1.
Bancroft, T. (1900). On the Morphology of the young form of *Filaria bancrofti* Cobb. in the body of *Culex ciliaris. Proc. Roy. Soc. N.S. Wales,* vol. XXIII. p. 48.
Cobbold (1879). The life-history of *Filaria bancrofti. Journ. Linn. Soc. Zool.* vol. XIV. p. 356.
Demarquay (1863). Note sur une tumeur de bourse. *Gaz. méd. Paris* (3), vol. XVIII. p. 665.
Le Dantec (1900). *Précis de pathologie exotique.* Paris.
Lewis, T. R. (1872). *On a Hæmatozoon inhabiting Human Blood.* Calcutta, 1872.
Linstow, v. (1900). Ueb. d. Art. d. Blutfil. d. Mensch. *Zool. Anz.* vol. XXIII. p. 26.
Low, G. C. (1900). A recent observation on *Filaria nocturna* in *Culex. Brit. Med. Journ.* I. p. 1456.
Manson, P. (1884). The metamorphosis of *Filaria sanguinis hominis* in the mosquito. *Trans. Linn. Soc. Zool.* vol. II. pp. 10 and 367.
—— *Tropical Diseases.* London : Cassell and Co.
Nuttall, G. H. F. *Encycl. Medica,* Edinburgh, vol. VIII.
Scheube (1883). *Die Filariakrankheit.* Volkmann's Samml. kl. Vortr. No. 232.

II. *Filaria immitis* (Leidy, 1856).

*Synonyms.* *F. canis cordis* Leidy, 1850. *F. papillosa, hæmatica canis domestici* Gruby and Delafond, 1852.

*General account.* This parasite occurs in the dog, in which it was first seen by Panthot in 1679 and afterwards by Peyronnie in 1778. It has also been found in the fox, and the wolf. Noè and Fülleborn shewed that *Anopheles maculipennis,* and also *Stegomyia fasciata,* serve as the intermediate hosts of this species.

*Distribution.* *F. immitis* is very common in China and Japan where most of the dogs are infected. It is also common in Italy, especially in the marshy districts round Pisa and Milan. It has also been recorded from England, France, Denmark, Germany, Australia, Fiji, the United States and Brazil.

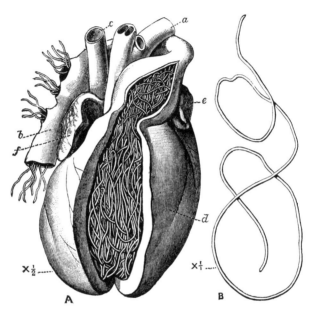

Fig. 57. *A*, view of the heart of a dog infested with *Filaria immitis* Leidy ($\times \frac{1}{2}$); the right ventricle and base of the pulmonary artery have been opened. *a*, aorta; *b*, pulmonary artery; *c*, vena cava; *d*, right ventricle; *e*, appendix of left auricle; *f*, appendix of right auricle. *B*, a female *F. immitis* removed from the heart to show its length. Natural size. (After Shipley.)

*Description.* The adult is a filiform whitish worm, tapering at both extremities, especially at the tail, and rounded anteriorly. The mouth is terminal, and surrounded by six, small, indistinct papillæ. The anus is near the end of the tail. The male is 12–18 cm. in length by 0·7–0·9 cm. in breadth, and possesses a spirally wound tail, bearing two small lateral ridges supported by papillæ. According to Schneider there are 11 papillæ, six of which are post-anal. From the anus arise two spicules of unequal length. The female is 25–30 cm. in length, by 1–1·3 mm. in breadth. The tail is short and blunt, and the vulva is situated near the origin of the intestine, a distance of about 7 mm. from the mouth. The eggs hatch in the uterus, liberating embryos about 285 to 295 μ in length, by 5 μ in breadth ; their anterior ends are somewhat tapered, whilst posteriorly the body tapers off into a long and delicate tail.

*Life-cycle.* As in the case of *F. bancrofti,* the embryos of *F. immitis* are liberated into the blood and appear in the peripheral circulation. According to Manson the embryos of this species, as in *bancrofti,* are more common in the blood during the night, thus exhibiting a nocturnal periodicity, but this is denied by Fülleborn. If the embryos are injected into the blood of a healthy dog, they will persist in the circulation for several months.

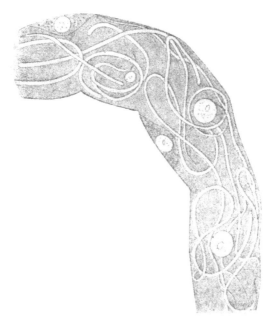

Fig. 58. Part of the Malpighian tubule of an *Anopheles claviger,* infected with the embryos of *Filaria immitis.* (After Noè.)

The further development of the embryos takes place in certain species of mosquito and has been carefully investigated by Noè and Fülleborn. The most efficient intermediate host was found to be *Anopheles maculipennis*, which invariably became infected by feeding on blood containing the embryos. On the other hand, under similar conditions only about 20 per cent. of *Stegomyia fasciata* shewed any development of the filariæ within their bodies. Noè found that development would also take place in a large number of Anophelines, including *Anopheles bifurcatus, Myzorhynchus pseudopictus* and *Myzomyia superpicta*, and also in the following Culicines : *Culex penicillaris, C. malariæ* and *C. pipiens*.

When a mosquito has fed upon an infected dog, three or four times as many filariæ are found in the stomach of the insect as in the blood of the dog. The reason for this apparent increase is the concentration of blood that takes place in the gut of the mosquito, most of the serum being excreted within an hour after a meal.

Within 20 to 40 minutes after being ingested by an *Anopheles*, the filariæ are found in the Malpighian tubules, in which site they undergo their further development. The worms are guided to the tubules by some chemiotactic influence, for they have been shewn to be attracted towards the mouth of an open capillary tube containing an emulsion of a Malpighian tubule in normal saline.

The embryos, during their development in the mosquito, cause a marked alteration in the character of the epithelium of the Malpighian tubules, which may be the cause of the high mortality amongst infected insects. The rate of development of *F. immitis*, as in the case of *bancrofti*, depends mainly upon the temperature, for at 26° C. the whole process is complete within ten days, whereas at 20° to 21° C., it is very much prolonged. When the development is complete, the young filariæ bore through the walls of the Malpighian tubule into the body-cavity of their host, and migrate towards the head. They usually come to rest within the sheath of the proboscis, but isolated examples may be found in the palps and legs.

When an infected *Anopheles,* containing filariæ in its proboscis, feeds on a dog, the worms escape through the fine membrane (Dutton's membrane) uniting the labellæ, and thus get on to the surface of the skin. If this is sufficiently moist they penetrate the epidermis, and may be found in the subcutaneous tissues. The young filariæ then make their way towards the heart and great vessels of the dog, and there develop into the adults. The worms may also be found in other regions of the body, but in any case the embryos, on being liberated, make their way into the circulation. According to Galeb and Pourquier the embryos may pass into the fœtal circulation, and therefore the disease may be transmitted hereditarily.

*The pathogenic effects* on the dog vary considerably ; weakness, anæmia, cough, icterus, ascites and lameness may be observed and a fatal result is frequent. No effective treatment is known.

*Filaria recondita* Grassi, 1890. This filaria, which also inhabits the dogs in many parts of the world, is closely related to *F. immitis.* Grassi and Calandruccio have shewn that the embryos develop in the body of the dog-flea (*Pulex serraticeps*), the cat-flea (*Pulex irritans*), and also in a tick (*Rhipicephalus siculus* Koch). Although infection experiments with fleas gave no positive results, it seems probable that these insects may serve as the intermediate hosts for this filaria.

REFERENCES.

Calandruccio (1892). Descrizione degli embrioni e delle larve della filaria recondita (Grassi). *Atti dell' Accad. Giornia,* vol. LXIX.
Fülleborn, F. (1908). Ueber Versuche an Hundefilarien und deren Uebertragung durch Mücken. *Arch. f. Schiffs. u. Tropenhyg.* vol. XII. Suppl. 8, 43 pp. 4 pls.
—— (1912). Untersuchungen über die chemotaktische Wirkung der Malpighischen Gefässe von Stechmücken auf Hundemikrofilarien. *Centralbl. f. Bakter.* vol. LXV. pp. 349–352.
—— (1912). Zur Morphologie der Dirofilaria immitis Leidy, 1856. *Ibid.* vol. LXV. pp. 341–349.
Grassi and Noè (1900). Uebertragung der Blutfilariæ ganz ausschliesslich durch den Stich von Stechmücken. *Centralbl. f. Bakt. Orig.* vol. XXVIII. No. 19.

Noè, G. (1901). Sul circlo evolutivo della Filaria bancrofti (Cobbold) e della *Filaria immitis* (Leidy). *Ric. f. n. laborot. d. anatomia normale d. R. Univ. di Roma*, vol. VIII. pp. 275–353.

—— (1903). Ulteriori studi sulla *Filaria immitis. Rend. Acc. d. Lincei.* vol. XII. pp. 476–483.

Shipley, A. E. (1896). Nemathelminthes and Chaetognatha, in *Cambridge Natural History*. London : Macmillan and Co.

# CHAPTER XIII

## ORTHORRHAPHA BRACHYCERA

The flies belonging to this series are characterised by the form of the antennæ, which, although variable, are never truly Nematocerous, nor yet like those of the Cyclorrhapha. They are usually composed of three dissimilar segments, of which the third is sometimes elongate and subdivided into a number of indistinctly separated segments. When an arista is present it is always terminal in position, and never superior as in the Cyclorrhapha. Rarely, as in the Leptidæ, the antennæ may be divided into more than three segments. The palpi are one- or two-jointed. Around the base of the antennæ there is no definite arched suture enclosing a small depressed space, as in the Cyclorrhapha Schizophora. The venation of the wings is usually more complex than that of any of the other divisions ; the second longitudinal vein is simple, but the third and fourth veins are often forked. The anal cell is closed before the border of the wing, or distinctly narrowed at the border. A discal cell is practically always present.

This group includes 16 families of flies, of which only one— the Tabanidæ—is of any interest from the present point of view. Two other families, the Leptidæ and Asilidæ, include a few blood-sucking species, but are of little importance. As, however, many of the species belonging to these and other families, are habitually predacious on insects, they have an economic interest, and therefore we append the following synopsis. The only one of these families that includes species known to carry disease is the Tabanidæ.

*Synopsis of the families of Orthorrhapha Brachycera[1].*

I. Third antennal segment composed of a series of indistinctly separated subsegments; empodia pulvilliform; third and fourth longitudinal veins forked.

(a) Costal vein extending all round the wing; squamæ large; the third antennal segment never has a style or arista .. .. *Tabanidæ.*

(b) Costal vein extending all round the wing; squamæ small; third antennal segment may have a style, or arista, or not, or the antenna may consist of a large number of segments .. .. .. .. *Leptidæ.*

(c) Costal vein not extending beyond tip of wing, longitudinal veins not crowded anteriorly; two sub-marginal and five posterior cells always present, the fourth closed. Third antennal joint composed of seven annuli, with a terminal style or arista .. .. .. .. .. *Acanthomeridæ.*

(d) Costal vein not extending beyond tip of wing; longitudinal veins usually more or less crowded anteriorly, posterior ones often weak; four or five posterior cells, the fourth rarely or *never closed* .. *Stratiomyidæ.*

II. Third antennal segment simple, with or without a terminal style or arista; empodia pulvilliform.

(a) Head small, formed almost entirely by the eyes; thorax large and humped; squamæ peculiarly large .. .. .. .. *Acroceridæ.*

(b) Squamæ small or moderate; venation of wings peculiarly intricate *Nemestrinidæ.*

(c) Squamæ small; wing venation more or less resembling that of *Tabanus* .. .. .. .. .. .. .. .. *Leptidæ.*

III. Third antennal segment simple, with or without a terminal style or arista; empodia, when present, bristle-like; third longitudinal vein, and often the fourth, forked.

(a) Crown of head concave between the eyes:
(i) Proboscis a rigid chitinous dagger; flies bristly and hairy *Asilidæ.*
(ii) Proboscis with fleshy labella; antennæ composed of four segments; flies without bristles .. .. .. .. .. .. *Mydaidæ.*

(b) Crown of head not excavated between the eyes:
(i) Wing with five posterior cells; third and fourth longitudinal veins curve forwards .. .. .. .. .. .. *Apioceridæ.*
(ii) Wing with five posterior cells; fourth longitudinal vein does not curve forwards; predaceous flies .. .. .. .... *Therevidæ.*
(iii) Wing with three or four (rarely five) posterior cells and often with dark markings; anal cell large; usually hairy bee-like flies, often with a long slender proboscis used for sucking the nectar from flowers *Bombyliidæ.*

[1] Modified from Alcock, *loc. cit.* p. 132.

(iv) Wing with three or four posterior cells, anal cell often small; femora and tibiæ often with combs of spinules; small dull-coloured predaceous flies usually with a stiff proboscis for impaling prey .. *Empididæ*.

(v) Wings with three posterior cells; proboscis not projecting; small flies often found on windows .. .. .. .. *Scenopinidæ*.

IV. Third antennal segment simple, with or without an arista; the empodia, when present, are bristle-like; third longitudinal vein not forked.

(*a*) Wings shaped like a lance-head, the venation somewhat as in the Psychodidæ .. .. .. .. .. .. .. *Lonchopteridæ*.

(*b*) Second basal cell confluent with discal cell; anal cell, if present, small; usually brilliantly coloured flies with metallic sheen .. *Dolichopodidæ*.

(*c*) Second basal and discal cells either confluent or distinct; anal cell, if present, small; not brilliantly coloured flies .. .. .. *Empididæ*.

(*d*) Antennæ apparently two-jointed, with a three-jointed arista; wings (rarely wanting) with several stout veins anteriorly and other, weaker ones apparently connected with them and running obliquely across the wing; small hunchbacked, quick running, bristly flies.. .. .. *Phoridæ*.

# CHAPTER XIV

## FAMILY TABANIDÆ (BREEZE-FLIES, CLEGGS, HORSE-FLIES, GAD-FLIES, SERUT-FLIES)

*Description.* The members of this extensive and important family are usually large and strongly built flies, the females of which feed on blood. The head is large; the antennæ are projecting, and the third joint is composed of four to eight indistinct segments, or annuli. The eyes are very large and laterally extended; in the male they meet along the middle line (holoptic), but in the female the eyes are smaller and a narrow streak is left between them (dichoptic). In the living insect the eyes are often iridescent and usually marked with green, purple, or brown bands, or spots.

The proboscis is projecting, sometimes as long as, or longer than, the body, and the mouth parts are adapted for piercing and cutting. Generally the labium is coarse and fleshy and the labella are large; the epipharynx and hypopharynx are strong dagger-shaped structures; the mandibles are sharply pointed and the maxillæ have serrate edges. The palpi are distinct and two-jointed; the terminal joint is inflated and hangs in front on each side of the proboscis. The thorax and abdomen are clothed with fine hairs, never with bristles, and are often striped or marked with dull colours. The abdomen is broad, never constricted at the base, and composed of seven visible segments. The legs are stout and the tibiæ sometimes dilated; the pulvilli and empodia are in the form of large membraneous plates. The venation of the wings is very constant; the third and fourth longitudinals are forked, so that two marginal and five posterior cells are always present; the basal cells are large and the anal cells usually closed. The marginal or costal vein encompasses the entire wing (Fig. 5). The squamæ are large.

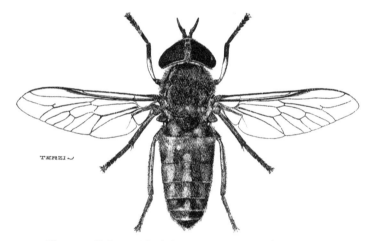

Fig. 59. *Tabanus kingi* Austen, ♀ (×3). (After Austen.)

*Habitat.* The members of this family are widely distributed throughout the world and about 1800 different species have already been described. They are especially evident on clear warm days, as soon as the sun has warmed the air, and are usually most active towards midday, but near Sedbergh, Yorkshire, the writer has been badly bitten by *Hæmatopota* in the early mornings.

The males live entirely on the juices of flowers, honeydew, etc., and, in the absence of other food, the female will also feed on these substances. By nature, however, the female feeds on blood, and is one of the most blood-thirsty of all insects. Its bite is painful, but usually is not followed by any marked inflammation, or swelling.

*Life-cycle.* The eggs of the Tabanidæ are commonly laid in large shapely masses on the leaves and stems of plants growing in marshy ground, or overhanging water. In some species they are deposited on stones or rocks above the water of streams, and are very difficult to discover.

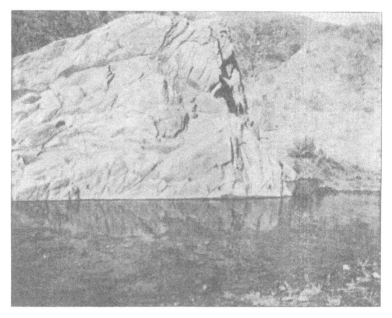

Fig. 60. A rock at Khor Arbat, Anglo-Egyptian Sudan, showing sites selected by *Tabanus kingi* for ovipositing (indicated by crosses); the three lower crosses represent freshly laid egg-masses. (After King.)

The eggs of *Tabanus par* were observed by King to be laid separately on the under surface of the leaves of water-plants. The colour of the eggs is usually brown or black, and at ordinary summer temperatures they hatch out in from seven to nine days

The larvæ may be found in rotting logs and stumps, in the soil at the edges of pools and streams, under stones in ditches, or swimming free in the water.  If kept supplied with a diet of angle-worms the larvæ can easily be reared, either in jars of moist earth, or in jars containing sand and water.  As a rule they are cannibalistic in habit and only one can be reared in each jar, but *T. biguttatus* is an exception to this rule, and in this species several can be reared together in the same receptacle. The larvæ are cylindrical in form, pointed at both ends ; the body is composed of eleven segments, each of which is usually encircled by a prominent fleshy ring, or row of protuberances,

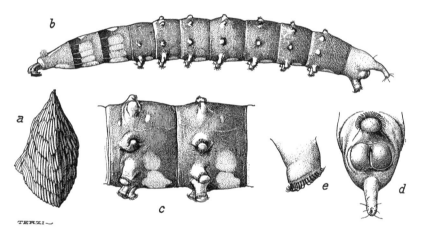

Fig. 61.  Egg-mass and mature larva of *Tabanus kingi* Austen.  *a*, egg-mass,  ×6 ;  *b*, lateral view of larva,  ×3 ;  *c*, lateral view of 4th and 5th abdominal segments,  ×6 ;  *d*, posterior view of anal segment (inverted), ×6 ;  *e*, lateral view of anal pseudopod.  (After King.)

which are most pronounced on the ventral side, where they serve as prolegs.  The head is small, but distinct, and the mouth parts are very peculiar ;  the mandibles are attached so as to move antero-posteriorly ;  when they are retracted the anterior ends point forwards, but when extended they point downwards and backwards, thus forming a pair of hooks that serve to hold prey. The duration of the larval stage depends upon the temperature. In temperate countries the larva usually lives through the winter and only pupates the following spring, but in Egypt King was able to rear *T. par*, from the freshly hatched larvæ to adults, in three and a half months. The pupal stage is usually completed in three to four weeks, and as the whole development generally takes about eleven months, the duration of the larval stage is very considerable. In some cases it probably takes more than one year for its development. When fully grown the larva buries itself in the sand, or earth, in its immediate neighbourhood, and then pupates.

*Classification.* The following synopsis of the genera of Tabanidæ is taken from Miss Ricardo's *Revision of the Family* ; the more important genera, which have a world-wide distribution, are printed in capitals :

### Synopsis of Genera of Tabanidæ.

#### I. TABANINÆ.

Ocelli absent ; hind tibiæ not spurred.

1 { Third antennal segment composed of four subsegments or rings, and not angulated or spurred at base .. .. .. .. = 2
{ Third antennal segment composed of five subsegments or rings = 5

2 { Rings so distinct that the antenna appears to consist of six segments
*Hexatoma* Meigen (Europe).
{ Rings not so distinct as to modify the appearance of the antenna = 3

3 { Wings with a profusion of ring-like and scroll-like markings
HÆMATOPOTA.
{ Wings without circles and scrolls.. .. .. .. .. = 4

4 { First and second antennal segments pubescent in the male, third segment longer than the first ; eyes hairy
*Dasybasis* Macquart (Chili and Australia).

5 { First antennal segment globose, situated on a frontal protuberance
*Bolbodimyia*, Bigot (Venezuela).
{ First antennal segment not globose .. .. .. .. = 6

6 { Third antennal segment not angulated or toothed at base .. = 7
{ Third antennal segment angulated or toothed at base .. .. = 9

7 { Body covered with metallic scales
*Lepidoselasa* Macquart (South America).
{ Body metallic in colouring *Selasoma* Macquart (South America)
{ Body not in any way metallic; first antennal segment longer than is usual in *Tabanus* ; wings commonly with brown markings = 8

8 { Antennæ long, the third segment cylindrical, and situated on a pro-jecting tubercle .. .. *Udenocera* Ricardo (Ceylon).
{ Antennæ not as in *Udenocera*
*Diachlorus* Osten Sacken (America and Philippines).

9　{ Abdomen short, stout, very convex　　　*Stibasoma* Schiner (America).
　　{ Abdomen not as in *Stibasoma*　..　..　..　..　..　= 10

10　{ Antennæ long and slender, first segment long
　　{ 　　　　　　　　　　*Acanthocera* Macquart (South America).
　　{ Antennæ not as in *Acanthocera*　..　..　..　..　..　= 11

11　{ Slenderer in build, usually with thorax and abdomen banded ; third
　　{ 　　antennal segment slender, wings mostly with brown markings
　　{ 　　　　　　　　　　*Dichelacera* Macquart (South America).
　　{ Stouter in build, third antennal segment stout　..　TABANUS Linn.


## II. PANGONIINÆ.

Ocelli usually present ; hind tibiæ spurred.

1　{ Third antennal segment composed of eight or seven subsegments or
　　{ 　　rings ; proboscis usually elongate　..　..　..　..　= 2
　　{ Third antennal segment composed of five rings ; proboscis short　= 14

2　{ Third antennal segment with a tooth　　*Dicrania* Macquart (Brazil).
　　{ Third antennal segment not toothed　..　..　..　..　= 3

3　{ Wings short ; body flat, elliptical　　*Apocampta* Schiner (Australia)·
　　{ Wings not short　..　..　..　..　..　..　= 4

4　{ Third antennal segment with each subsegment branched
　　{ 　　　　　　　　　　*Pityocera* Tos (Central America).
　　{ Third antennal segment not branched　..　..　..　..　= 5

5　{ Upper corner of eye terminating in an acute angle
　　{ 　　　　　　　　　　*Goniops* Aldrich (North America).
　　{ Upper corner of eye not terminating in an acute angle ..　..　= 6

6　{ Antennæ deep-seated, inclined downwards ; palpi very large
　　{ 　　　　　　　　　　*Cadicera* Macquart (South Africa)
　　{ Antennæ and palpi not as in *Cadicera*　..　..　..　..　= 7

7　{ Antennæ awl-shaped ; end of proboscis hatchet-shaped ; anal cell
　　{ 　　open and anal vein curved
　　{ 　　　　　　　　*Pelecorhynchus* Macquart (Australia and S. America).
　　{ Antennæ, proboscis, etc., not as in *Pelecorhynchus*　　= 8

8　{ Proboscis scarcely extending beyond palpi
　　{ 　　　　　　　　　　*Apotolestes* Williston (California).
　　{ Proboscis extending beyond palpi　　　　　　= 9

9　{ Wings with fourth posterior cell closed　..　..　..　= 10
　　{ Wings with fourth posterior cell open　..　..　..　= 11

10　{ Eyes bare　..　..　..　*Dorcalæmus* Austen (South Africa).
　　{ Eyes not bare　　*Scione* Walker (South America, Seychelles, Australia).

11　{ Wings with first posterior cell closed　..　..　..　= 12
　　{ Wings with first posterior cell open　..　..　..　= 13

12　{ Eyes bare　..　..　PANGONIA Latr. (subgenus *Pangonia*).
　　{ Eyes hairy　..　..　PANGONIA Latr. (subgenus *Erephrosis*).

13　{ Eyes hairy　..　DIATOMINEURA Rond. (subgenus *Diatomineura*).
　　{ Eyes bare　..　DIATOMINEURA Rond. (subgenus *Corizoneura* Rond.)

14　{ First and second segments of antennæ short　..　..　= 15
　　{ First and second segments of antennæ long　..　CHRYSOPS Meigen.

15 { Second segment of abdomen unusually large, spurs of tibiæ small
                                              *Pronopes* Loew (Cape Colony).
    Abdomen and tibiæ not as in *Pronopes* ..    ..    ..    ..    = 16

16 { Face concave in the middle *Rhinomyza* Wied. (Cape Colony and Java).
    Face not concave    ..    ..    ..    ..    ..    ..    = 17

17 { Wings with first posterior cell open SILVIUS Meigen (subgenus *Silvius*).
    Wings with first posterior cell closed
                    SILVIUS Meigen (subgenus *Esenbeckia* Rond., Brazil).
    Third segment of antennæ with an acute spine
                                  *Gastroxides* Saunders (India).

*Tabanidæ and disease.* It must be admitted that the evidence in support of the view that Tabanidæ act as disease carriers is rather unsatisfactory. Their voracious blood-sucking habits and conspicuous size have given the flies a bad reputation in many parts of the world, and natives frequently assign various ill-effects to their bites.

Most of these accusations, however, have not yet been justified, although it seems probable that certain trypanosomiases of animals, especially Surra, may be carried by Tabanidæ.

There are many difficulties in the way of conducting experiments with these flies. They are always very impatient of captivity and spend most of their time attempting to escape. As a result it is difficult to make them feed on any particular animal, and the flies soon die. Up to the present time hardly a single experiment has been recorded in which the possibility of a cyclical mode of transmission of trypanosomes by Tabanidæ has been investigated, for in no case have the flies lived a sufficient length of time to decide the point[1]. Possibly the best way of testing whether Tabanids act as the true invertebrate hosts for any disease, would be to capture large numbers of wild flies and feed them on susceptible animals. In this manner, the presence of any naturally infected insects might be detected. The occurrence of flagellates in the alimentary canal of a large proportion of Tabanids is certainly rather suspicious, for in many cases it is difficult to distinguish

[1] Mitzmain has recently conducted experiments on the transmission of Surra by *Tabanus striatus* and has definitely excluded the possibility of a cyclical development, but has succeeded in obtaining direct transmission.

between developmental forms of ingested trypanosomes and the various insect flagellates.

It has been shown repeatedly that when Tabanidæ, interrupted in a feed on an infected animal, are at once transferred to a healthy one, the latter may become infected as a result of their bites. In these cases the parasites, present in the blood, are simply mechanically transferred from the first animal to the second by means of the proboscis of the insect. Almost any blood-sucking insect is capable of such transference of infection, but the importance of this mechanical transmission should not be under-estimated.

With the exception of El Debab (*T. soudanense*), there now seems little doubt that the pathogenic trypanosomiases of Africa are all transmitted by various species of *Glossina*, which serve as the true invertebrate hosts and, once infected, remain so for considerable periods. On the other hand, there is evidence to shew that these diseases, once started, may continue to spread in the absence of tsetse-flies.

In this connection the outbreak of *Trypanosoma pecorum* infection in a herd of cattle belonging to the Uganda Sleeping Sickness Commission is of some interest, for there seems to be little doubt that in this case *Tabanus secedens* Walk. was responsible for spreading the infection. The herd contained a few animals that had been experimentally infected with *T. pecorum*. Shortly after the appearance of swarms of *Tabanus*, large numbers of the cattle, that had remained healthy for a year, shewed signs of infection with *T. pecorum*. It should be noted, however, that *Glossina palpalis* were also found in small numbers after the Tabanids had disappeared, and their presence might have been overlooked previously.

Jowett made some experiments near Cape Town with a cattle trypanosome of the *Dimorphon* type, obtained near Beira, Portuguese East Africa. As this infection seems to spread in the absence of tsetse-flies, transmission experiments were made with *Hæmatopota* and *Stomoxys*.

" Numbers of *Hæmatopota* and *Stomoxys* were collected at frequent intervals and placed in large glass lamp chimneys, the ends of which had been closed with mosquito netting. After having shaved and damped a patch of skin on the trypanosome infected subject, one end of such a tube was then applied to the latter. As soon as it was seen that a number of flies had commenced to feed on this animal, the tube was removed and without delay applied to the skin of a healthy animal, the flies being allowed to finish their meal on the latter. At the conclusion of the experiment the flies in most instances were killed. Occasionally they were dissected. Only on two or three occasions were they kept and used for feeding a second time during the following days. The experiment therefore, permitted only of mechanical transmission."

Only one positive result was obtained out of five experiments. In this case 122 *Stomoxys* were fed in the course of 14 days on an infected sheep and afterwards on a healthy sheep. After an interval of six days three *Hæmatopota*, of which one was seen to bite, fed similarly. Trypanosomes were found in the blood of the sheep 13 days later, and it died after another 10 days. The experiment shews that this trypanosome can be conveyed mechanically by one of these species, and Jowett thinks that the *Hæmatopota* were responsible.

Hart records an experiment in North-Eastern Rhodesia supporting the view that *Pangonia* and *Stomoxys* may transmit trypanosome infections.

An outbreak of trypanosomiasis (*T. dimorphon*, or *pecaudi*) occurred on a farm fifty miles from Fort Jameson. The owner stated that tsetse-fly had never been seen, but *Pangonia* had been numerous. Two bullocks infected with trypanosomes were kept at the farm and the remainder sent away. Then three healthy cows were brought from Fort Jameson and kraaled with the two bullocks, and to eliminate the chance of their being bitten by a stray tsetse-fly, the animals were fed close to the house. The experiment began on April 11th and the animals were at once bitten by *Pangonia* and *Stomoxys nigra*. On May 27th trypanosomes were seen in one of the cows, and the remaining two died of trypanosomiasis at the beginning of July. It is impossible to decide whether the infection was due to *Pangonia* or *Stomoxys*, or both, and the possibility of stray tsetse-flies having bitten the animals is also not excluded.

Captain Hadow sent to the Wellcome Research Laboratories blood smears from two sick bulls at Kadugli, Kordofan. These were examined by Dr Balfour and found to contain numerous trypanosomes, the species probably being *T. brucei* (or *pecaudi*). These bulls could not have been bitten by tsetse-flies, for the only tsetse area in Kordofan is at Kawalib, sixty miles from Kadugli. The infection was attributed by the Arabs to the serut fly (*Tabanus* or *Pangonia*).

The circumstantial evidence in support of the view that El Debab, a disease affecting dromedaries in the North of Africa, is mainly carried by Tabanids, is much stronger than in the case of the other African trypanosomiases. The natives of North Africa from time immemorial have accused the serut flies of inoculating this disease into the dromedaries. When these animals remain during the summer in regions where Tabanids are numerous, the mortality from El Debab in the following months is very great. On the other hand, if Tabanids are few or absent, the disease seems to be unable to become established.

In Algeria the majority of the Tabanids appear between the 1st and 15th of June; they last for about forty days and then disappear, as soon as their enemies the Asilids begin to hatch out. The Tabanids live in the damp valleys and often frequent the tufts of *Thapsia*, appearing as soon as this plant flowers, and disappearing after it has withered.

Experimentally, Drs Edmond and Etienne Sergent, in Algeria, have been able to transmit *T. soudanense*, the pathogenic agent of El Debab, by the bites of *Tabanus nemoralis*, Mg. and *T. tomentosus* Macq.

The flies were first allowed to bite heavily infected rats or mice and subsequently fed on healthy animals. When there was no interval between the two feeds, five successful transmissions were obtained, and in one case after an interval of 22 hours the flies were still infective. Throughout these experiments only rats and mice were employed, never the natural host of the trypanosome.

These results are in harmony with what is known about the history of the disease.

Generally the infection lasts at least one year in camels, and in the month of June practically every herd contains several individuals with numerous trypanosomes in the blood. These animals would act as centres from which the infection could be spread by the Tabanids. These latter feed during the sunny hours of the day and usually attack the herd in swarms. As a result of the active movements of the camels, the insects are continually flying from one animal to another, and the conditions are very favourable to the spread of any infection.

Horses may also be infected by the agency of these same insects, but such cases are rare, as horses are not usually kept in the neighbourhood of herds of camels.

Three other trypanosome diseases, viz. Nagana, Mal de la Zousfana and Dourine, have been transmitted experimentally by the bites of various species of Tabanidæ in Algeria.

Transmission was only effected when the insects fed on the healthy animals immediately after having bitten an animal containing a great many trypanosomes in its blood. In no case was any infection produced if there was an interval of more than a few minutes between the two bites. A single bite was sometimes sufficient to cause inoculation of the disease, and therefore, under suitable conditions, it is probable that this mode of transmission can assume great importance.

According to Cazalbou, the disease of dromedaries at Timbuctoo known as Mbori, and also Souma (*T. cazalboui*) at Ségou, a disease affecting horses and cattle, are both propagated by *Tabanus tæniatus*, Macq. and *T. biguttatus*, Wied.

There is evidence showing that Tabanidæ are agents for the transmission of Surra (*T. evansi*). Thus Rogers, in the Federated Malay States, invariably produced the infection in dogs and rabbits by the successive bites of many Tabanids. A dog bitten by 12 flies that had just previously sucked blood from another dog, heavily infected with *T. evansi*, shewed parasites after an incubation period of seven days.

Fraser and Symonds repeated these experiments employing various species of *Tabanus*, *Hæmatopota* and *Stomoxys*. With four species of *Tabanus*—*T. fumifer*, *T. partitus*, *T. vagus*, and

*T. minimus*—they had four successes, three when there was no interval between the two feeds, and one after a five-minute interval. Ten experiments were performed and in each case only one or two flies were used. Five experiments with *Stomoxys* and two with *Hæmatopota* under similar conditions gave negative results. A number of Tabanidæ were then fed on infected animals and, at varying intervals, emulsions of the body contents of the flies inoculated into susceptible animals. It was found that the trypanosomes in the alimentary canal of *Tabanus* remained infective for 24 hours, but after longer periods lost their virulence.

Leese studied the natural transmission of Surra at Mohaud, India, and made experiments with mosquitoes, *Stomoxys, Tabanus, Hæmatopota* and sand-flies. Four *Tabanus*, which were fed on camels, in two of which trypanosomes were numerous, and transferred immediately to a white rat, produced infection in the latter, and under similar conditions ten *Hæmatopota* produced infection in a guinea-pig. Of three similar experiments, employing *Stomoxys*, only one gave positive results, so it seems that *Tabanus* is able to transmit Surra better than *Stomoxys*. On the other hand, Leese is strongly of the opinion that *Tabanus* and *Hæmatopota* are not specific transmitters, for outbreaks of the disease have occurred under circumstances that precluded the possibility of their being the carriers. Nevertheless, in the Punjab the worst " Surra zones " seem to be in places where *Tabanus* is most numerous. Baldrey has also performed some experiments on the transmission of Surra by various Tabanids and found that the trypanosomes remained virulent in the gut for not longer than 24 hours. An attempt was made to test the possibility of a cyclical mode of transmission, but all the Tabanids died by the end of the nineteenth day. Up to this date the inoculation of their body contents into susceptible animals gave negative results.

In America, Mohler and Thompson noted an outbreak of Surra following the importation of zebus from India. This herd consisted of 51 cattle that had been imported from Poona, where their blood was examined twice with negative results. On arrival in New York they appeared to be in good condition, but 2 ccs. of blood from each animal were injected into rabbits. Three of these rabbits showed *T. evansi* in their blood, and after some delay the three cattle thus shewn to be infected were destroyed and the remainder screened. At this time there were many *Tabanus atratus* present, together with other Tabanidæ and *Stomoxys calcitrans*.

In subsequent series of inoculations, 13 more animals were found to be infected and removed ; finally, the remainder were put in fly-proof box-stalls in a fly-proof stable, and these cattle all remained healthy. The authors are of the opinion that *Tabanus atratus* was responsible for the spread of the infection amongst the herd, but the results are not very conclusive, as the cattle may have been infected before they arrived.

In the Philippines, Mr M. B. Mitzmain informs me that he has succeeded in obtaining the direct transmission of Surra by means of *Tabanus striatus*. The flies were bred in captivity and transmission was successful from guinea-pig to monkey, and from horse to horse. In addition, this observer states that *T. striatus* is undoubtedly the carrier of Surra in extensive epidemics throughout the Philippines, and that there is a " very decided correlation between the predominance of this fly and outbreaks of Surra."

On the whole, the available evidence supports the view that Surra may be directly transmitted by the bites of various Tabanidæ, and that in nature they play a very important part in the spread of the infection. It is doubtful, however, whether the transmission is always mechanical, and further experiments on this point are much to be desired.

Since the above account was written, Leiper, in West Africa, has discovered that two species of *Chrysops* serve as the intermediate hosts of *Filaria loa*. At present no details are available, but this discovery is especially interesting, as it is the first record of any Tabanid having been shewn to be responsible for the transmission of a human disease.

REFERENCES.

Alcock, A. (1911). *Entomology for Medical Officers.*
Austen, E. (1909). *African Blood-sucking Flies.* British Museum.
Cazalbou (1904). *Recueil de Méd. Vétérinaire,* vol. LXXXI. p. 615.
—— (1906). *Rev. Générale de Méd. Vét.* Nos. 89–90.
Fraser and Symonds (1908). *Studies from the Institute for Medical Research.* Federated Malay States, No. 9.
Hart, R. (1911). *Journ. Comp. Path. and Therap.* Dec. 1911, p. 354.
Jowett, W. (1911). *Ibid.* vol. XXIV. p. 21.
King, H. H. (1908). *Third Report Wellcome Research Laboratories, Khartoum.* London : Baillière, Tindall and Cox, p. 213.
Leese, A. S. (1909). *Journ. Trop. Vet. Sci.* vol. IV. p. 107.
Mohler, J. R. and Thompson, W. (1911). *26th Annual Report (for* 1909), *Bureau Animal Industry.* Washington, p. 81.
Montgomery and Kinghorn (1907). *Ann. Trop. Med. and Parasit.* vol. II. p. 130.
Ricardo, G. (1901–1904). *Ann. and Mag. Nat. Hist.*
Rogers, L. (1901). *Proc. Roy. Soc.* B. vol. LXVIII. p. 163.
Sergent, Ed. and Ét. (1905). *Ann. Inst. Pasteur,* vol. XIX. p. 17.
—— (1906). *Ibid.* vol. XX. p. 665.

# CHAPTER XV

## CYCLORRHAPHA SCHIZOPHORA

*General description.* All the members of this series are distinguished by the presence of a distinct frontal lunula and frontal suture. The antennæ are composed of three segments of which the terminal bears an arista, almost invariably dorsal in position, and never thickened into a terminal style. There are never more than three posterior cells present (Fig. 63) the first of which may be closed or narrowed in the margin, but the others remain open. None of the longitudinal veins are forked ; the marginal and sub-marginal cells are never closed ; and the anal cell very rarely extends towards the margin of the wing. The flies are all more or less bristly.

This very large division, including several families, is termed by Williston, the Myodaria. It may be divided into two groups, the Acalyptratæ and Calyptratæ, which are distinguished as follows :

## (1)  Acalyptratae.

The squamæ are always small, or vestigial, so that they do not conceal the halteres when viewed from above. The auxiliary vein is often indistinct or vestigial, or close to the first longitudinal, with which it may be fused. The basal cells are small, and the posterior ones indistinct or wanting. The males are never holoptic and the front is never markedly constricted. The thorax is without a complete transverse suture and the posterior callosity is usually absent. The members of this group are never large flies, but usually small, or very small. None of them are known to suck blood, but certain species, e.g. Sepsis, are probably concerned in the transmission of disease[1].

## (2)  Calyptratæ.

The squamæ are well-developed, never vestigial, and generally conceal the halteres when viewed from above. The auxiliary vein is always distinct along its whole course and the first longitudinal is usually of considerable length, never very short. The males are often holoptic or the front markedly constricted. The thorax has a complete transverse suture in front of the wings and a posterior callosity is present. The members of this group are generally flies of moderate or considerable size and are never very small. The house-fly and tsetse-fly are two well-known examples of this large and important group, which is of the highest economic importance. Williston divides them into six families, of which the only one that we shall consider is the Muscidæ.

### Synopsis of Families of Calyptratæ.

1 { Mouth and mouth-parts small or vestigial; first posterior cell closed or narrowed (except in Gastrophilus). Bot-flies   .. = Oestridæ
   Mouth of usual size, mouth-parts not vestigial   ..   ..   .. = 2

2 { Hypopleuræ with a tuft of bristles; first posterior cell narrowed or closed   ..   ..   ..   ..   ..   ..   ..   .. = 3
   Hypopleuræ without a tuft of bristles; first posterior cell narrowed or fully open in the margin   ..   ..   ..   ..   .. = 6

[1] Vide Graham-Smith, G. S. (1913), Flies and Disease. Non-bloodsucking Flies (Cambridge University Press).

3 $\begin{cases} \text{Antennal arista bare or somewhat pubescent} & \quad = Tachinidæ. \\ \text{Antennal arista plumose or distinctly pubescent} & \quad .. \quad .. \quad = 4 \end{cases}$

4 $\begin{cases} \text{Antennal arista bare on the distal half; bristles rarely present on the} \\ \quad \text{dorsal surface of the anterior segments of abdomen} = Sarcophagidæ. \\ \text{Antennal arista plumose or pubescent to the tip} \quad .. \quad .. \quad .. \quad = 5 \end{cases}$

5 $\begin{cases} \text{Dorsum of abdomen usually bristly on anterior part ; legs usually long} \\ \quad = Dexiidæ. \\ \text{Abdominal segments without bristles, except more or less near the tip ;} \\ \quad \text{legs not markedly elongated} \quad .. \quad .. \quad .. \quad = \text{MUSCIDÆ.} \end{cases}$

6 $\begin{cases} \text{First posterior cell narrowed or closed ; arista plumose to the tip} \\ \quad = \text{MUSCIDÆ.} \\ \text{First posterior cell very slightly or not at all narrowed in the margin ;} \\ \quad \text{arista plumose, pubescent or bare} \quad .. \quad .. \quad = Anthomyidæ. \end{cases}$

## Family MUSCIDÆ.

The various individuals of this family are distinguished by the absence of bristles on the abdomen, except at the tip, and by the narrowed first posterior cell. The antennal arista is usually plumose to the tip, sometimes only on the upper side, and rarely bare. The eyes of the male are approximated or contiguous, and the front of the female broad. The eyes may be either bare or hairy. With the exception of *Glossina*, the abdomen is composed of four visible segments. The members of this family are generally of moderate size, and are never elongate, very hairy, or bare flies.

For the sake of convenience, we have followed Alcock in dividing the Muscidæ into two artificial groups according to whether the adults suck blood or not. The importance of the latter group (including house-flies, blowflies, etc.) as carriers of disease, has been described by Graham-Smith (*loc. cit.*) and it is unnecessary to give any further description of them in the present account. On the other hand, the blood-sucking Muscidæ include some of the most formidable biting-flies that carry disease.

### Blood-sucking Muscidæ[1].

In the majority of blood-sucking Muscidæ the proboscis is strongly chitinized and rigid, is slightly or not at all retractile, and is more or less slender and tapering, and the labella are small, rigid and strongly chitinized, and serrated or spinose, so

[1] After Alcock, *loc. cit.*

that the proboscis forms a very efficient apparatus for piercing the skin. ˙˙Occasionally the proboscis is only partly chitinous and is retractile, and the labella are large and fleshy, but even in these cases strong teeth, capable of cutting through the skin, are present. In other respects the proboscis resembles that present in the non-biting Muscidæ, being longitudinally grooved on its dorsal surface, so as to ensheathe the epipharynx and hypopharynx, which together form a tube, by apposition and basal interlocking. The blood-sucking habit is equally well developed in both males and females.

Although *Glossina* and *Stomoxys* are the only two genera that have been proved to carry infection, there is every possibility that other members of the group may suddenly acquire unenviable notoriety from this point of view, and therefore we include the following table of the genera, taken from Alcock:

*Genera of Blood-sucking Muscidæ.*

1 { Arista feathered only on the dorsal surface, individual hairs being also feathered. Proboscis with a bulbous base and very slender shaft. Maxillary palps long and slender, forming a sheath round the proboscis. Fourth longitudinal vein curved in its proximal portion so as to enlarge the anterior basal cell distally and to contract the discal cell basally; and sharply bent forward in its distal portion in line with the posterior cross-vein so as to nearly close the first posterior cell at a point much anterior to the tip of the wing. Abdomen composed of seven visible segments .. .. =*Glossina.*

Individual hairs of arista not feathered. Shaft of proboscis not remarkably slender. Maxillary palps not forming an obvious sheath for the proboscis. Fourth longitudinal vein not markedly sinuous in its proximal portion and bending forwards in its distal portion at a point considerably beyond the posterior cross-vein. Abdomen composed of four visible segments .. .. .. .. =2

2 { Maxillary palps slender, less than half the length of the proboscis. (Arista feathered dorsally only. Third longitudinal vein with some bristles on its proximal part.) .. .. .. .. =*Stomoxys.*

Maxillary palps more or less spatulate, almost as long as the proboscis, always much more than half its length .. .. .. =3

3 { Proboscis chitinous in all its extent, the labella small .. · .. =4

Proboscis with the distal part, and large labella, fleshy. Terminal fleshy part of proboscis reflexed beneath the chitinous part in repose. Arista feathered dorsally and ventrally; third longitudinal vein not bristly; fourth longitudinal vein abruptly bent so as nearly to close the first posterior cell

=*Philæmatomyia* (including ? *Pristorhynchomyia*).

4 {
    Arista feathered only on dorsal surface    ..    ..    ..    ..    $=5$
    Arista feathered on both dorsal and ventral surface    ..    ..    $=6$
}

5 {
    Proboscis long and tapering ; fourth longitudinal vein gently curved distally so as to leave the first posterior cell wide open; third longitudinal vein without bristles    ..    ..    ..    $=Lyperosia.$
    Proboscis short and stumpy ; first posterior cell narrowly open ; third longitudinal vein with some bristles proximally    $=Stygeromyia.$
}

6 {
    Fourth longitudinal vein strongly curved distally, so as to leave first posterior cell narrowly open. Third longitudinal vein without bristles    ..    ..    ..    ..    $=Hæmatobosca.$
    Fourth longitudinal vein slightly curved distally. so as to leave first posterior cell widely open    ..    ..    ..    ..    ..    $= 7$
}

7 {
    Third longitudinal vein with some bristles proximally    $=Hæmatobia.$
    Third longitudinal vein without bristles    ..    ..    $=Bdellolarynx.$
}

# CHAPTER XVI

## THE TSETSE-FLIES—GENUS *GLOSSINA*, WIED., 1830

*Diagnosis.* The genus *Glossina* is sharply distinguished from all other members of the Muscidæ by its viviparous mode of reproduction, which resembles that of the Pupipara, and also by certain peculiarities in the structure of the antennæ and in the wing venation. Austen gives the following diagnosis of the genus :

" Narrow-bodied, elongate, dark brown, blackish, yellowish-brown, or yellowish flies belonging to the Family Muscidæ, ranging in size from about 6 or 8 mm. in the case of *Glossina tachinoides*, Westw., to as much as 13 or 13·5 mm. in that of a large female of *G. brevipalpis*, Newst., or *longipennis*, Corti ; recognisable when alive and at rest by the wings being closed flat one over the other above the abdomen (beyond which they project considerably), instead of divaricate (as in the case of *Stomoxys*) or tectiform (as in *Hæmatopota*), and by the proboscis (*i.e.* proboscis ensheathed in the palpi), projecting horizontally in front of the head ; palpi, as seen in the natural position, extending slightly beyond the proboscis, their inner sides grooved so as to form a sheath for the latter, to which in life they are applied so closely as entirely to conceal it ; base of proboscis suddenly expanded beneath into a large onion-shaped bulb."

*General description.* In addition to the above-mentioned characters, there are certain others which aid in the differentiation of the genus. The antenna, in both sexes, contains in the

16—2

second and third segments a curious sense-organ, consisting of a number of sacs lined with sensory epithelium and opening to the exterior by a well-marked pore on the inner surface of the third segment. From the structure of this organ it is supposed to be auditory in function. The arista of the antenna is three jointed, the first two joints being very small, the terminal one broad and compressed, and feathered on its upper side with about 22 or 23 fine branching hairs.

The eyes are large and in both sexes are well separated ; the anterior facets towards the inner margin are much larger than those behind.

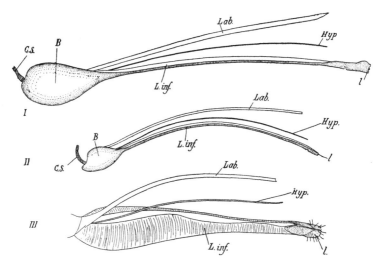

Fig. 62. Comparative morphology of the proboscis of *Glossina* (I), Melophagus (II) and *Stomoxys* (III).

B, proboscis bulb ; G.S., common salivary duct ; Hyp., hypopharynx ; L., labellæ ; Lab., upper lip (labium) ; L. inf., lower lip. I, *Glossina palpalis* ; II, *Melophagus ovinus* ; III, *Stomoxys calcitrans* ; × 35. (After Roubaud.)

The horizontally projecting proboscis is strongly chitinized and consists of a bulbous base contracting to a long and very slender shaft. The base of the proboscis, or proboscis bulb, is surrounded posteriorly by a fold of skin forming the hind-wall of the buccal cavity. The proboscis is grooved dorsally to contain the stylet-like epipharynx and the tubular hypopharynx which, by apposition, form a suctorial tube.

The maxillary palps are slender and as long as the proboscis, round which they form a loose sheath when the insect is resting.

The wings possess a very striking venation which is quite sufficient in itself to distinguish the genus. The fourth longitudinal vein is strongly curved in its proximal portions. The anterior basal transverse vein, at the base of the discal cell, is very short, and this first curve of the fourth longitudinal vein reduces the basal half of the discal cell, whilst the anterior basal cell is correspondingly increased. The fourth vein then bends upwards to join the anterior transverse vein, after which

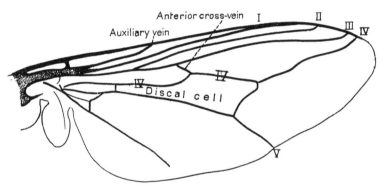

Fig. 63. Wing of *Glossina palpalis* to shew the venation.

it runs obliquely downwards almost at right angles to its former course. After joining the posterior transverse vein it again bends upwards and reaches the margin of the wing some distance before the apex. The second, third and fourth longitudinal veins all turn upwards at their tips and the anterior transverse vein is very oblique.

The sexes of *Glossina* can be readily distinguished, as in the male the external genitalia form a large oval swelling, the hypopygium, lying beneath the ventral surface of the seventh abdominal segment. The anus forms a median slit in the front part of this hypopygium and anteriorly on the venter of the sixth abdominal segment is a pair of smaller swellings, termed hectors. When the hypopygium is turned back a system of complicated appendages is displayed, the arrangement and structure of which have been shewn by Newstead to be of great use in classification. These appendages are briefly as follows : the superior claspers, whose chief function is apparently to grip the abdomen of the female ; the editum ; the inferior claspers, which present very striking morphological differences

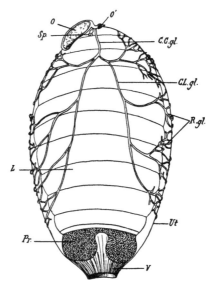

Fig. 64.   Gravid uterus of *G. palpalis* containing a larva at an advanced stage of development.   Dorsal view × 10.

    *C.G.gl.*, common excretory duct ;  *CL.gl.* principal lateral trunk of the uterine glands ;  *L*, body of the larva ;  *O.O.*, ovary ;  *Pr.*, caudal protuberances of larva ;  *R.gl.*, ramifications of uterine gland ;  *Sp*, spermatheca ;  *Ut*, uterus ;  *V*, vagina.  (After Roubaud.)

in the various groups ; the harpes, small bilateral appendages most highly developed in the *fusca* group and rudimentary or absent in the remaining groups ; the juxta, or penis sheath ; the penis ; the median process, present only in the *fusca* group, lying in the middle line between the inferior claspers ; and the connecting membrane, present in the *palpalis* and *morsitans* groups, but absent in the *fusca* group.

The method of reproduction, discovered by Bruce, is very remarkable, resembling that of the Pupipara, and is probably the result of their exclusively blood-sucking mode of life. The female lays a single larva at a time, which is retained and nourished in the oviduct until it is full grown. After the larva is born, it at once burrows into the ground and pupates. The larva is generally of a yellowish-white colour and bears at its posterior extremity a pair of large dark-coloured protuberances and between them is a depression into which open the spiracles (Fig. 70). The pupa is dark brown in colour with a slight sheen. It is broadly ovoid in shape and the larval protuberances are equally conspicuous, forming, together with the size and shape of the depression between them, a means of identifying the immature stages of different species.

*Distribution.* The members of this genus are entirely restricted to Africa and the south-west corner of Arabia, together forming the Ethiopian region, and range between the latitudes of 18° N. and about 31° S. Within these limits the tsetse-flies are not found continuously but are generally confined to belts or patches of forests, bush, and warm and damp situations where shade can be obtained. The areas in which the tsetse-fly occurs are commonly known as " fly-belts " and are well exemplified in the case of *G. morsitans*. Tsetse-flies are said to be absent from dry open plains without shade.

*Determination of the species of* GLOSSINA.

It seems probable that most, if not all, of the species of the genus *Glossina*, are of importance as carriers of disease and therefore we include the following table for their determination. In the classification, the important work of Austen has been followed throughout, and according to his scheme the species may be divided into four groups :

## *Synopsis of species of* GLOSSINA, *after Austen*[1].

Tarsi of hind-legs entirely \ *Glossina palpalis Group* (*I*), also *G. morsitans*
dark brown or black      /        var. *paradoxa* (*vide infra*).

Only the two last joints of hind tarsi are dark-coloured, thus forming a conspicuous contrast with the remaining joints which are pale.

{ Species of small size, length not exceeding 10·5 mm., usually much less; wing expansion not greater than 22·5 mm. Upper surface of abdomen distinctly banded, with conspicuous dark brown transverse marks on a pale ground colour.    ..    ..    ..    *Glossina morsitans Group* (*II*).

Species of large size, exceeding 10·5 mm. Wing expansion at least 25 mm.

{ Wings fairly dark. Palpi long and slender (except in *tabaniformis*).    *Glossina fusca Group* (*III*).

Upper surface of abdomen not marked with distinct bands as in the previous group.

{ Wings pale. Palpi short.    *Glossina brevipalpis Group* (*IV*)

### I. GLOSSINA PALPALIS *group*.

Dorsum of abdomen ochraceous-buff or buff; third and following segments exhibiting sharply defined, dark brown or clove-brown interrupted transverse bands. Length not more than 8 mm. ..    .. *tachinoides*, Westw. (p. 253).

Closely resembling *tachinoides*, but distinguished by its bright ochraceous colour and relatively narrow head. Length of ♀ (only specimen known) 7 mm.

*austeni*, Newstead.

Third joint of antennæ pale, clothed with long and fine hairs, forming a conspicuous fringe on front and hind margins. Length 8 to 9 mm.

*pallicera*, Bigot.

Dorsal surface of abdomen dark sepia-brown; median paler area on second segment broad and more or less quadrate or irregular in outline. Hypopygium of male buff or ochraceous-buff ..    .. *caliginea*, Austen.

Dorsal surface of abdomen blackish-brown; median pale area triangular in outline. Hypopygium of male grey. Length of male always exceeding 8·5 mm. ..    ..    ..    ..    ..    .. *palpalis*, Rob. Desv. (p. 256).

---

[1] Handbook of the Tsetse-Flies, 1911.

## II. Glossina morsitans group.

1. Last two joints of front and middle tarsi with sharply defined, clove-brown or black tips .. .. .. .. .. .. .. .. = 2.

Last two joints of front and middle tarsi either entirely pale or, at most, faintly brownish at the tips, never so dark as to form a sharp contrast with the remaining joints .. .. .. .. = *pallidipes*, Austen (p. 271).

2. Third joint of antennæ fringed with fine hairs on front margin. The dark brown transverse abdominal bands extending close to the hind margins of the segments .. .. .. .. .. = *longipalpis*, Wied. (p. 274)

Third joint of antennæ not fringed with fine hairs on front margin. Transverse abdominal bands not extending close to the hind margins of the segments. = *morsitans*, Westw. (p. 276).

(a) Markedly paler than typical *morsitans*, but more or less agreeing in its general characters .. .. .. .. *morsitans* var. *pallida*, Shircore.

(b) Resembling *morsitans* but distinguished by having all the joints of hind tarsi dark as in *palpalis group* .. *morsitans* var. *paradoxa*, Shircore.

## III. Glossina fusca group.

1 ⎰ Third joint of antennæ fringed with fine hairs on anterior and posterior margins. Fringe on anterior margin conspicuous under a hand lens ( × 15) when fly is examined in profile .. .. .. .. = 2
Third joint of antennæ with fringe of hairs on anterior margin so short as to be scarcely noticeable under a hand lens, the longest hairs not exceeding one-sixth the width of the third joint. Palpi long and slender = 3

2 ⎰ Length of longest hairs on anterior margin of third joint of antennæ equal to from one-fourth to one-third of the width of joint. Palpi of moderate length. Number of hairs on arista 18 to 23 = *tabaniformis*, Westw.

3 ⎰ Pleuræ drab-grey or isabella-coloured ; hind coxæ buff or greyish-buff = *fusca*, Walk.
Pleuræ dark grey ; hind coxæ mouse-grey .. = *fuscipleuris*, Austen.

## IV. Glossina brevipalpis group.

1 ⎰ Dorsum of thorax with four sharply defined, dark brown, more or less oval or elongate spots, arranged in a parallelogram, two in front of and two behind the transverse suture. Proboscis bulb with a sharply defined brown or dark brown tip .. .. = *longipennis*, Corti (p. 286).
Dorsum of thorax without such spots. Proboscis bulb not dark or brown at tip .. .. .. .. .. .. .. .. = 2

2 ⎰ Wings with upper, thickened portion of anterior transverse vein much darker in colour than adjacent veins and thus standing out conspicuously against the rest of the wing = *brevipalpis*, Newstead (p. 288).
Wings with the part in question not darker than the adjacent veins, the wings being practically unicolourous .. = *medicorum*, Austen.

## GLOSSINA and Disease.

The more common members of this genus have all been proved to be capable of serving as the invertebrate hosts of various species of trypanosomes, and in addition may carry infection directly from one animal to another, when there is no long interval between the bites.  Some species of trypanosomes seem to be mainly spread by only one species of *Glossina*, as in the case of sleeping sickness (*T. gambiense*), which seems to be restricted to regions where *G. palpalis* is present.  Nevertheless, *G. morsitans* has been shewn experimentally to be capable of transmitting *T. gambiense* and it is difficult to see why such transmission does not take place in nature.  Fortunately, this trypanosome seems to be unable to readily adapt itself to development in more than one species of *Glossina*, but some of the cattle trypanosomes, *e.g. T. cazalboui* and *T. dimorphon*, seem to be able to develop in any species of *Glossina*, though not with equal facility in all of them.

Probably the most important factor restricting the spread of trypanosomiases is the difficulty with which the tsetse-flies become infected.  When several *Glossinæ* are fed on an animal containing trypanosomes in its blood, only a relatively small proportion of the flies become infected, the number depending on a variety of conditions which are not thoroughly understood.

Attention may be called to Miss Robertson's experiment with *T. gambiense* and *G. palpalis*, reproduced in tabular form on page 309, from which it appears that the percentage of flies in which the trypanosomes develop, depends to some extent on the stage of the infection in the vertebrate host.  Yet another important condition is the interval that elapses between an infective and the subsequent feed.  In the case of *T. gambiense* and *G. palpalis*, the trypanosomes that may have developed in the gut of the fly after the first feed are frequently swept out by the next influx of blood and thus no infection is produced.  Strange as it may seem, from Miss Robertson's experiments there can be little doubt that when flies are fed every two or three days there is much less chance of them becoming infective than if they are starved after a meal of infected blood.

Probably temperature exercises a greater influence than any other known factor on the development of trypanosomes in the tsetse-fly. Kinghorn and Yorke have shewn that *T. rhodesiense* can only complete development in its invertebrate host, *G. morsitans*, at a temperature of at least 75° to 80° F. Similarly Kleine and Fischer on Lake Victoria were quite unable to transmit *T. gambiense* by means of *G. morsitans*, whilst on the warmer shores of Tanganyika, Taute, employing the same species, succeeded without much difficulty (*vide* p. 306).

The observations on the natural infections of tsetse-flies have shewn that flies of different species frequenting the same district are not infected in the same proportions, nor in the same manner. Moreover these proportions, even for the same species, vary in different localities, as for example in West Africa. Thus Bouet and Roubaud found that in Lower Dahomey *T. cazalboui* predominated in *G. longipalpis* and *palpalis*, *T. dimorphon* in *longipalpis* and *tachinoides*, and *T. pecaudi* in *longipalpis*. On the other hand, in Upper Dahomey, *T. pecaudi* was most predominant in *G. morsitans*, and in Casamance *T. dimorphon* in *morsitans*. The number of *G. palpalis* becoming infected with *T. cazalboui* when fed on an animal suffering from this infection, was 40 per cent. in Middle Dahomey, and *nil* in Upper Casamance, although repeated attempts were made to infect the flies. These experimental results were confirmed by an examination of natural infections. In Middle Dahomey one fly in thirty was naturally infected with *T. cazalboui*, whilst in Upper Casamance out of 560 flies examined only one shewed infection of the proboscis.

Souma (*T. cazalboui*) exists in both regions, but it is evident that some other species of tsetse besides *palpalis* must be responsible for its transmission in Casamance. From these data Roubaud deduces that the receptivity of a given species of *Glossina* for any particular virus, is not uniform throughout the region of the flies' distribution. In other words a virus is only endemic where there are receptive races of tsetse-flies.

From this point of view it is worthy of notice that, in spite of numerous experiments, up to the present no one has succeeded in transmitting *T. gambiense* by *G. palpalis*—or any other tsetse-fly—on the west side of Africa. It seems that the West African races of *G. palpalis*, are more or less refractory to infection with *T. gambiense*, for the climatic conditions in Dahomey, Casamance and in Uganda, do not differ sufficiently to explain the difficulty of transmission in the two former districts.

Thus the evolution of trypanosomes in the invertebrate host is a very complex problem and, before commencing prophylactic measures in any particular district, it is first of all necessary to determine, by careful experiments with the local races of *Glossina*, which species are responsible for the spread of the local strains of trypanosomiasis. If this is not done, there is a great danger of administrative efforts being wasted in the attempt to destroy a comparatively harmless species of *Glossina*, whilst the more important carrier escapes. The results of experiments in other neighbourhoods are of very little use, for, as mentioned above, in one district *T. cazalboui* is carried by *G. palpalis*, whereas in another all attempts to infect this tsetse with the same trypanosome have been unsuccessful.

In the following pages we have summarized the available information concerning the bionomics of all species of *Glossina* that have been proved to carry any infection, together with a brief mention of the infections they are known to transmit. Further details of the experiments and observations on the latter point will be found under the heading of the various species of trypanosomes (Chapter XVIII).

REFERENCES.

Austen, E. (1911). *Handbook of the Tsetse-Flies.* British Museum, (Nat. Hist.) London.
Newstead, R. (1911). *Bull. Ent. Research,* vol. II. p. 9.
—— (1912). *Ann. Trop. Med. and Parasit.,* vol. VI. p. 129.

## Glossina tachinoides Westwood, 1850.

*Synonyms.*  G. *palpalis* var. *tachinoides* Austen, 1903.  G. *decorsei*
Brumpt, 1904.

*Description.*  *Glossina tachinoides* is one of the smallest of
the known tsetse-flies, the length of the female being from
6·8 to 8·4 mm. and of the male 6·0 to 6·75 mm.  Among those
species having all the tarsi of the hind-legs dark, it may easily
be recognised by its small size and its very distinctly banded
abdomen.  On the dorsum of the second segment of the
abdomen there is a median quadrate pale area, which is very
conspicuous and is one of the distinctive characters of the
species.

*Distribution.*  G. *tachinoides* is widely distributed throughout West Africa having been recorded from the Senegal to the
French Congo, including Gambia, Gold Coast, the Northern
Territories, Togoland, French Guinea, Ashanti, German Cameroons, and Nigeria, where it is especially abundant in the north.
In addition the species occurs in the French Sudan, on the shores
of Lake Chad, and has been recorded from Southern Arabia
and German East Africa.  According to Neave, the *tachinoides*
recorded from the last named locality may prove to be
G. *austeni*, Newstead.

*Bionomics.*  G. *tachinoides* closely resembles *palpalis* in its
habits, being found in the vicinity of water, especially along the
banks of rivers.  It generally prefers rather more open wooded
tracts than *palpalis* and is not found in the groves of wild
palms along the small streams.  According to Simpson, the
species is most abundant where the country is open, vegetation
sparse, the dry season well-defined and the rain-fall slight.
It is the predominant tsetse-fly occurring along the rivers in
the region bordering on the Sahara and seems to have come
from the north.

Dr Alexander, in Northern Nigeria, found *tachinoides* in a
large marsh consisting of elephant grass, with occasional
clumps of palm trees and thick undergrowth, though he failed
to find the fly on the banks of a river about three quarters of a
mile away.

Although usually confined to the vicinity of water, in Southern Arabia G. *tachinoides* occurs in thick belts of euphorbia, tamarisk and cactus, often some distance from the edge of any water, but is never seen in the date groves or along the patches of cultivation.

Moiser has recently given an interesting account of the habits of G. *tachinoides* in the Bornu Province, Northern Nigeria, where the flies have existed for an indefinite period confined to the thick bush. In order to study the vertical range of the flies, men were posted up trees at heights varying from 10 to 25 feet, but in no case were any of the insects seen, although there were several on the ground. As a result of his observations Moiser comes to the following conclusions :— Deep shade and proximity to water appear to be the main factors influencing the distribution of the flies. Their natural resting place is on the lower side of twigs and branches of undergrowth, under the shade of large trees, at a height usually not greater than a foot above the ground. The flies are very restless and the observer is of the opinion that during the day they are continually moving about from place to place within the fly-belt and only for short periods rest on the under surface of twigs and small branches and perhaps on the ground. They do not usually travel higher than four or five feet and probably never as high as ten feet, therefore it is unlikely that the flies feed on monkeys or birds, but on the ground animals, *e.g.* the warthog, duiker or bushbuck.

G. *tachinoides* requires a meal fairly frequently and according to Moiser cannot withstand starvation without water for longer than 24 to 30 hours. On the other hand Roubaud kept ten flies in saturated air and all were alive after three days, and three after ten days. In captivity they will feed on the bodies of other tsetse-flies and it is not improbable that in nature they feed on other insects, ticks, grasshoppers etc. Certainly in Arabia, Carter noticed this fly in localities where the chance of getting a feed of mammalian blood must be very slight indeed. The flies feed voraciously on human beings and are very troublesome, as they are quite active in dull weather and in the very early hours of the morning, when *palpalis* is usually quiescent. Moreover, according to Dr Alexander the flies bite after dark, at 7.0 p.m. he having had to take refuge in his mosquito net, and his boys remarked that the flies were more troublesome than mosquitoes.

*G. tachinoides* is very resistant to heat, an exposure of one and a half hours in a stove at 40° C. being well borne. As a result the species is able to exist in very warm regions and occurs in the Sudan in localities that are too hot for *G. palpalis*.

*Reproduction.* The flies copulate immediately after hatching and at 25° C. the larvæ are deposited at intervals of about eight days. The duration of the pupal stage in Dahomey (at 24° to 25° C.) was found by Roubaud to be from 28 to 35 days.

Like *palpalis*, the pupæ will resist immersion in water for a period of 20 hours, and are able to withstand a temperature of 35° C. for ten hours in the day, so long as the experiment is only continued for a few days ; if it goes on for a month, all the pupæ die.

## G. TACHINOIDES *and Disease.*

This species is one of the main carriers of Souma (*T. cazalboui*) and *T. dimorphon*, in West Africa. Moreover, although direct experimental evidence is lacking, it is likely that *tachinoides* is able to transmit sleeping sickness. In Togoland on the Oti River, a tributary of the Volta, Zupitza believes that it takes the place of *G. palpalis* as a carrier of this disease.

*Prophylaxis.* The methods that will be described for *G. palpalis* (see p. 315) are also applicable to *tachinoides*, and in Northern Nigeria experiments have been made on the effect of cutting down the undergrowth on the banks of rivers. One month after the clearing very few *tachinoides* could be found and pupæ were sought without success.

### LITERATURE.

Carter, R. Markham (1906). *Brit. Med. Journ.* Nov. 17, 1906, p. 1393.
Moiser, B. (1912). *Bull. Ent. Research*, vol. III. p. 195.
Neave, A. S. (1912). *Ibid.* p. 275.
Roubaud, E. (1911). *Compt. Rend. Acad. Sci.* pp. 406 and 637.
Simpson, J. J. (1912). *Bull. Ent. Research*, vol. III. p. 301.
Zupitza (1909). Cf. *S. S. Bulletin*, vol. II. p. 149.

## Glossina palpalis Rob. Desv. 1830.

*Synonyms. Nemorhina palpalis* Rob. Desv. 1830. *Glossina longipalpis* Walker (*nec* Wiedemann), 1873. *G. ventricosa* Bigot, 1885. *G. tabaniformis* Bigot, 1885. *G. maculata* Newstead, 1907. *G. fuscipes* Newstead, 1910.

*Description*[1]. "Length, ♂ 8 to 9 mm., ♀ 8·6 to 10·2 mm., width of head ♂ 2·4 to 2·6 mm., ♀ 2·5 to just under 3 mm.; width of front of vertex, ♂ 0·6 mm., ♀ 1 mm; length of wing, ♀ 7 to 8·4 mm., ♂ 8·4 to 9·2 mm.

"Abdomen clove-brown or blackish-brown ; thorax usually paler, with dark brown markings on a greyish ground ; abdomen generally with at least an indication of a pale or slate-grey longitudinal median stripe, with pale lateral triangular markings, and usually the hind margins of the segments narrowly pale. Femora in typical race more or less mouse-grey, greyish-brown, or dark slate coloured ; tibiæ, extreme tips of femora, and first three joints of front and middle tarsi buff or ochraceous-buff, hind (or middle and hind) tibiæ sometimes infuscated in ♂ ; hind tarsi blackish-brown or clove-brown above ; wings strongly tinged with sepia-brown, but not quite so dark as in *G. caliginea.*

"*Head.*—*Face* and *jowls* cream-coloured or cream-buff ; posterior surface of head (*occiput*) entirely cinereous ; *frontal stripe* varying from ochraceous to dark chestnut ; frontal margins (sides of front or parafrontals) greyish, seen from the side with a dark brown elongate area below ; ocellar triangle smoke-grey, enclosing the dark brown ocellar spot, which is joined posteriorly to a sharply defined dark brown band, uniting the vertical bristles and very conspicuous except in the darkest specimens ; second joint of *antennæ* more or less yellow at the apex in front, third joint narrowly buff at extreme base on outer side, otherwise entirely mouse-grey ; arista buff, dark brown beneath ; palpi mouse-grey, blackish on upper side, proboscis bulb dark brown.

"*Thorax.*—Dorsum in most clearly marked specimens bluish-grey or greyish olivaceous, with brown markings. These markings when fully visible are as follows : a narrow stripe on each side of the median line, interrupted before reaching the transverse suture and again before reaching the hind margin ; the section of each stripe behind the suture is expanded posteriorly, and the terminal portion of the stripes immediately in front of the hind margin takes the shape of a pair of more or less confluent ill-defined spots, sometimes confluent with the stripes in front ; next to the two admedian stripes on each side of the suture itself a more or less sharply defined oval spot ; on the out-side of this a longitudinal stripe, more or less interrupted and sometimes obsolete in the middle, but in front curving round outwards behind the humeral callus and then running backwards along the lateral margin of the dorsum nearly to the post-alar callus ; in the area thus enclosed is a broad ill-defined patch in front of and behind the suture while the lateral stripe itself sends off two prolongations, which run inwards for a certain distance on each side of the suture. Humeral callus with a spot on its upper portion, confluent with the curved stripe behind it ; a more or less ill-defined spot on the post-alar callus also. Pleuræ olive-grey or smoke-grey in male, drab-grey or olive-grey in female, a more or less distinct brown patch in the centre of the meso-pleura. Scutellum buff or cream-buff, olive-grey at the base, the usual dark

[1] Taken from Austen, *Handbook of the Tsetse-Flies,* 1911, p. 24.

brown patch on each side of the median line more or less conspicuous ; apical
scutellar bristles in the female variable in length—(sometimes as in specimens
from the Congo Free State and Uganda) short, sometimes (as in specimens
from Liberia, Sierra Leone, and the Gambia) nearly as long as in the male.

*Abdomen.*—Dorsum clove-brown or blackish-brown ; first segment and a
median triangular area on the second (its base resting on the front and its
apex on the hind margin of the second segment) buff-coloured or cinereous,
the pale triangle continued backwards as a narrow, more or less well-defined
median stripe, usually reaching at least so far as the hind margin of the fifth
segment ; lateral margins of the segments from the second onwards grey,
expanded on the apical angles into triangular markings, extreme hind margins
of the segments from the second to the sixth usually narrowly pale or grey ;
seventh segment, as also the hypopygium in the male, entirely grey.

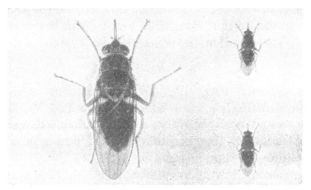

Fig. 65. *Glossina palpalis.* Photographs taken by Dr Graham, on the Gold
Coast, shewing the flies in a position of rest. The fly to the left is magnified
3½ diameters, those to the right are of natural size. (From the *Sleeping
Sickness Bulletin.*)

*Legs.*—Last joint of front and middle tarsi dark brown, often more or less
buff at base, sometimes distal third alone dark brown, remainder buff ;
penultimate joint of front and middle tarsi dark brown, more or less buff at base.

*Wings* as described above. *Squamæ* waxen-white, border of the antisquama
darker, fringed with short, darker hairs.

*Halteres* cream-buff.

## Glossina palpalis var. wellmani Austen (1905).

*Synonym. G. bocagei* França, 1905.

" ♂, ♀ —Distinguishable from typical *G. palpalis*, Rob.-Desv., by a peculiar
reduction in the markings of the dorsum of the thorax.

"*Frontal stripe* pale ochraceous ; thoracic markings much reduced, so
that *the thorax in a well-preserved specimen appears spotted*, the antero-lateral
markings taking the form of spots or blotches ; the *spot immediately behind
the inner extremity of the humeral callus* on each side small, ovoid, or nearly
circular, and especially conspicuous when the insect is viewed from above and
slightly from behind ; femora pale, the dark area much reduced."

*Distribution.* *Glossina palpalis* is widely distributed throughout the western equatorial tropical region of Africa. Along the west coast it extends from the Senegal to Angola, where the variety *wellmani* predominates. Inland it extends as far as Bahr el Ghazal and, according to Brumpt, Lake Rudolf. Proceeding southward the eastern boundary of the species includes the shores of Lake Victoria in British and German East Africa, and Tanganyika together with its rivers. In N.E. Rhodesia the fly is common in the valley of the Luapula River and its southern limit of distribution follows the boundary between N.W. Rhodesia and the Congo, and across Angola to the town of Benguela. *G. palpalis* has never been found in Nyasaland or the region of Lake Nyasa.

## Internal Anatomy.

*The digestive tract* (Fig. 66). The internal anatomy of *Glossina palpalis* has been carefully described by Minchin, whose account of the digestive tract is closely followed in the present work, with the exception that the term proventriculus is substituted for that of stomach.

Commencing with the œsophagus (*Oes.*), this portion of the alimentary canal runs first of all upwards from the pharynx, then bends sharply round and passes backwards through the brain. After bending round, the œsophagus becomes extremely narrow, but gradually widens after passing through the brain. Immediately after entering the thorax it opens ventrally into the proventriculus, a dilatation of the gut which marks the commencement of the digestive region. From the point at which the œsophagus opens into the proventriculus, the duct of the sucking stomach, or crop, begins.

The intestine arises from the proventriculus about the middle of its dorsal side and runs backwards through the thorax as a straight tube of even calibre until it enters the abdomen, where the intestine swells out into the more strictly digestive portion of the alimentary canal,

The abdominal intestine is of great length and forms a number of complicated coils, which are represented in Fig. 66. It may be divided into thirteen limbs, for purposes of description, each limb being separated from the following one by a more or less sharp bend. The fifth, sixth and seventh limbs together form a well-marked loop, which is generally the most dilated portion of the intestine and is sometimes regarded as the true

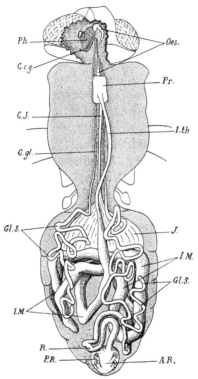

Fig. 66. Internal Anatomy of *Glossina palpalis*. (After Minchin, from Roubaud.)

 *A.R.*, rectum ; *G.c.g.*, junction of the two salivary ducts (*G.gl.*) ; *Gl.S.*, salivary glands ; *G.J.*, duct of sucking stomach ; *I.M.*, intestine ; *I.th.*, thoracic intestine ; *J.*, sucking stomach ; *Oes.*, œsophagus ; *Ph.*, pharynx ; *Pr.*, proventriculus ; *P.R.*, rectal papillæ ; *R*, hind-gut.

stomach. Posteriorly the intestine passes into the capacious rectum which has four rectal glands, each supplied by a bunch of small tracheæ.

The appendages of the alimentary tract are the salivary glands, the sucking stomach or crop, and the Malpighian tubules.

The salivary glands (Fig. 66, *Gl.S.*) commence as two long coiled tubes, occupying a superficial dorsal position in the abdomen, on each side of the heart. The coils of the glands may extend as far backwards as the fourth or fifth abdominal segment. After many twists and turns each tube runs forward to the waist and after passing into the thorax diminishes rapidly in diameter, becomes more or less straight, and at the same time passes to the ventral side of the body. From this point the salivary gland becomes the salivary duct. In the thorax the ducts run on each side of the duct of the crop and passing under the proventriculus, reach the neck, where they become so extremely attenuated that their course is difficult to follow. As they enter the neck the ducts curve over towards each other and pass under the brain and then under the pharynx, uniting in a median duct shortly before opening in the hypopharynx.

The crop, or sucking stomach (Fig. 66, *J.*), is morphologically a ventral diverticulum of the hinder end of the œsophagus, arising from the point at which the latter communicates with the proventriculus, in such a way as to appear as a direct continuation of the œsophagus. It consists of a slender tube or duct running backwards below the first part of the intestine and expanding distally into a large sac, occupying the first two abdominal segments. Usually the crop is filled with gas but shortly after feeding it is found filled with blood.

The Malpighian tubules arise by a pair of main stems given off from opposite sides of the tenth limb of the intestine. Each of these stems soon divides into two, and the four tubules thus formed ramify throughout the body of the insect.

*Bionomics. Glossina palpalis* is only to be found at the edge of water, or water courses. It especially frequents the banks of rivers and lakes that are surrounded by overhanging trees, or scrub, but occasionally it occurs in regions where there is practically no shade, as for example, on Lake Tanganyika, where the shore is bare but for the presence of a few reeds. In the Congo the fly frequents those parts of the rivers that are surrounded by dense forest and, according to Roubaud, this locality is determined by the necessity of two conditions—a high and constant temperature, and an almost saturated atmosphere. The same observer remarks on the predilection of the fly for the neighbourhood of fords and those parts of the river most frequented by man.

There is no record of *G. palpalis* from a greater altitude than 4000 feet, but it is common on the shores of Lake Victoria at a height of 3700 feet. Such an altitude is exceptional, however, and in most parts of Africa it is not found at so high a level, probably owing to the unsuitable climatic conditions.

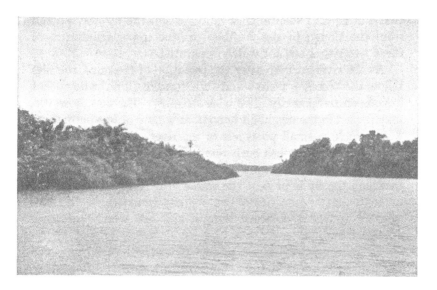

Fig. 67. View on the River Gambia beyond Barijali shewing the dense nature of the vegetation, which consists of Ferns, Palms, Pandani, etc., and is a typical haunt of *Glossina palpalis*. (After Simpson.)

Hodges distinguishes a natural range and a " following range." By the former is meant the distance from water within which the flies naturally wander in search of food, and in most cases this natural range does not exceed 30 yards. By following range is meant the distance to which flies will follow victims who have passed through the natural range. It rarely exceeds 300 yards, although flies have been caught at distances of 1500 yards from any water. Native water carriers are sometimes accompanied for long distances, the flies resting on their persons or on the water pail. On the other hand Bagshawe has shewn that the fly may travel at least a mile along the banks of water, and the observations on seasonal distribution suggest that *G. palpalis* is capable of travelling for very considerable distances.

During the rainy season the flies ascend to the upper limits of the rivers and thus may appear in valleys that are dry for the greater part of the year. In this manner the range of *G. palpalis* may be considerably extended and there is a danger that during an exceptionally rainy season the fly may spread from the Congo to the Zambesi, as the upper tributaries of these two rivers are not widely separated.

As the rivers dry up after the cessation of the rains, the flies follow the receding waters and thus forsake those valleys that have been temporarily filled with streams. The flies, however, may persist in the neighbourhood of any more or less permanent water, such as small pools left in the river-bed. It is possible therefore to distinguish such temporary haunts, only occupied by the fly during the rainy season, from the permanent haunts in which the fly is present the whole year round. Needless to add, the latter constitute the sources from which the flies migrate to the temporary haunts and are worthy of more careful attention.

In addition the flies are subject to seasonal variations even in their permanent haunts, the numbers greatly diminishing during the dry summer and increasing during the rainy season. The reason for this decrease in numbers during the dry season has not been satisfactorily explained, but it may depend to some extent on the breeding habits of the insect (*vide infra*).

The habits of *G. palpalis* are fairly well known and its presence can readily be detected when the flies are abundant. The peculiar buzzing noise made by the insects whilst flying and also the quick darting manner in which they flit from place to place when not actually feeding, enable experienced observers to identify the flies without actually catching specimens. The best way of detecting the presence of flies is to coast along slowly in a canoe, when if the weather is favourable, the insects, if present, soon appear in the boat. The attraction of moving bodies for this species is very marked and has been noticed by many observers.

Thus Simpson, while travelling in a river-launch up an infested river in Nigeria, noticed that as long as the boat remained stationary at the landing stage, no tsetse-flies attempted to come on board, although swarms of them were flying about near the banks of the stream. But as soon as the launch moved away, the flies rose in swarms and flew after the boat, many settling on the bows and deck and being carried up the stream for very considerable distances.

The fly is not seen until after sunrise, the insects usually appearing about 7 to 7.30 a.m. on bright still mornings. The time of appearance, however, varies with the locality and in densely shaded regions may be considerably later. In the afternoon the numbers diminish about 4 to 4.30 p.m. and on the approach of sunset most of them disappear ; only very exceptionally have they been known to feed at night. In cloudy or rainy weather very few flies are to be seen, and wind at once drives all of them into shelter. Although the presence of the sun seems necessary for the fly's activity, it prefers the shade, and indeed, if exposed to the direct rays of the sun dies in a very short time.

It has been noticed by all observers that the tsetse-fly prefers a dark skin to a white, and dark clothes to light ones. Europeans when accompanied by natives are rarely molested to any great degree. Ensor states that white clothing confers the greatest degree of immunity from the attacks of these insects, and this statement is supported by all travellers in fly regions. Dutton and Todd write as follows : " One day while coming down the Kasai the Captain put on a blue cloth jacket. Many more tsetses were found to settle on his coat than on the white duck suits of the European passengers and of the negro steersman." As a rule *palpalis* does not bite through clothes but it is easily able to pierce socks and ordinary white drill suits.

When feeding the fly spreads out its front pair of legs, and then lowers its proboscis into the skin (Fig. 68). It then begins to gorge and its abdomen swells visibly and the insect may

ingest more than twice its own weight of blood.  The excess
of fluid is got rid of very quickly, yellow liquid being excreted
from the anus.

There is no evidence that *G. palpalis* can exist without
vertebrate blood, but it will readily feed on both warm- and
cold-blooded animals.  It is not dependent upon any particular
species for its food, but the experiments of Kleine shew that
the flies thrive much better on mammals and birds than on
reptiles.  In one case three batches of 232 female *palpalis*
were fed respectively on wethers, fowls, and crocodiles, between
July 8th and August 6th.  During this period there died
no less than 190 of the flies that fed on crocodiles, whereas
the numbers of flies that died in the other two batches were
respectively 25 and 35.  Moreover, those nourished on the
reptilian blood never laid any larvæ, whilst the flies fed on
wethers gave birth to 82, and those on fowls to 89 larvæ.

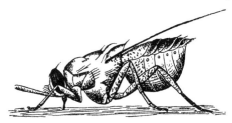

Fig. 68.  *Glossina palpalis* in the act of feeding.  (After Roubaud.)

From these results it is evident that crocodile blood is a
very unfavourable diet for *G. palpalis*, in spite of the large
numbers of flies that may be seen feeding on these reptiles.
Koch stated that on Lake Victoria the blood of the crocodile
formed the staple diet of the tsetse-flies, but the experiments
of Kleine, confirmed by Roubaud, shew that the fly must also
derive its food from some other source in order to be capable
of breeding[1].

[1] This is a very good instance of the danger of introducing prophylactic
measures without a careful examination of every possible factor that might
influence the results.  After Koch's observation, numerous persons advocated
the destruction of the crocodiles as a means of diminishing the number of
*palpalis*, whereas it is probable that the only effect of this host instead of
increasing, is to *reduce* the numbers of flies, by adversely affecting their reproductive powers.

Minchin thought that the fish-eating birds of this region might furnish a constant supply of food and this view is supported by the fact that in captivity the flies readily feed on fowls and moreover thrive on this diet. *G. palpalis* has been observed to feed on lizards, chameleons, snakes, frogs and mudfish, in addition to birds and mammals, but the latter constitute the most important hosts. There is little doubt that the fly prefers man to any other host and in captivity it thrives better when fed on human blood than on that of experimental animals.

As the fly feeds only during the daytime, it is evident that the various larger animals, such as antelopes, buffaloes, etc., that visit the water only at night time, or in the early morning must be excluded as a probable source of food, and it is generally agreed that *palpalis* is not dependent on the presence of big game.

Roubaud found that at 26° C. under ordinary conditions the female flies, if permitted to gorge themselves, fed once every three days, whereas the males would feed after two days, even when they had not digested their previous food. If the temperature was raised to 28° C. the females could be induced to feed more often, and at this temperature digestion was practically complete after 48 hours. In captivity the most favourable temperature for the flies was found to be about 28° C., but this is near the limit ; an alternation of 26° C. by day and 30° C. by night was well borne, but a continuous temperature of 30° C. was rapidly fatal. The degree of humidity has a marked effect on the ability of the fly to resist starvation, for at 33° C. in a saturated atmosphere insects were found to live six times longer than in one of moderate humidity, and twelve times longer than in a perfectly dry atmosphere. Similar results were obtained in the case of flies kept at 26° C., for in a saturated atmosphere a male and female were observed to live 10 and 13 days respectively, whereas in a dry atmosphere most of the flies were dead after one day and only one, a male, lived two days.

It follows, therefore, that dryness of the air accelerates nutritive changes and causes the fly to feed more frequently ;

the results also explain the necessity to the flies of a humid atmosphere such as the neighbourhood of shady rivers.

The length of life of the fly is very considerable. In the laboratory, Kleine observed one female to live for 227 days, which is the record up to the present. Carpenter has recently tried to ascertain the length of life of the fly by marking large numbers and then liberating them in order to see how long marked specimens could be caught at the same spot. One female was recaptured 182 days and one male 199 days after they had been marked.

*Reproduction.* As in all tsetse-flies *G. palpalis* does not lay eggs, but deposits the fully formed larva, after it has undergone a period of gestation within the uterus.

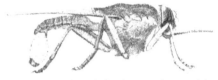

Fig. 69. *Glossina palpalis.* Female in the act of parturition. ( × 4.) (After Newstead.)

The first larva is dropped three to four weeks after copulation, the gestation being exceptionally long because the uterine glands are not well developed. Afterwards larvæ are dropped at intervals of nine to ten days, so long as the temperature remains at about 25° C. and the fly has abundant food. Roubaud found that one female produced eight larvæ in 13 weeks ; when dissected, the uterus of this fly contained one egg, but the ovary was empty. It is possible that the female may go on producing larvæ for a very considerable period, but the observations on this subject are too few to be of any use. Although in the laboratory the fly breeds all the year round, it is probable that in nature the seasonal effects may be very great, for in cold weather the tsetse does not bite readily and food has a marked influence on its reproductive activities. The female feeds readily at the commencement of gestation, but as the larva approaches maturity ceases to feed until it is born, when she again becomes hungry.

The pregnant flies are liable to certain accidents of gestation, for in captivity they frequently abort after being disturbed. Sometimes the larva pupates whilst still within the uterus, and in this case both the mother and its offspring invariably perish, as the former is unable to feed and the latter cannot emerge from the pupal case. A high degree of humidity is very unfavourable to reproduction, for Roubaud noticed that when flies were exposed to a saturated atmosphere they either aborted or did not develop larvæ. These results would explain why the females sometimes avoid the immediate neighbourhood of water, whereas the males generally seek the damp places where they require less food. The effect of this difference is to cause that separation of the sexes of the flies, that has been noticed by many observers.

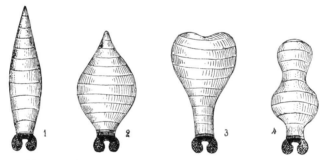

Fig. 70. Freshly laid larva of *Glossina palpalis* shewing the changes in the body form. (After Roubaud.)

When the larva is born it is a white cylindrical maggot, with two black protuberances at its posterior extremity. Its dimensions vary from 7 to 7·4 mm. in length by 2·8 to 3·5 mm. in diameter. At first the larva is very active, presenting curious alternate contractions and expansions of its body (Fig. 70) causing it to assume very varied forms. These movements enable the larva to bore its way into any fissures or loose soil, and are peculiar to the members of the genus *Glossina*. In loose sand the larva usually comes to rest at a depth of about half an inch to an inch and then pupates. The duration of the free larval stage does not exceed an hour to an hour and a half, but depends to some extent on the sur-roundings.  If the ground is soft and dry the larva very soon comes to rest and often pupates within half-an-hour, whereas in hard or damp soil it may be unable to find a suitable place for some little time.   In any case, the larva ceases to move after a comparatively short period of active life and then pupates.

The pupa is of the usual cylindrical form, but at its posterior extremity, it bears the two caudal protuberances that are present in the larva.   It darkens rapidly after its formation and within four hours becomes dark brown in colour.   The dimensions of the pupa are 6·5 to 6·6 mm. in length by 3·5 mm. in diameter.

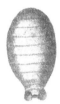 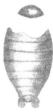

Fig. 71.  *Glossina palpalis.*  Puparia before and after the escape of the imago.  ( × 4).  (After Newstead.)

The duration of the pupal stage depends mainly on the temperature, and may vary from 17 to 72 days.  In the laboratory pupæ kept at 25°–27° C. hatch out in from 32 to 33 days, but at slightly lower temperatures Brumpt found that the nymphal period lasted from six to seven weeks. The optimum temperature is probably about 27 °C., for Roubaud found that pupæ exposed to higher temperatures either did not hatch, or produced unhealthy flies.  If placed in damp sand the pupæ are soon killed, and immersion in water, for periods exceeding 24 hours, is also fatal.  Moreover, a pupa exposed to the action of the sun's rays for four hours on two successive days, failed to hatch, although protected throughout the experiment by a layer of earth 5 cms. in thickness.

*Breeding localities.*  In 1906 pupæ of *G. palpalis* were discovered by Bagshawe on the shore of Lake George and subsequently on the shores of Lake Albert and the Victoria

Nile. The pupæ were all found within 10 to 25 yards of water, and were in the shelter of banana plants, or of shrubs, or of trees and tangled undergrowth, etc., where the soil consisted of crumbling vegetation. The pupæ lay at a depth of from half to a little more than an inch, and the site was always moderately dry. Zupitza in the Cameroons found the pupæ lying somewhat superficially in the humus and moss in the forks of branches, and cracks in the bark of trees, especially in the angles of the leaf-sheaths of palms, at a height of a few inches up to about 12 feet above the ground.

On the Sesse Islands, Fraser and Marshall found that the most favourable site for the pupæ was the loose dry sand on the shore of the water, close to the undergrowth that edged the forest and sheltered to some extent by the trees. The distance from high water mark was usually five yards and never more than 15. Later Fraser found that the pupæ were very numerous in sandy parts of the lake shore, as many as 800 being collected in one day.

Carpenter, in Uganda, has confirmed these observations and found that the locality where most pupæ were obtained (2000 to 3000 monthly) is formed of small pebbles mixed with coarse sand, four or five feet above the present level of the lake and about four to five yards from the water's edge. The pupæ are found at the edge of the belt of vegetation, which faces south-east and is shaded after mid-day.

Carpenter's conclusions are as follows :

" 1. Favourite sites for depositing pupæ are those which are in shade, but where there is free air circulation.

" 2. The soil, commonly gravel or coarse sand, must be dry and loose.

" 3. The fly does not extrude its larva until the middle of the day, always selecting a shady spot."

*Natural enemies.* The peculiar mode of reproduction of the tsetse-flies renders the immature stages to a great extent immune from the attacks of many insectivorous animals.

Nevertheless, the pupæ must be devoured by many species of birds, although up to the present there are no observations on this point. Bagshawe observed pupal cases with a small hole in the side; the contents had been devoured evidently by parasitic insects, probably belonging to the Chalcididæ.

The adult fly possesses numerous enemies, none of which, however, seem to be of very great importance in checking its numbers. Doubtless numerous insectivorous birds and reptiles must prey on the fly, but again precise information is lacking. The gorged insects are often carried off by a large species of wasp (*Bembex*), in order to furnish its burrows. Carpenter found no less than 31 tsetse-flies in the burrow of a species of *Bembex* occurring in Uganda. Roubaud often observed *G. palpalis* captured by spiders of the genus *Dolomedes*, which live on aquatic plants at the edge of streams and hunt both Diptera and Neuroptera. Ants are said to be very dangerous enemies, and when tsetse-flies are kept in cages they are frequently attacked and destroyed by swarms of a very small species, *Pheidole megacephala* F. The tiny ants seize hold of the legs and wings of the flies, which soon succumb to the attacks of these redoubtable foes.

It is possible that in nature various species of *Cincindela*, the tiger-beetle, prey on the tsetse-fly, for they are common on the banks of streams.

## G. PALPALIS *and Disease.*

It is well known that in nature sleeping sickness (*T. gambiense*) is mainly, if not entirely, transmitted by *G. palpalis*. Although it may be possible to infect other species of tsetse-flies in the laboratory, the distribution of sleeping sickness coincides so closely with that of *G. palpalis*, that there can be no doubt of its importance in the spread of the disease.

In addition a number of the trypanosomiases of animals have been shewn to be spread by this species. Thus it is the " host of choice " for *T. cazalboui*, and moreover has been proved capable of transmitting *T. brucei*, *T. dimorphon*, *T. pecaudi*, *T. nanum* and *T. pecorum*. It is probable that the trypanosome of crocodiles is also carried by *G. palpalis*.

REFERENCES.

Austen, E. (1911). *Handbook of the Tsetse-Flies.*
Bagshawe, A. G. (1909). *Sleeping Sickness Bulletin,* vol. I. p. 89.
(An excellent summary of all previous observations on *G. palpalis,* together with original notes and suggestions.)
Carpenter, G. D. H. (1912). *Rep. S. S. Comm. Roy. Soc.* p. 79.
Dutton and Todd (1906). Memoir XVIII. *Liv. School Trop. Med.*
Kleine (1909). *Deutsche Med. Wochenschr.* 1909, p. 1956.
Minchin, E. A. (1905). *Proc. Roy. Soc.* vol. LXXVI. p. 531.
Newstead, R. (1912). *Bull. Entom. Research,* vol. III. p. 355.
Roubaud, E. (1909). *La Glossina palpalis. Thèse de Doctorate ès Sci. Nat. Paris.*
——— (1911). *Compt. Rend. Acad. Sci.* 1911, p. 406.
Simpson, J. J. (1911). *Bull. Entom. Research,* vol. II. p. 187.

### Glossina pallidipes Austen, 1903.

*Description.* This species seems to be the eastern form of *G. longipalpis* which it resembles in most of its features. It may be distinguished from the other members of its group by the pale colour of the last two joints of the front and middle tarsi. It is a medium-sized or rather large species, the length of the female varying from 9·75 to 11·25 mm. and of the male from 8·5 to 10·4 mm.

*Distribution.* *G. pallidipes* is essentially an East African species and has been recorded from Zululand in the south to Uganda and British East Africa in the north. It is possible that its range has become more restricted in modern times for it is probable that it used to occur in the Transvaal, but disappeared after the rinderpest.

*Bionomics.* *G. pallidipes* resembles *morsitans* in its habits, but according to Neave is not so completely independent of water. In British East Africa it is especially abundant in certain belts along the coast, but also occurs inland, whilst in Portuguese East Africa it is found at higher altitudes than *morsitans,* going up to as much as 5000 feet. Generally speaking the fly seems to require a moderate degree of humidity, but is more or less independent of cover.

The late Dr W. A. Densham, as recorded by Austen, found the flies near and in a narrow belt of true forest at Kibero,

Uganda. "They were numerous along the native path, in long grass with scattered trees, for a quarter of a mile before reaching the forest. They attacked freely at 8.30 a.m. on a summer morning, were easily caught with the hand, and were observed to bite through a worn blue service puttee. They were seen and caught along the native path after entering the forest, and for two miles the other side of the belt, which is only about 300 yards in width, occasional flies being seen until the village was reached. Half-an-hour after arrival two were captured by my boys in camp and brought to me. On returning from the village next day no flies were seen until nearing the forest, so that the ' occasional ' flies mentioned above may all have been ' following' flies. If so, they follow much further than *G. palpalis.* There are many rhino, pig, and buffalo in the forest, and *Colobus* monkeys are numerous. There are no natives nearer than two miles, but a well-trodden path connects two villages, and passes through the fly. The natives know of the fly but do not consider it dangerous to animals. They keep sheep and goats, and drive them along this path. No cattle are kept for many miles round."

In British East Africa, Dr P. H. Ross found that *G. pallidipes* generally occurs on the edge of the bush or in open spaces where animals, chiefly goats, graze, but never at any great distance from water. It is easily found from July to October, the dry season, but during the rest of the year is practically absent. In this locality the fly is frequently attracted by the lights of trains, etc., and has been observed to enter railway carriages and be transported a distance of at least 150 miles.

In Mozambique, Dr Sant' Anna found several areas infested with fly. These areas consist of forests of low trees with poor foliage and of somewhat short and scattered herbaceous vegetation, with few shrubs. The tsetse-flies are usually very rare but in some regions they occur in large numbers. In the largest of these areas, known as Maganja da Costa, to the east of the river Licugo, the flies occurred in enormous numbers in the native huts. Although the species is stated to be *morsitans* all the flies sent from this locality were determined by Austen as *G. pallidipes.*

## G. PALLIDIPES and Disease.

As mentioned below Austen has shewn that it is almost certain that Bruce, in his Zululand experiments on the transmission of *T. brucei*, employed *G. pallidipes* and not *G. morsitans*. In addition, Dr P. H. Ross has found *G. pallidipes* in British East Africa naturally infected with a trypanosome that seems to belong to the *dimorphon* group. In one case a dog naturally infected with trypanosomes on Mombasa Island, is stated to have been almost certainly infected by the bites of *G. pallidipes* on the island.

In another case wild *G. pallidipes* from the neighbourhood of Kibwezi (British East Africa) were fed on a healthy monkey. In all "209 flies were fed between July 15 and December 10. The animal died on January 11, and it was only after death that trypanosomes were found. Inoculation of blood from the dead monkey into a fresh monkey resulted in infection, but inoculation of a dog at the same time failed. In this case infection was suspected nine days after feeding began, but repeated examinations of the blood during five months were always negative. The monkey became very thin, and had all the appearance of a trypanosome-infected monkey, and the temperature chart was also very suggestive of trypanosomiasis. The trypanosomes found in this animal were 17–18 microns in length, including a short, free flagellum, and had rather a blunt posterior end."

In further experiments with this trypanosome, goats and sheep were found to be immune against infection and two monkeys that became infected were alive after five months and a year respectively. With regard to the immunity of goats and sheep, the author notes that the Wakamba natives move their cattle to the hills in August when *G. pallidipes* is about to reappear, stating that the fly would kill them, but they do not move their sheep and goats.

From these observations it is evident that *G. pallidipes* is capable of transmitting other infections in addition to *T. brucei*, but up to the present there is no very precise information as to the manner in which it is effected. Presumably the transmission is usually indirect, as in the case of most other species of tsetse-flies.

REFERENCES.

Austen, E. (1903). *Monograph of the Tsetse-Flies.*
Neave, S. A. (1912). *Bull. Entom. Research*, vol. III. p. 275.
Ross, P. H. (1909–10). *Reports of the Nairobi Bacteriological Laboratory.*
Sant' Anna, J. F. (1911). Quoted in *S. S. Bulletin*, vol. III. p. 143.

## Glossina longipalpis Wied., 1830.

*Description.* This species closely resembles *G. pallidipes* in its general appearance. It is slightly larger than *G. morsitans* and may be distinguished by the possession of a fringe of fine hairs on the anterior margin of the third joint of the antennæ. In addition the dark brown, transverse, abdominal bands extend close to the hind margins of the segments, and the last two joints of the front and middle tarsi have sharply defined, clove-brown or black tips. The length of the male varies from 8·4 to 9·0 mm. and of the female from 9·0 to 10·0 mm.

*Distribution.* *G. longipalpis* is essentially a West African species, its range extending from Senegal to the south-eastern corner of the Congo Free State. In addition a single specimen was collected in 1864, by Sir John Kirk in the Zambesi valley, between Tete and the Victoria Falls. There are no other records, however, of its occurrence further south than the Congo Free State and it seems to have disappeared from the valley of the Zambesi. Between the limits of its distribution the species is fairly common and it is one of the most important tsetse-flies of the West Coast of Africa.

*Bionomics.* *G. longipalpis*, although not closely restricted to the immediate vicinity of water, is not found as far distant from it as *G. morsitans*. In southern Nigeria, Simpson states that the species is associated with a moister climate and is especially found in denser vegetation of the mixed deciduous forest type. On the other hand, Kinghorn states that in Ashanti *G. longipalpis* is essentially an open country fly and is not found in the forest belt. The only grass country in which it was rare was Banda and its absence from this locality was attributed to very large stretches of land being under cultivation. The most important observations on the bionomics of this species are those of Roubaud in Dahomey. In this region *G. longipalpis* is found near the streams and large rivers. The separation of the sexes is well marked, the males being met with only in the tufts of bushes along the edge of the forest near the water courses, while the females are found in open clearings where there are acacias and mimosas. The fly is especially abundant during the rains, but seems to disappear almost completely in the dry season, especially after the bush is burnt. During the rainy season the fly extends its range very considerably and may be found more and more outside its usual haunts, individuals occurring in the savannahs far from any water course. The period of the north-east wind (Harmattan) is very unfavourable to them.

*G. longipalpis* feeds mainly on wild mammals, accompanying them in their movements; it especially frequents paths recently trodden by hippopotamus and elephant.

*Reproduction.* *G. longipalpis* has never been observed to copulate in captivity. Moreover, it is very susceptible to the influence of physical conditions, a temperature of 35°–37° C., with either saturated or dry air, interfering with reproduction.

At 25° C., Roubaud found that the females deposited larvæ at intervals of about ten days, and the pupal stage, at an average temperature of from 24° to 25° C., was found to last from 26 to 35 days. The pupæ hatch out all the year round, including the cold season, and the diminution of flies in the dry season cannot be explained by the assumption that during this period the pupal stage is prolonged.

## G. LONGIPALPIS *and* Disease.

This species is a most important carrier of animal trypano-somiasis. Thus in Dahomey, Bouet and Roubaud found that the wild flies were frequently naturally infected with *T. dimorphon*, and that on the Ouémé River a very large pro-portion of the flies were infected with *T. pecaudi*. *G. longipalpis* is said to be the "host of choice" for this latter trypanosome.

In addition, this species is an efficient intermediate host for *T. cazalboui*.

REFERENCES.

Austen, E. (1911). *Handbook of the Tsetse-Flies*, p. 63.

Bouet and Roubaud (1910). *Ann. Inst. Pasteur*, vol. XXIV. p. 658 ; *Bull. Soc. Path. Exot.* vol. III. pp. 599, 722.

Kinghorn, A. (1911). Cf. *S. S. Bulletin*, vol. III. p. 136.

Roubaud, E. (1911). *Compt. Rend. Acad. Sci.* vol. CLII. p. 406.

Simpson, J. J. (1912). *Bull. Entom. Research*, vol. III. p. 137.

### Glossina morsitans Westwood, 1850.

Synonym. *Glossina submorsitans* Newstead, 1911.

♂, ♀. Length ♂ 7·2 to 9 mm., ♀ 8·6 to 9·6 mm. ; width of head, ♂ 2·4 to 2·75 mm., ♀ 2·5 to 3 mm. ; width of front at vertex, ♂ 0·6 mm., ♀ 0·8 to 1 mm., length of wing, ♂ 7·6 to 8·2 mm., ♀ 8·2 to 9·5 mm.

" Dorsum of thorax light grey, olivaceous-grey, or smoke-grey in ♂, drab-grey in ♀, the thoracic markings in both sexes incompletely developed, and reduced to brownish or mouse-grey longitudinal streaks ; dorsum of abdomen buff to ochraceous-buff (in pinned specimens sometimes mouse-grey or olivaceous owing to post mortem changes), with a larger or smaller clove-brown blotch (sometimes indistinct or almost wanting) near each basal angle

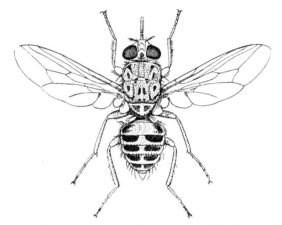

Fig. 72. *Glossina morsitans.* Dorsal view of female. ( × 4.)

of the second segment, and the third to the sixth segments inclusive each with a very conspicuous clove-brown transverse band, interrupted in the median line, not reaching the lateral margins, and not extending beyond the basal three-fourths of the segment, if so far ; legs buff, last two joints of hind tarsi clove-brown or black, last two joints of front tarsi and penultimate joint of middle tarsi conspicuously tipped with clove-brown or dark brown, last joint of middle tarsi entirely dark brown above in typical race, otherwise distal half or third of last joint of middle tarsi alone dark brown or clove-brown, re-mainder of joint merely brownish or even entirely pale." (Austen.)

## *Glossina morsitans* Westw., var. *pallida* Shircore.

" *Thorax* slate-grey, pattern indistinguishable ; scutellum with two dark triangular areas which are contiguous at their upper inner angles. *Abdomen* with the darker blotches on each side of the second segment very faint ; on the other segments the banding is not a prominent feature, as it is in the typical form ; the bands olive-grey, their margins being distinct and defined from the ground-colour, which is a few shades lighter. In the middle line the banding is cut off square, leaving a very narrow straight line down the centre of the segments ; the outer margins of the bands sloping away from below upwards and leaving light areas on each side. *Legs* with all the joints of the front and middle tarsi pale,'except the distal end of the latter which has a faint darkish ring ; the last two joints of the hind tarsi faintly dark, but nothing like so dark as in *G. morsitans. Wings* tinged with light yellowish-brown.

NYASALAND : 1 ♂, Dowa district, 6. v. 1912.

*Type* in the British Museum.

This fly was picked out at a glance from more than a hundred *G. morsitans*, and is distinctly and remarkably paler throughout." (Shircore.)

## *Glossina morsitans* Westw., var. *paradoxa* Shircore.

" Superficially resembles *G. morsitans* in appearance and size, but *the hind tarsi are entirely dark*, as in the *palpalis* group. The superior claspers of the male genitalia resemble those of *G. submorsitans*, as figured by Prof. Newstead, but are more deeply pigmented throughout, and especially along the lateral and posterior borders.

NYASALAND : 1 ♂, Nyamsato, near Chunzi, Dowa district, 4. vi. 12.

*Type* in the British Museum.

If casually observed, this tsetse would probably be taken for an ordinary *G. morsitans* ; but if the abdomen had become discoloured it might well be mistaken for *G. palpalis*. The superior claspers have only been looked at with a hand-lens ( × 12) ; they were prized open and examined *in situ*." (Shircore.)

*Distribution. G. morsitans* is by far the most widely distributed of all the tsetse-flies, occurring from Abyssinia and Senegambia in the north to Zululand in the south. In all cases the fly is restricted to very definite regions known as " fly-belts " or " fly-areas," and does not occur spread over large tracts of country. It is therefore difficult to give an accurate idea of its distribution without going into great detail, but the fly has been recorded from the following countries :

Southern Abyssinia, Anglo-Egyptian Sudan, Bahr el Ghazal, Uganda, British, German, and Portuguese East Africa, Zululand, the North Eastern Transvaal, Bechuanaland, S., N. E. and N. W. Rhodesia, Nyasaland, the Congo Free State, Upper

Ubangi, Northern and Southern Nigeria, Dahomey, Togoland, Gold Coast Colony, Ashanti, Northern Territories, Ivory Coast, French Guinea, Gambia and Senegal.

*Bionomics.* In the present place it is only possible to give a brief account of the more important observations on this subject. The reader desirous of further information will find an excellent summary of all the earlier observations on *G. morsitans* in Austen's *Monograph of the Tsetse-flies*.

As a general rule, *G. morsitans* is confined to certain restricted and often very well-defined tracts of country, known as "fly-belts," the boundaries of which, however, are liable to variation; for Hall found that in North Eastern Rhodesia the fly considerably extended its range of distribution between the years 1904 and 1909, and Neave is of the opinion that the flies are now recovering the ground lost at the time of the rinderpest, when *G. morsitans* disappeared from the Transvaal.

Usually the fly prefers a region in which there is sufficient vegetation to provide a moderate but not excessive cover, and a hot and moderately dry climate. It seems to be almost independent of surface water and is most active in a dry atmosphere ; though in some districts the flies seem to be more common in the neighbourhood of rivers.

In Nyasaland they are never found in open grass country, but only in bush, especially in those portions of the forest where Sanya trees and antelope are most abundant. Dense forest is generally avoided by the flies, but they prefer regions scattered with trees that give shade. Sir Alfred Sharpe's observations in this region are of considerable interest, especially on the effect of cultivation on the prevalence of the fly. He states " I am acquainted with villages which are situated inside fly-areas and wherever the natives build their villages in such localities, and clear ground for their food-gardens, tsetse immediately disappear from the cleared ground. I have often noticed that, when approaching those villages from the bush, fly which are following the carriers, or are actually upon their persons biting them, will gradually disappear after entering the cleared ground, and by the time the village is reached, no fly can be seen. On the other hand, I have known cases where villages have

been abandoned, and after a time, as the natural bush has
grown up, the flies have reappeared in places where the native
food-plantations formerly were." The same observer is also
of the opinion that the tsetse is not entirely dependent for its
existence upon the blood of wild mammals. In Nyasaland,
enormous numbers of tsetse occur in districts that are almost
destitute of game and at the north end of Lake Nyasa, before
the advent of rinderpest, there were many thousands of buffalo
but no *morsitans*. On the other hand, it is the opinion of

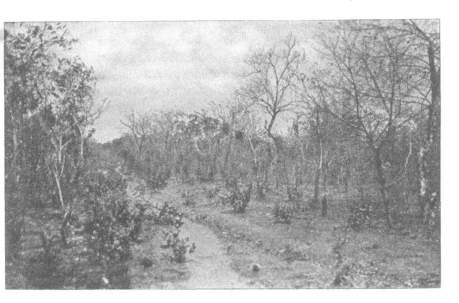

Fig. 73. Path through thin deciduous bush between Yallol and Fula Fara-
feni, Bathurst, to shew a typical haunt of *G. morsitans*. (After Simpson.)

many observers that when game and especially buffaloes are
abundant, the fly also appears in large numbers and that after
the epidemic of rinderpest, following which in many regions
there was very little game and practically no buffaloes, the
fly disappeared. Amongst these conflicting statements it is
difficult to arrive at the truth, but certainly Sharpe's observation that the tsetse may occur in the absence of wild mammals,
shews that any scheme of game destruction would be both rash

and premature at the present time, considering our incomplete knowledge of the subject. No direct evidence has yet been published, supporting the view that *morsitans* takes in any food other than blood, but the flies have been observed apparently drinking dirty water at the edges of puddles. If placed in a bottle with ripe water-melon the flies may be seen to thrust their proboscides into it, but there is no evidence of any food being ingested.

The effect of climate on the numbers of flies is very marked. Within a " fly-area " the tsetse will not necessarily be found there at all times of the year. It is often possible to go through such a region without seeing a single fly. For example, in Nyasaland, between the settlement of Zomba and the Mlange Mountains, a distance of about 40 miles, lies an extensive plain. During the months of May or June flies are practically absent, whereas in October, it is necessary to pass through about 25 miles of " fly." On the advent of the first rains in November, they begin to disappear, but may still be found until the arrival of the cold weather in April and May. In the Luangwa Valley, North Eastern Rhodesia, Lloyd observed that the fly was very common during the early part of the dry season, but the numbers diminished until the commencement of the rains, when the numbers at once increased. At Nzoa, in the higher ground of the Congo Zambesi watershed (altitude 4000 ft.), the fly only became numerous after the rains had ceased. It is evident, therefore, that within any particular fly-area, the number of tsetse may vary according to the season of the year.

Although many observers state that *G. morsitans* is more or less independent of moisture, Dr J. O. Shircore, who has devoted a great deal of attention to this question, has clearly shewn that in Nyasaland, and probably in other regions, the fly is greatly affected in its distribution by the presence or absence of moisture. At the height of the dry season the tsetse is only found in certain restricted areas to which the term " Primary Fly Centres " has been applied. These primary centres are the only regions where, in the dry season, water is actually above the earth's surface, or at no great distance below it.

In these places there is light forest with fairly short grass and occasionally open glades, whilst game is abundant, a combination which is ideal for the flies.  From these regions they extend into the surrounding country along connecting forest as soon as the conditions become suitable, and this extension may easily be observed.

Dr Shircore, therefore, advocates the destruction of the primary centres by means of clearing and bush-fires, during the height of the dry season, when there are very few tsetse-flies in the surrounding country.  As these primary centres are often of very limited area, the destruction of the fly in these regions is a prophylactic measure that might easily be adopted, instead of the game destruction and wholesale clearance of the country which is being advocated by certain individuals.

The fly will feed with avidity on almost any large mammal or bird, and does not seem to be dependent on any particular species for its food-supply.  In Nigeria, Simpson noticed that these insects seem to have a great predilection for baboons, enormous swarms accompanying the herds of these animals, and in the Bahr el Ghazal, Selous has noticed the same peculiarity.

Usually G. *morsitans* becomes active about sunrise, disappears during the hottest hours of the day and recommences to bite when it becomes cooler and also after the sun has set. Other observers, however, state that it is most aggressive during the hottest hours of the day.  Occasionally they will feed at night, especially if a bright moon is shining, and sometimes even in its absence.  As a rule the flies disappear during a shower, but they have been known to bite during heavy rain.

Like G. *palpalis*, the present species is especially attracted by moving objects, but quickly leaves them as soon as all motion ceases.  Thus Montgomery and Kinghorn note that even in its natural haunts, G. *morsitans* will quickly retreat from a person coming to a halt, although they may have been pestilent immediately prior to this.

In addition to being attracted by dark colours, Newstead found that the shades most preferred by this species were khaki and yellowish-green, whilst white was the least attractive of all. The flies will readily bite through one thickness of clothing and if the bottoms of the trousers are open they frequently creep up the legs and bite above the socks.

The males feed on blood as readily as the females, and the large swarms of tsetse are mainly composed of the former. The females seem to be more hardy than the males, for in certain transmission experiments with G. *morsitans*, Fischer employed 636 males and 766 females ; 70 days later only 135 males had survived, whilst 265 females were still alive.

In captivity moisture is rapidly fatal to this species ; moreover it is very intolerant of high temperatures, for Roubaud, in Dahomey, observed that specimens exposed to 40° C. died within an hour. The fly, however, occurs in districts, *e.g.* the Luangwa Valley, where the thermometer frequently registers 42° C. in the shade.

Practically nothing is known about the natural enemies of G. *morsitans*, but Newstead in Nyasaland has found examples of the fly in the food contents of two species of birds, viz. : the common African Drongo (*Dicrurus afer*) and a small Bee-eater. It is possible that the fly is susceptible to rinderpest for it is difficult to explain the disappearance of this insect from South Africa and the Transvaal on any other hypothesis.

The well-known hunter, Mr F. C. Selous, has published some interesting observations relating to this question. It is well known that after the great epidemic of rinderpest in 1896, G. *morsitans* disappeared from practically all the country south of the Zambesi. Throughout this region the buffaloes were exterminated, but although there seems to have been a very close association between these animals and G. *morsitans*, it is well known that the tsetse-fly can thrive on the blood of other animals, and as zebras, giraffes, antelopes, etc. were all left in considerable numbers it is difficult to understand why the fly also disappeared.

It is possible, of course, that the tsetse-fly had become so restricted in its feeding habits, that when its usual host, the buffalo, disappeared, it was unable to adapt itself to feeding on other animals and simply died out through lack of food, but it seems more reasonable to suppose that the rinderpest had a directly injurious action on the fly. Further observations on this question are necessary in order to explain the disappearance of *G. morsitans* from certain parts of Africa in recent times.

*Reproduction.* Most of the observations on the breeding habits of *G. morsitans* have been made during the past two or three years and are still very incomplete. Unlike *G. longipalpis*, *morsitans* readily copulates in captivity and in consequence the flies can be raised in the laboratory without much difficulty.

Fischer found that on Lake Victoria, bred flies began to drop larvæ about the twentieth day after hatching. Kinghorn, in Northern Rhodesia, states that 14 to 15 days is the usual gestation period under laboratory conditions (temperature 58·5° to 77·8° F.), but much irregularity was displayed by the females, and after the first larva had been born, many of them did not produce a second one for a considerable time. In Upper Dahomey, Roubaud found that the interval between successive deposits of larvæ, at a temperature of about 32° C., was usually eight to nine days.

Newstead found the pupæ in three separate spots in the forest, about one and a half miles from the banks of the Shire River, at a place lying about 18 miles due north of Liwonde, Nyasaland. The pupæ were found buried in soil at the foot of various trees. In Rhodesia, Jack has found the pupæ in several localities, *e.g.* under a clump of Mubula trees ; on a high ant-heap ; under the exposed roots of a Baobab ; at the base of a Mopani tree, etc. The author writes : " In all places except two, where pupæ were found, the soil was either sandy and easily worked, often rich in humus, or covered with leaves which afforded an easily penetrable shelter. In two instances cases were taken from hard soil, in one instance one and a half inches below the surface, but the chitin which forms the case is an enduring substance in a dry situation, so that the age of these cases is difficult to judge. The soil may have been soft when the larvæ entered or they may have penetrated along a crack. It is in the highest degree improbable that a larva could penetrate one and a half inches of hard baked ant-heap.

In every instance the ground was well drained and often the slope was very sharp.   All the pupa cases except four were from trees near the bank of a river or wet vlei, where there was shade and where the " fly " congregates in the dry weather. The four excepted were taken from the base of a large Baobab tree on the summit of a hill not far from a river (the Sinyama)

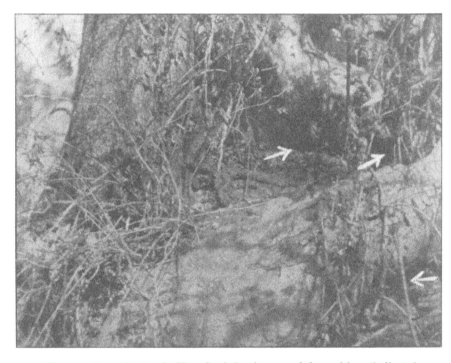

Fig. 74    Base of a tree in Nyasaland shewing one of the positions (indicated by arrows) in which the pupæ of *Glossina morsitans* may be found.  (After Jack.)

it is true, but away from the influence of the water, there being no shade about the roots in August.   This points to the fact that the larvæ are deposited in any convenient situation, when the fly is scattered during the wet weather....

" The summary of the investigations into the breeding haunts is therefore, that in the dry weather the larvæ are deposited in sheltered positions about the bases of big shady trees, such as are at that time of the year practically confined to the banks of rivers, pools, and vleis, dry or otherwise on the surface. Generally the soil is easily worked, and often humus is abundant, and the drainage is usually good. The selection of a well drained situation may not seem necessary in the dry weather, but the instinct to select such would doubtless be of great value, when the pupal period extends into the rains. During the wet weather it is probable that the young are deposited more generally through the bush."

Mr R. S. Harger, late of North Eastern Rhodesia, in a letter published in *The Field* states that he had often watched *G. morsitans* depositing its eggs (= larvæ) in the damp soil, thrown up by the digging of a trench round his tent.

In captivity, when the freshly laid larva is placed on powdered earth it immediately commences to burrow until it is from one to two centimetres below the surface, when it at once proceeds to pupate. Apparently the larvæ are capable of secreting a slightly viscid fluid, for in glass tubes they were often observed to adhere to the side and Kinghorn suggests that the purpose of this fluid is to gather the earth around the pupa.

As in all species of *Glossina*, the duration of the pupal stage varies according to the temperature. In Rhodesia, at a temperature of 15° to 25° C., Kinghorn found that the pupal period varied from 47 to 53 days. On Lake Victoria, according to Fischer, the period lasts on an average from 35 to 40 days, whilst Roubaud, in the Upper Dahomey, found that at a temperature of about 32° C. the duration of the pupal stage was only 23 to 28 days. Lloyd, at Nawalia, obtained similar results, for at temperatures ranging from 17° to 28° C., the average duration of the pupal period varied from 22 to 51 days.

As in the case of *G. palpalis*, intra-uterine pupation has been observed occasionally.

### G. MORSITANS *and Disease.*

*G. morsitans* is known to be the carrier of more trypanosome diseases than any other species of *Glossina*.

In the first place it has been proved to be the main, if not the only, carrier of *T. rhodesiense*, the pathogenic agent of the human trypanosomiasis of Rhodesia, Nyasaland and certain parts of German East Africa (Rovuma River). Moreover Fischer's experiments on the Victoria Lake, clearly shew that under experimental conditions *T. gambiense* may be transmitted by this species of tsetse, in which it undergoes a cyclical development.

In addition *G. morsitans* has been proved to be the intermediate host of the following infections : *T. brucei, T. pecaudi, T. cazalboui, T. dimorphon, T. pecorum, T. congolense* and *T. simiæ*, each of which is described below, together with the manner in which the fly conveys the infection.

REFERENCES.

Austen, E. (1903). *Monograph of the Tsetse-Flies.*
—— (1911). *Handbook of the Tsetse-Flies.*
Fischer, W. (1913). *Arch. f. Schiffs u. Trop. Hyg.* vol. XVII. p. 73.
Hall (1910). *Bull. Ent. Research,* vol. I. p. 183.
Jack, R. (1912). *Ibid.* vol. II. p. 357.
Kinghorn, A. (1912). *Ibid.* vol. II. p. 291.
Lloyd, Ll. (1912). *Ibid.* vol. III. p. 233.
Montgomery and Kinghorn (1909). *Ann. Trop. Med. and Parasit.* vol. III. p. 322.
Neave, S. A. (1912). *Bull. Ent. Research,* vol. III. p. 275.
Newstead, R. (1910). *Ann. Trop. Med. and Parasit.* vol. IV. p. 369.
Roubaud, E. (1911). *Compt. Rend. Acad. Sci.,* No. 14, p. 637.
Sharpe, Sir A. (1910). *Bull. Ent. Research,* vol. I. p. 173.
Simpson, J.J. (1912). *Ibid.* vol. II. p. 301, and vol. III. p. 137.
Selous, F. C. (1910). *African Nature Notes and Reminiscences,* London.
Shircore, J. O. (1914). *Bull. Ent. Research,* vol. V. p. 87.

### Glossina longipennis Corti, 1895.

*Description.* This species resembles *G. brevipalpis* in its size and general appearance, but may easily be distinguished by the presence of four sharply defined, dark brown, more or less elongate spots on the thorax arranged in a parallelogram, two in front and two behind the transverse suture. The proboscis bulb has a sharply defined brown, or dark brown, tip. The length of the male varies from 10·2 to 11·6 mm., and of the female from 11·9 to 13·0 mm.

*Distribution.* G. *longipennis* seems to be restricted to the north east corner of Africa for it has only been recorded from Somaliland and British East Africa. It probably also occurs in Southern Abyssinia.

*Bionomics.* Dr P. H. Ross states that the present species is found all the year round in the same haunts as G. *brevipalpis.* It is most easily caught after 4 p.m. resting on the red soil of paths or caravan tracks, and seems to resemble G. *brevipalpis* in its feeding habits. G. *longipennis* is attracted by lights at night and is probably the commonest tsetse-fly caught in the railway carriages. On one occasion for a night and a day the station master's house at Kenani was occupied by these flies in such numbers that during the night the lamps were extinguished, and Ross suggests that this may be an instance of migration. Incidentally it may be mentioned that Peel, who captured this species in West Somaliland, found that it occurred in a definite fly-belt extending from Biermuddo to Boholo Deno. The species seems to be independent of water and most active in a dry atmosphere. Brumpt found that in Somaliland it generally fed at night, attacking both man and animals.

## G. LONGIPENNIS *and Disease.*

Brumpt is of the opinion that Aïno, a cattle disease of Somaliland caused by a trypanosome probably identical with *T. brucei,* is transmitted by G. *longipennis,* and brings forward evidence in support of his hypothesis. Dr P. H. Ross is the only one who has succeeded in obtaining any experimental proof of the disease-transmitting capabilities of this species. A large number of freshly caught flies from the neighbourhood of Kenani were kept in an incubator at 25° C. The flies were then fed on a monkey between 5th December, 1912, and January 11th, 1913, the animal being bitten 577 times. Trypanosomes were found in its blood on January 13th and the author for the present would class them in the *T. dimorphon* group.

### REFERENCES.

Austen, E. (1911). *Handbook of the Tsetse-flies.*
Brumpt, E. (1902). *Arch. de Parasitologie,* vol. v. p. 158.
Ross, P. H. (1904–10). *Nairobi Laboratory Reports,* vol. i. also *Tropical Diseases Bulletin,* 1913, vol. i. p. 505.

### Glossina brevipalpis Newstead, 1910.

*Synonyms.* *G. fusca* Austen, 1903 (*nec* Walker). *G. tabaniformis* Stuhlmann, 1902 (*nec* Westwood).

*Description.* Owing to an unfortunate error in Austen's Monograph, *G. brevipalpis* was there described under the name *G. fusca*, as with the scanty material at the author's command it was very difficult to form correct conclusions as to the characters of the species. As a result the majority of writers following Austen, have described the habits and occurrence of the present species under the name *G. fusca*.

*G. brevipalpis* is the common large tsetse-fly of many parts of Eastern, Central, and Southern Africa. The most striking casual feature of the species is the darkening of the wings in the region of the anterior and posterior transverse veins, so as to appear as dark spots on the otherwise pale wings. It may be distinguished from *G. longipennis* by the absence of a dark brown ocellar spot, of a brown tip to the proboscis bulb and of the characteristic dark spots on the thorax. In addition, it may be distinguished from *G. fusca* by having the proboscis and palpi much shorter ; the head distinctly wider, and closer to the thorax ; the thoracic markings and general colouration much less distinct ; also, the size is often larger.

The length of the male varies from 10·2 to 12·25 mm. and of the female from 11·0 to 13·5 mm.

*Distribution.* This species has been recorded from British, German and Portuguese East Africa, Uganda, Nyasaland, Northern Rhodesia, the Katanga district of the Congo Free State and Angola. Although occurring in the two latter districts, *G. brevipalpis* has not hitherto been found on the west coast of Africa, but is essentially an East African species.

*Bionomics.* The many descriptions of the habits of this species have nearly all been given under the name of *G. fusca* and this point should be remembered in looking up references on the subject. *G. brevipalpis* requires only a moderate degree of humidity and is generally found where there is fairly heavy timber and bush. It is more adaptable to external conditions than *G. palpalis*, and Stuhlmann notes that it requires an average yearly temperature of 23° to 26° C., with a maximum of 36° to

37° C. and a minimum of 10° to 12° C., and an average humidity of 66 to 83 %. In British East Africa it occurs at varying levels from the sea coast to Fort Hall, a height of 4000 feet. According to Dr P. H. Ross, in the valley of Kibwezi it is generally found among rocks on the hills, resting on the slightly damp black cotton soil between boulders. It may be caught in quantities all the year round, but is more abundant during the wet season. It is said to be markedly nocturnal in its feeding habits and on one occasion was met with in numbers resembling a swarm of bees. On the other hand Milne states that the fly generally bites between three and five in the afternoon, and in the Kibwezi valley is more prevalent during May and June than any other time of the year.

In German East Africa, Stuhlmann found that the fly was present at Anami all the year round, but Keysselitz and Mayer state that very few females could be captured during December, January and February. Like many other species of tsetse-fly, *G. brevipalpis* occasionally follows animals to some distance from its actual haunts and Stuhlmann notes that in this way, especially during the hot weather, isolated examples were frequently found amongst the mountains at altitudes up to 3250 feet, whilst during December to April the flies were often met with in the settlements.

In Nyasaland, Davey recorded the capture of a few individuals belonging to this species, all of which, with one exception, were caught within 900 yards of the edge of Lake Nyasa. Sanderson was informed by the natives that during the rains (January), at which time practically the whole country is under water, *G. brevipalpis* is very prevalent in North Nyasaland all over the grassy plain lying between the shore of the lake and a line of foot-hills some ten miles away. In June and July this species was found, sometimes in very large numbers, in the beds of all the streams between Karongo and Sougive, although many of them were dry. It was occasionally caught in the native villages.

According to Dr Sanderson, *G. brevipalpis* is active and desirous of feeding only in the early morning before 8.0 o'clock and in the evening after about 4.0 o'clock. During the daytime the fly remains sheltered under the leaves of bushes, or in the grass, always near the ground, or low down on the trunks of trees, not more than two or three feet from the base.

At Kaporo, near the north end of Lake Nyasa, Davey found that they preferred to rest on trees surrounded by creepers and undergrowth, and hidden away in crevices in the bark or under the branches. While thus resting motionless Sanderson states that the flies are very difficult to discover and their presence would be entirely unsuspected.

About 4.0 p.m. when the fly is ready to feed, it emerges from its hiding-place and settles on dried leaves, sticks or dust on paths, apparently lying in wait for a meal. As the wild animals on their way to the water in the evening often stand for a time on emerging from the forest on to a path, the flies would thus have an opportunity of feeding. According to Davey, although *G. brevipalpis* as a rule seems ready to bite human beings in the evening, it does not set to work with the same rapidity and voracity as *G. morsitans*.

Stuhlmann kept large numbers of the flies in captivity at Amani, German East Africa, and found that they required a meal of blood at least every six or seven days, and by feeding them every fourth or fifth day, individual females were kept alive for upwards of four months.

Sanderson writes : " The flies bite through dark clothes, but have never been seen to settle on white surfaces " and Stuhlmann frequently noticed that when a light and a dark-coloured mule were walking side by side, only the latter was attacked.

In Nyasaland, Davey found that wherever he met with this fly game was abundant. Once during the wet season, having shot two bush-pigs about sunset, on going up to them he found several *G. brevipalpis* apparently trying to suck blood from the carcases, although for some time previously he had been unable to find any of the flies.

Although in captivity approximately equal numbers of males and females are obtained from pupæ, there is an enormous preponderance of males among the captured specimens.

Stuhlmann found that in order to catch females it was necessary to use some animal as a decoy, but even then they were much more difficult to catch than males. The gravid females are probably much more wary and move about less than the males, and are consequently more rarely caught.

*Reproduction.* In nature the flies have occasionally been observed *in coitû* on tree-trunks. Stuhlmann noticed that in captivity only freshly hatched females received the males, but possibly the behaviour of the flies was modified by the artificial conditions.

Stuhlmann has. given a very complete account of the breeding habits of this species in German East Africa and the following observations are taken from his report.

When females were kept at a temperature of 23° to 25° C., they gave birth to larvæ at intervals of about 12 days, but by varying the temperature the interval could be varied from 10 to 21 days. In three and a half months one female gave birth to eight larvæ, of which, however, two were dead. The extrusion of larvæ apparently proceeds uninterruptedly the whole year round, but the intervals are prolonged during the cold season.

The freshly extruded larva is of the usual *Glossina* shape and its behaviour previous to pupation has been well described.

" If the new-born larva be placed in a glass dish or on blotting-paper, it crawls about for a time exactly like an ordinary fly-maggot, after which it becomes stationary and soon contracts, its chitinous integument thickens and darkens, and in about three-quarters of an hour it has assumed the appearance of a coarctate pupa. If, however, the larva be transferred to moderately damp sand, it at once burrows into it, making a straight tunnel ; thus in one case a larva penetrated to a depth of 8·5 cms. Under such conditions, from an hour and a quarter to an hour and a half elapsed before the change to the pupal state was completed. In dry sand a larva did not burrow so deeply, since, as it burrowed, the sand continually fell in, but nevertheless it reached a depth of 2 to 3 cms. We may assume that in nature the larvæ behave in a similar way ; the fly will deposit its offspring on a spot which is sheltered and slightly damp, and the larva will at once burrow beneath the surface."

The average duration of the pupal stage at 30° C. was found to be about 36 days, but by varying the temperature it could be shortened to 30 days or prolonged to as much as 65 days.

There is some evidence to shew that this species may reproduce parthenogenetically, for on two occasions Stuhlmann observed fully developed larvæ laid by virgin females that had been bred in captivity.

## G. BREVIPALPIS and Disease.

Although there is little doubt that the present species is an important carrier of cattle trypanosomes precise information is lacking. According to Stuhlmann, in German East Africa it is one of the chief disseminators of Nagana among domestic animals. Both Koch and Stuhlmann fed G. brevipalpis on animals infected with T. brucei and attempted to trace the development of the parasite within the vertebrate host. The latter author gives an interesting description of the various supposed developmental changes undergone by the trypanosomes, but in no case did any direct inoculation experiments give positive results and therefore the transmission of T. brucei by G. brevipalpis remains as yet unproven.

Similarly in the case of T. gambiense, Koch observed a commencement of its development in the gut of G. brevipalpis and Fischer is of the opinion that this species may occasionally act as an intermediate host for sleeping sickness.

Dr P. H. Ross has shewn that the fly is able to transmit mechanically T. gambiense from infected to healthy monkeys. During 91 days, 51 flies were fed first on an infected monkey and eight hours later on a healthy one. The latter shewed parasites in its blood on the ninety-fifth day.

Later the same investigator had two positive results in the transmission of T. gambiense by G. brevipalpis employing the " interrupted " method of feeding, but as the flies were caught in nature there is a slight doubt as to whether the trypanosome was really gambiense.

REFERENCES.

Austen, E. (1903). *Monograph of the Tsetse-Flies*, p. 95.
—— (1911). *Handbook of the Tsetse-Flies*, p. 85.
Davey, J. B. (1910). *Bull. Entom. Research*, vol. I. p. 143.
Koch, R. (1905). *Deutsche Med. Wochenschr.* vol. XXXI. Nov. 23.
Milne, A. D. (1910). *S. S. Bulletin*, vol. II. p. 37.
Neave, S. A. (1912). *Bull. Entom. Research*, vol. III. p. 275.
Newstead, R. (1910). *Ann. Trop. Med. and Parasit.* vol. VI. p. 372.
Ross, P. H. (1908). *Colonial Report East African Protectorate*, No. 6490.
—— (1910). *Nairobi Laboratory Reports*, vol. I.
Sanderson, M. (1911). *Bull. Entom. Research*, vol. I. p. 292.
Stuhlmann, F. (1907). *Arb. Kais. Gesundheitsamle*, vol. XXVI. p. 301.

# CHAPTER XVII

## GLOSSINA AND DISEASE

### THE TRYPANOSOMES

*Diagnosis, etc.* The trypanosomes constitute a well-defined group of flagellates inhabiting the blood of vertebrates, and with few exceptions the known pathogenic species are mainly transmitted by various species of *Glossina*. As many of them are carried by more than one kind of tsetse-fly, it will be convenient to discuss them collectively, instead of describing each trypanosome separately under the heading of one of its carriers.

The genus *Trypanosoma* includes all those flagellates characterised by the possession of a more or less elongated fusiform body and a single anterior flagellum, which, at least during some part of the life-cycle, arises near the posterior end of the body, and for the greater part of its length is attached to a fold of the periplast, known as the undulating membrane. Occasionally the flagellum does not become free anteriorly but is attached to the undulating membrane along its whole length.

The dimensions of different species, or even of different stages of the same species, may range from as small as 12 microns in length by 1·5 microns in breadth, up to more than

100 microns in length by 10 microns in breadth ; but the great majority of them are between 20 and 30 microns in length, by 1·5 to 2·5 microns in breadth.

*General description.* The body of a trypanosome consists of an elongated fusiform mass of cytoplasm containing two nuclei and bounded by a more or less distinct periplast. The cytoplasm may stain uniformly, but frequently contains numbers of chromatic granules, the presence or absence of which is sometimes of use for classificatory purposes. The larger of the nuclei is usually situated about the middle of the length of the body and is known as the trophonucleus. Typically it consists of an oval, lightly-staining vesicle, containing a deeply-staining, central karyosome. The smaller nucleus, known as the kinetonucleus, is generally situated at, or near, the posterior, non-flagellate extremity of the trypanosome. The kinetonucleus is also known as the centrosome, blepharoplast, or micro-nucleus, but all these terms are liable to lead to confusion. The term blepharoplast, or centrosome, should be reserved for the small basal corpuscle, or end-bead, situated close to the kinetonucleus, from which arises the flagellum, running forward attached to the surface until it reaches the anterior extremity of the body. In its course along the body the flagellum is attached to the surface by means of a transparent membrane, the undulating membrane, which varies considerably in its development in different species, but is always distinct. The parasite mainly progresses by the aid of wave-like motions of this undulating membrane, accompanied by wriggling of the whole body. The movements of the living trypanosome are sometimes of use in identifying the species, the very quick darting motions of *T. lewisi* and *T. cazalboui* being very characteristic.

The relative positions of the two nuclei serves as a means of distinguishing *T. rhodesiense*, and the size of the kineto-nucleus is a character of considerable value, but the dimensions of the parasite probably constitute one of the most useful means of identifying the various species.

In giving the dimensions of any particular species it is necessary to give the measurements of a moderately large

number of individuals, and the most convenient way of presenting the result of such a series of measurements is by means
of a Galtonian curve. With this graphic method it is possible
to detect whether the species is dimorphic or monomorphic,
and Bruce has shewn how it is possible to distinguish species
that have the same range of dimensions, e.g. T. brucei and
T. evansi.

*Mode of division.* In the blood, the parasites multiply by
longitudinal fission, the details of which are essentially the same
in all species of trypanosomes. The first sign of division is
usually seen in the kinetonucleus, which seems to swell up,
resulting in the formation of an oval vesicle, throughout which
the .chromatin is evenly distributed. The chromatin then
aggregates together in the form of a band lying across the middle
of the vesicle, which now becomes slightly elongated. This
band then divides transversely and the two halves move apart,
one of them usually approaching the trophonucleus, and apparently without any further changes, beyond the disappearance
of the vesicle, these two bands constitute the two daughter
kinetonuclei. The details of this process can only be observed
in those trypanosomes possessing a comparatively large
kinetonucleus and have not been followed in the case of those
species with excessively small ones.

The end-bead, often with the basal part of the flagellum,
divides at the same time as the kinetonucleus. In some forms
the flagellum together with the undulating membrane divides
along a considerable part of its length, so that the new flagellum
is formed by splitting of the old one, whilst in other cases an
entirely new daughter flagellum develops from one of the daughter end-beads.

The trophonucleus usually divides shortly after the division
of the kinetonucleus is complete. The central karyosome
divides, and the two halves move apart until they are situated
one at each pole of the nucleus, still remaining connected,
however, by a fine line. In some species the chromatin may
become arranged in the form of an equatorial plate, which then
splits transversely, each half moving up towards its respective
pole. In other species no equatorial plate is formed, but the

chromatin merely becomes aggregated around each pole and division is more or less direct. In either case the connecting line eventually disappears and the two daughter nuclei gradually assume the usual form. Meanwhile the new flagellum has become nearly as long as the old one. The animal then splits longitudinally, the fission commencing at the anterior end and extending down until the two halves are connected merely by their posterior extremities, in which position they may remain for some little time before finally separating.

In some species, e.g. T. lewisi, the trypanosomes multiply by a process of schizogony, and multinucleate forms are not infrequently found in many other species. The presence or absence of such forms occasionally gives some help in the determination of the species.

*Biological characters.* Certain trypanosomes will only live in one particular vertebrate host and when injected into other species are unable to survive. None of the pathogenic trypanosomes, however, are restricted to one species, the nearest approach to it occurring in the case of T. simiæ, which only affects monkeys and goats.

The great majority of trypanosomes have little or no effect upon the health of their hosts and accordingly are termed non-pathogenic. On the contrary, the most important parasites from the present point of view—the pathogenic trypanosomes—have a marked injurious effect on the health of the animals they inhabit.

The effect of these parasites on their hosts is of help in distinguishing the various forms, as the incubation period, duration of the disease, symptoms, etc, etc., all furnish useful indications.

Yet another means of distinguishing these pathogenic trypanosomes is furnished by the results of inoculating the parasites into various experimental animals. The smaller animals are refractory to certain trypanosomes that are pathogenic to ruminants, and on the other hand some parasites have a much more pathogenic effect on small animals than on large ones.

The method of infection is another important character.

Some trypanosomiases are transmitted entirely by coïtus others by tsetse-flies, and yet others by *Stomoxys* and Tabanids. In those few cases in which the life-cycle of the trypanosome in the tsetse-fly (*Glossina*) has been followed, the evolution of the flagellate within the body of the fly is found to differ in different species, and in future this may furnish an important means of distinguishing them. At present it is possible to distinguish those trypanosomes which infect the whole length of the alimentary canal of the fly (*infection totale*), from those that are restricted to the proboscis.

*Cross immunity reactions.* The most certain method of distinguishing any two races of trypanosomes is by means of their immunity reactions. Thus, given two races of trypanosomes *A* and *B*, an animal having recovered from *A* is inoculated with *B*, in order to determine whether or not it possesses immunity against the latter, and *vice versa.* If an animal which has recovered from *A* is still susceptible to *B*, one assumes that *A* and *B* constitute distinct species. On the other hand if an animal which has recovered from *A*, and therefore is immune against this strain, is also immune against *B*, the two are considered to be identical.

This method is only capable of application in the laboratory and cannot be used during expeditions in the tropics.

*Sero-diagnostic methods.* Laveran and Mesnil have also called attention to the possibility of employing sero-diagnostic methods in the identification of trypanosomes. The serum of an animal which has acquired immunity against any particular trypanosome, is often active when mixed with blood containing this trypanosome, and inactive when mixed under similar conditions with other species of trypanosomes. Unfortunately the activity of the immune sera is too variable to give any very certain results, and this method, therefore, only gives useful *indications.*

The production of agglutination by means of the addition of immune serum of the same species of trypanosome is also of use in some cases, but is very inconstant.

*Classification.* The identification of the various species of trypanosomes has become a matter of great difficulty, especially in the case of the numerous cattle trypanosomes of Africa, and at the present time there is no simple method by which the different varieties can be distinguished with any certainty. In some cases the morphology is sufficiently distinctive, but in most cases the trypanosomes are chiefly distinguished by their biological characters, and these are often very difficult to observe even in well equipped laboratories. In every case, therefore, species should be distinguished as much as possible by morphological characters, for the present practice of giving specific names to merely " physiological varieties " is of questionable value.

In the following table we have adopted Laveran and Mesnil's method of sub-dividing trypanosomes into three groups, according to the presence or absence of a free flagellum, or those strains in which both forms occur. It has been found necessary to omit many so-called species that have been insufficiently described, and whose identification is very uncertain, if not impossible.

### Key to the pathogenic trypanosomes of Africa.

A. Trypanosomes in which the flagellum always possesses a free part anteriorly.

1 ⎰ Living trypanosome extremely active, frequently darting across the field
⎱ of the microscope. Dogs, monkeys, rats and mice all refractory to infection ; ruminants and horses susceptible
= *cazalboui*, Laveran ( = *vivax*, Bruce etc. *nec* Ziemann).
Dogs, rats and mice susceptible to infection   ..   ..   ..   = 2

2 ⎰ Monkeys and ruminants more or less refractory to infection. Horses
⎱ susceptible   ..   ..   ..   ..   .. = *equiperdum*, Doflein.
Monkeys and ruminants susceptible to infection   ..   .. = 3

3 ⎰ Parasite more or less dimorphic   .. = *brucei*, Plimmer and Bradford.
⎱ Parasite monomorphic   ..   ..   = ⎰ *evansi*, Steel.
⎱ *evansi* var. *mbori*, Laveran.
*togolense*, Mesnil and Brimont.
*soudanense*, Laveran.

The latter four trypanosomes are distinguished by their cross immunity reactions.

B.   Trypanosomes in which the flagellum does not become free anteriorly.

1 { Parasite distinctly dimorphic   ..     =*dimorphon*, Laveran and Mesnil.
  { Parasite monomorphic ·   ..     ..     ..     ..     ..     ..     =2

2 { Monkeys, dogs, rabbits, etc., refractory to infection   =*nanum*, Laveran.
    Monkeys and goats susceptible; dogs, rabbits, etc., refractory to infection
              =*simiæ*, Bruce, Harvey, Hamerton, Davey, and Lady Bruce *.
    Monkeys, dogs, rabbits, etc., susceptible to infection
              = { *congolense*, Broden.
                { *pecorum*, Bruce, Hamerton, Bateman, and Mackie.

The latter two species are distinguished by cross immunity reactions.   In addition *T. pecorum* is more virulent than *T. congolense.*


C.   Trypanosomes having forms with a free flagellum and forms without a free flagellum.

1 { Trypanosomes immobilised by human serum   ..     =*pecaudi*, Laveran.
  { Trypanosomes unaffected by human serum   ..     ..     ..     =2

2 { In rats, trypanosome shewing a variable proportion of forms with the
        trophonucleus at the posterior end of the body
                        =*rhodesiense*, Stephens and Fantham.
    Trypanosomes never shewing any posterior nuclear forms
                        =*gambiense*, Dutton.

   * In this species the extreme tip of the flagellum may sometimes become free for a length of 2–3 microns.


### REFERENCES.

Laveran and Mesnil (1912).   *Trypanosomes et Trypanosomiases*, 2nd edition.   Masson et Cie.   Paris.   (Contains a very complete account of the literature on the subject.)

# CHAPTER XVIII

## GLOSSINA AND DISEASE (*continued*)

### SLEEPING SICKNESS (*T. gambiense*)

*Synonyms.* African Trypanosomiasis (*pro parte*) ; African Lethargy ; Trypanosome Fever ; Sleeping Dropsy ; Morbus Dormitious ; Maladie du Sommeil ; Schlafkrankheit ; Doença de Sonno ; Letargia dei Negri ; Malattia del Sonno. Also a very large number of native names.

*Definition.* Sleeping Sickness is an acute or chronic infection with *Trypanosoma gambiense* Dutton, characterised by an inflammatory condition of the lymphatic system, leading to a meningo-encephalitis and a meningo-myelitis. The disease is usually transmitted by *Glossina palpalis* Rob.-Desv., but *G. morsitans* and probably some other species of the same genus are capable of becoming infective.

*History.* The first mention of this disease occurs in 1734, when John Atkins, a Naval Surgeon, gave a clear description of cases of the disease on the Guinea Coast. In the appendix to his book, entitled *The Navy Surgeon*, occurs the following passage : " The *Sleepy Distemper* (common among the negroes) gives no other previous Notice, than a want of Appetite two or three days before ; their sleeps are sound, and Sense and Feeling very little ; for pulling drubbing or whipping will scarce stir up Sense and Power enough to move ; and the Moment you cease beating the smart is forgot, and down they fall again into a state of Insensibility, drivling constantly from the Mouth as if in deep salivation ; breathe slowly, but not unequally nor snort.

" Young People are more subject to it than the old ; and the Judgement generally pronounced is Death, the Prognostick seldom failing. If now and then one of them recovers, he certainly loses the little Reason he had, and turns Ideot...."

" In Searching for the Cause of this Distemper it will be necessary to repeat what I have observed, that the Bulk of

Slave-Cargoes mostly consist of Country People, as distinguished from the Coast People, apparently if the principal Way of Supply be considered.  At Whydah more Slaves are brought than on the whole Coast besides ; and why ?  The King of that Country, and his next neighbours, understand sovereignty better than others, and often make War (as they call it), to bring in whole villages of those more simple Creatures inland, to be sold at Market, and exchanged for the Tempting Commodities of *Europe*, that they are fond and mad after.

"The immediate cause of this deadly sleepiness in the Slaves is evidently a Super-abundance of Phlegm or Serum, extravased in the Brain, which obstructs the Irradiation of the Nerves ; but what the procatartick Causes are, that exert to this Production, eclipsing the Light of the Senses, is not so easily assigned....

"The cure is attempted by whatever rouses the Spirits ; bleeding in the jugular, quick purges, Sternatories, Vesicatories, Acu-Puncture, Seton, Fontanels, and Sudden Plunges into the Sea ; the latter is most effectual when the Distemper is new, and the Patient as yet not attended with a drivling at Mouth and Nose."

From this account there can be no doubt that the author had observed cases of sleeping sickness, but no further mention of the disease occurs until 1803, when Winterbottom gave a fairly clear account of the malady as he saw it on the west coast of Africa, near Sierra Leone.  Whilst the slave trade was in progress, some of the natives infected with sleeping sickness were carried across to the West Indies, and in 1808 Moreau de Jonnès recorded its presence amongst the negro slaves in the Antilles.

In 1840, Clarke wrote a more complete account of the disease, based upon observations made at Sierra Leone, and during the next twenty years a number of English and French doctors published various descriptions of sleeping sickness.

In 1869, Guérin met with the disease in the island of Martinique among the slaves who had been imported from the west coast of Africa.  The disease never spread in these countries to which it had been imported, and Guérin was able to shew that in Martinique the infection was certainly not contagious. Dr Corré, in 1876, gave a good description of the disease as observed in the Senegal and attributed it to a kind of ergotism, or scrofula, and to the moral condition of the people. In addition he describes the ravages of sleeping sickness in the Senegambia, where whole villages had been swept away and many towns abandoned as a result of " Nelavane," the local name for the disease.

Mense, in 1885 to 1887, found sleeping sickness widely distributed throughout the navigable reaches of the Congo as far up as the Stanley Pools, and the disease had not been lately introduced into this region for it was well known by the natives. In 1871, the first case of this disease appeared on the banks of Quanza, in Angola, and since that date thousands of victims have been claimed and numerous villages abandoned.

Until this outbreak in Angola, for many generations sleeping sickness seems to have been confined to certain parts of the west coast of Africa, especially the Congo, which also formed its southernmost limit, and the Senegambia. Although the disease has now spread to the south into Angola, up to the present the region of the Gambia still forms its northern limit, and it is interesting to note that the natives of this region have a superstition that sleeping sickness came from the provinces to the south of them.

In the eighties of the last century, the malady was still restricted to the west of Africa, but after this date began that opening up of Africa, that has resulted in sleeping sickness spreading inland as far as Uganda and the great lakes. It is believed that unwittingly Stanley, the African Explorer, was responsible for the introduction of the disease into the lake region during his expedition for the relief of Emin Pasha. In 1887, Stanley travelled up the Congo with a large force and eventually reached the shores of Lake Albert Nyanza where he found Emin Pasha. Regarding this expedition Mense states : " Stanley's expedition for the relief of Emin Pasha, which travelled in 1888 from the Congo to the Nile, and which hired carriers from the Lower and Middle Congo, must certainly have brought many infected men along with it to the

Lake region, and possibly introduced the disease there. I myself was the witness of sick men regardlessly abandoned, of dead and dying, who marked the way even in the Cataract region."

After Stanley had met Emin they eventually proceeded to Zanzibar but a large number of soldiers and followers were left behind in a district to the west of the Lake Albert Nyanza. When Captain (now General Sir Frederick) Lugard arrived in Uganda in 1908, after deposing Kabarega, he went to Albert Nyanza and recruited a body of Sudanese, the remnants of those left behind by Stanley and Emin Pasha. About 400 to 500 able-bodied men were enlisted as soldiers and they, with their rabble of 7000 wives, children and followers, were settled in South Toro in 1891. A year later it was found advisable to move them to Busoga where they could be under better control, and for some years there continued recruiting of Sudanese soldiers brought to this province.

Sleeping sickness was then unknown in this part of Africa for none of the chiefs or missionaries had ever seen it and the symptoms are so evident that cases could hardly have been overlooked. In 1901 the disease was first recorded from Busoga and on investigation Dr Hodges found that sleeping sickness had occurred in one district of this province for six years previously and that many hundreds of natives had already died of it. As many of the settlers in Busoga had originally come from the Congo with Stanley's force, there can be little doubt that they were responsible for the introduction of the disease. In the next seven years the epidemic assumed such proportions that in Busoga alone no less than 200,000 people· out of a total population of 300,000 died of sleeping sickness. The disease was also prevalent in Uganda, occurring along the shore of Lake Victoria and on the islands.

In 1901, Forde noticed some peculiar parasites in the blood of a patient who was admitted into the hospital at Bathurst, suffering from an unknown type of fever. The following year Dutton examined the blood of this patient and found the peculiar parasites noted by Dr Forde, and recognized that they were trypanosomes. Subsequently trypanosomes were also

observed in the blood of a native in the Gambia and therefore
Dutton considered that it was probably a new parasite and
gave it the name of *Trypanosoma gambiense.* In 1902, Dutton
and Todd proceeded on an expedition to the Senegambia in
order to make further investigations into the nature of this
infection. They came to the conclusion that trypanosome
fever, or trypanosomiasis, was in natives a particularly mild
disease for many of those whose blood contained the parasites
appeared to be in perfect health, and none of them were seriously ill. Owing to the fact that these investigators had to
travel about, the cases could not be kept under observation for
any length of time and the relation between trypanosome fever
and sleeping sickness was not discovered.

In 1901, an epidemic of sleeping sickness broke out in
Uganda and the number of cases increased so rapidly that in
1902 the Royal Society sent out a Commission to investigate
the causes of this outbreak. This Commission composed of
Drs Castellani, Christy and Low, arrived in Uganda in 1902,
and at once commenced to work on the etiology of the disease.
Whilst Castellani was examining the brains and spinal cords of
persons who had died of sleeping sickness in the attempt to
find the cause of the malady, the other two members of the
Commission travelled about and eventually proved that the
area of infection was confined to a narrow strip of country
surrounding the lake shores and on the islands of Lake
Victoria. This restricted distribution had previously been
noticed by Hodges, and clearly shewed that there was no
relation between sleeping sickness and *Filaria perstans,* as
suggested by Manson, for the areas of infection were quite
different. In 1903, Castellani noted the presence of trypanosomes in the cerebro-spinal fluid of patients infected with
sleeping sickness, and the same year Bruce and Nabarro
arrived in Uganda to continue these investigations. Bruce
at once recognised the possibility that this trypanosome might
be the cause of sleeping sickness and on further examination
Castellani found that 70 per cent. of the cases contained these
parasites in the cerebro-spinal fluid.

The parasite was described under the name of *Trypanosoma*

*ugandense,* as Castellani considered that it was distinct from *T. gambiense* Dutton. Subsequently Bruce and Nabarro found trypanosomes in the cerebro-spinal fluid of practically all cases, but were puzzled by the fact that some natives shewed these parasites in their blood without presenting any very serious symptoms. Later, when patients suffering from trypanosome fever were kept under observation, it was found that this was merely an early symptom of sleeping sickness and that in the later stages the parasites appear in the cerebro-spinal fluid and the characteristic lethargic symptoms follow. The identity of *T. gambiense* and *T. ugandense* was also established by means of inoculating animals with the two strains, when they were found to produce exactly similar effects.

In 1903, Bruce and Nabarro shewed that sleeping sickness was carried by means of *Glossina palpalis,* and the manner in which they arrived at this discovery is of some interest. When it was proved that sleeping sickness was caused by the presence of a trypanosome in the blood, Bruce at once considered the possibility of the transmitting agent being a tsetse-fly as he had already proved to be the case in Zululand for another trypanosome disease, Nagana. Large numbers of tsetse-flies were found in the neighbourhood of Entebbe, but these belonged to a different species, *Glossina palpalis,* from the tsetse-fly of Zululand, *G. pallidipes.* The Commission, however, decided to find out the distribution of *Glossina palpalis,* in order to determine whether it bore any relation to that of sleeping sickness, and with this object tsetse-flies were collected from all parts of Uganda together with any records of the disease. When all the information was put together the evidence in favour of the tsetse theory of transmission was almost overwhelming, for in every locality from which sleeping sickness had been recorded the tsetse-fly was found to be present.

The final proof of this theory was obtained by feeding tsetse-flies on patients suffering from sleeping sickness, and subsequently, after various intervals, on healthy monkeys. The latter were found to become infected with *T. gambiense,* thus proving that *Glossina palpalis* can convey trypanosomes from sleeping sickness patients to healthy individuals. It was next shewn that if large numbers of the wild tsetse-flies in the neighbourhood of Entebbe were caught and fed on healthy monkeys the latter became infected with sleeping sickness. The discovery that the tsetse-fly is the carrier of the disease explained why sleeping sickness had not spread in the West Indies in spite of the frequent importations of infected negroes. In the absence of its invertebrate host the disease could not be transmitted from the patients to other persons.

In 1909, Kleine discovered the very important fact that *T. gambiense* undergoes a cyclical development in the body of *Glossina palpalis*, and that once infected the tsetse-fly may remain infective for a considerable period of time. In 1911, Taute, whilst experimenting on the shore of Lake Tanganyika, shewed that *G. morsitans* was also capable of acting as the invertebrate host for *T. gambiense*, and that the trypanosome underwent a cycle of development within the body of the insect resembling that in *G. palpalis*. Finally, Bruce, Hamerton and Bateman, in 1911, shewed that the wild game served as a reservoir for sleeping sickness, as antelopes and reed-bucks could remain infected, and *infective*, for long periods without presenting any signs of disease. The importance of this discovery from a prophylactic point of view cannot be over-estimated.

*Distribution.* At the present time sleeping sickness extends along the west coast of Africa from St Louis in the Senegal, to Benguella in the province of Angola, and inland as far East as the Omo River (Brumpt) and the Victoria Nyanza. The main centres of the disease are the Congo Free State, French Congo, Cameroons, Angola, Senegal and Senegambia, Uganda and along the shores of Lake Victoria and Tanganyika.

*Life history within the vertebrate host—Endogenous cycle.—* The life-cycle of *T. gambiense* has been elucidated by the researches of Minchin, Roubaud, Bruce, Kleine, and Miss Robertson. The last named investigator has given a complete description of all stages in the development, from which the following account is taken.

In the blood the short forms (so-called female forms) about 13 to 20 microns in length (Fig. 75) are the adult type. They have the longest duration in the circulation and appear to be the type from which the individuals capable of carrying on the cycle in the intermediate host, are derived. The blood of a monkey is infective to *Glossina* only as long as this form is present in sufficient numbers and moreover in a healthy state, for at times, in very heavy infections, the flagellates seem to become exhausted. These short forms grow up into the so-called intermediate or "indifferent" forms, that are an ill-defined and artificial group, chiefly to be recognised by their increased length and longer free flagellum. The intermediate forms are merely a step in the development of the division forms, which are the culminating stage of this process. The long slender forms that have been known as the male forms, are merely the individuals that are about to divide. It is, therefore, incorrect to speak of male, female, and indifferent forms, as these are all stages in the development of the short forms. Multiplication takes place in the circulating blood and the details are as follows : the first sign of division is the doubling of the kinetonucleus together with the end-bead, situated at the posterior end of the trypanosome. The flagellum then splits longitudinally, but only for about two-thirds of its length, when it becomes free. Previous to division the trophonucleus shews two well-marked dark granules, one at each pole, and these are joined together by a fairly thick line to the karyosome. The nucleus then divides, the chromatin becoming aggregated about each pole. By this time the body has become long and slender in form and eventually this long trypanosome separates into two daughter individuals that are of the short form.

No other mode of multiplication within the blood is known, although at times the nuclei may divide repeatedly without division of the cytoplasm. In such cases large multinucleate forms may be produced but they are merely the result of delayed division and not examples of true schizogony. In addition, certain authors have described various latent bodies or spores, small rounded nonflagellate forms, that are supposed to be capable of remaining dormant in the internal organs for considerable lengths of time and thus be the cause of the relapses. It is possible that some latent forms are produced, but up to the present the evidence for their existence is inconclusive.

One of the most noticeable features of the infection in the blood is the periodic increase and decrease in the number of trypanosomes in the peripheral circulation. It was formerly believed that the parasites completely disappeared from the circulation at certain times, but Ross and Thomson have shewn that when once a person becomes infected trypanosomes are constantly present in the blood. During the so-called negative periods the parasites are in such few numbers that their presence can only be detected by the examination of large quantities of blood, either by centrifuging or some similar means. These alternating periods of increase and decrease in the circulating blood are of irregular duration, and the circumstances which bring about the disappearance of the majority of the parasites are not thoroughly understood. After a period of depression the following increase in the number of flagellates is always accompanied by division in the peripheral blood.

These variations in the number of trypanosomes are accompanied by differences in their infectivity when ingested by the tsetse-fly. Thus it has been shewn that monkeys infected with *T. gambiense* have negative periods during which they are not infective to the fly, and moreover the percentage of flies that become infected after any particular feed varies with the stage of infection.

From this point of view, the following table, given by Miss Robertson, is of considerable interest. Monkey 113 was infected by wild *G. palpalis* from the shore of Lake Victoria, and first shewed trypanosomes in its blood on July 25th. From August 23rd up to the time of its death, fresh lots of flies were fed on this monkey and the percentage number of these flies that became infected is shewn in the table.

It is evident, therefore, that there is a marked difference in the infectivity of the parasite at different stages of its development, but in addition, different strains vary considerably in this respect. Thus, another monkey was infected by the direct injection of blood from a bush-buck which had been

## Monkey 113.

| Date | Condition of blood examined alive | + or − laboratory bred flies | Number of flies fed | Percentage of flies becoming infected |
|---|---|---|---|---|
| Aug. 20–22 | No trypanosomes seen in blood | No flies fed | — | — |
| ,, 23 | Few    ,,    ,,    ,,    ,, | − | 101 | 0 |
| ,, 24 | Numerous trypanosomes in blood | + | 45 | 11·1 |
| ,, 25 | ,,    ,,    ,,    ,,    ,, | + | 53 | 3·7 |
| ,, 26 | Very numerous trypanosomes in blood | − | 89 | 0 |
| ,, 27 | Very few trypanosomes in blood | No flies fed | — | — |
| ,, 28 | ⌠ No trypanosomes seen in blood | Flies fed | | |
| ,, 29 | ⌡ | both days | 25 | 0 |
| ,, 30 | Few trypanosomes in blood | − | 34 | 0 |
| ,, 31 | ,,    ,,    ,,    ,, | + | 107 | 1·8 |
| Sept. 1–3 | Not examined | | | |
| ,, 4 | Very few trypanosomes in blood | − | 32 | 0 |
| ,, 5 | ,,    ,,    ,,    ,,    ,, | No flies fed | — | — |
| ,, 6 | Moderate number of trypanosomes, dimorphism of broad and narrow forms very marked | − | 49 | 0 |
| ,, 7 | Moderate number of trypanosomes | No flies fed | — | — |
| ,, 8 | Trypanosomes very numerous indeed | + | 95 | 2·1 |
| ,, 9 | Fair number of trypanosomes but much fewer than on 8th | No flies fed | — | — |
| ,, 10 | Not examined | No flies fed | — | — |
| ,, 11 | Few trypanosomes | | | |
| ,, 12 | Trypanosomes very numerous indeed | + | 70 | 1·4 |
| ,, 13 | Trypanosomes very numerous indeed | No flies fed | 70 | 1·4 |
| ,, 14 | Trypanosomes very numerous indeed | ,, | — | — |
| ,, 15 | Blood swarming with trypanosomes | + | 20 | 10 |

infected with *T. gambiense* by laboratory bred flies. The bush-buck had harboured the trypanosome for about fifteen months. This monkey shewed infective and non-infective periods in exactly the same way as other infections, but the infective periods gave a remarkably large percentage of flies harbouring trypanosomes. Out of 150 *G. palpalis* that were fed on this monkey, 16 became infected, a percentage of 10·6 per cent., which is remarkably high, for Bruce, Hamerton, Bateman and Mackie found that the normal proportion of infected flies produced by the Uganda strain of *T. gambiense* in monkeys was only about one in 40.

*Life history within the invertebrate host,* G. palpalis—*Exogenous cycle.*—In addition to the initia linfectivity of the trypanosome mentioned above, several other conditions have a marked effect upon the development of *T. gambiense* in its invertebrate host, the tsetse-fly. A certain degree of warmth is essential and the more favourable results obtained on Tanganyika than in Uganda, in the transmission of *T. gambiense* by *G. morsitans,* can be explained by the differences in temperature between these two localities.

One of the most important conditions affecting development is the interval that elapses between the feed of infected blood and the following meal. When a newly-hatched fly is fed, it usually ingests sufficient blood to fill both its crop and gut. The next feed, taken in two or three days later, may either entirely replace the undigested remains of the first meal, or some of the first feed may remain in the crop and the fresh blood be taken on top of it. Occasionally the blood may be taken directly into the gut without even going into the crop.

If a fly has ingested trypanosomes at its first feed, the result of subsequent clean feeds varies in different individuals. The trypanosomes may be digested and disappear from the alimentary canal of the *Glossina* during the first 50 to 72 hours, without the intervention of a second feed. In other cases the flagellates survive in the gut in small numbers but disappear during the early stages of digestion of the new blood. It is evident from these two results that all trypanosomes cannot withstand the digestive processes and, of course, in such cases the fly does not become infected. In some flies the trypanosomes may survive and multiply in the gut in the blood retained from the first feed, although a second feed has been taken in on top. In these cases the trypanosomes may be swept out when the original blood is digested, and thus no infection be produced. The trypanosomes may survive and develop in the crop for as long as 12 days, providing that blood is constantly present. The gut of these flies may often shew no signs of flagellates, in which case the insect will not become infected, as there is never a permanent infection of the crop. When trypanosomes persist in greater or less numbers in the gut and crop of the same fly, the issue is somewhat doubtful as the flagellates may be swept out by subsequent clean feeds.

A permanent infection of the fly is obtained when the whole material of the first feed has been displaced from the gut by the second feed, and the trypanosomes still persist. Once parasites are well established in the new blood the rate of multiplication is such that there is little chance of their being destroyed at the next influx of blood.

There is no doubt that the critical time for the parasite is this influx of fresh blood after an infected feed. This is shewn by the very much larger percentage of infected flies found amongst those individuals that had only one feed and this the infecting one, than among those that had been subsequently fed every two or three days in the usual way. Out of 103 starved flies trypanosomes were found in 22 between the 6th and 12th day. 16 or 15·5 per cent. of these starved flies shewed a well developed infection of the gut, whereas under ordinary feeding conditions only about 3 per cent. of these flies became infected.

In the early days of the cycle in the alimentary tract of the fly many forms of parasites may be observed, depending on the various conditions. The trypanosomes may persist without multiplying, under which circumstances they degenerate and disappear within three to four days. In other cases the parasites persist in small numbers and begin to multiply, but when the adverse conditions of a new feed come upon them, they are unable to withstand them, and dividing and degenerating specimens may thus be found side by side. Persistence and quite normal development may occur in the crop and continue till the 10th or 12th day, so that it is evident that the stimulus to development in the fly is not dependent upon the digestive action of the gut fluid upon the blood.

The very large number of cases where the attempted multiplication fails to establish an infection, indicates the presence of a general inhibiting property in the *Glossina* and is a fairly constant factor in experiments with freshly hatched flies.

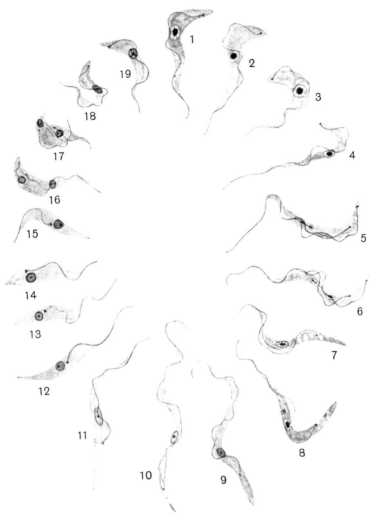

Fig. 75. (1–19). *Trypanosoma gambiense.* × about 2000 diameters. (After Muriel Robertson.)

1–4.    Trypanosomes from the blood of a monkey.
5–6.    Division of blood-types.
7–8.    Trypanosomes in the middle intestine of *Glossina*, 36–48 hours after ingestion.
9–10.   Slender proventricular types, final form of the gut development.
11–12.  Specimens newly arrived in the salivary gland.
13–15.  Typical salivary gland form, shewing the crithidial condition.
16–17.  Division of salivary gland forms.
18–19.  Final trypanosome types in the salivary glands, probably the infecting form.

Individual strains of *T. gambiense* vary greatly in the percentage of infected flies they produce, this being due to the greater
or less vigour of the trypanosomes interacting with the inhibiting forces of the fly. The negative blood periods, during which
the parasite is not in a fit state to carry on the cycle, are as
well marked in very vigorous strains as in those of lesser
vitality.

When the conditions are favourable to development in the
fly, the trypanosomes first become established in the posterior
region of the mid-gut. Here multiplication takes place and
trypanosomes of very varying sizes are produced, though the
parasites rarely surpass a length of 34 to 35 microns.

About the tenth day numerous trypanosomes are present,
and the characteristic slender forms may begin to appear, but
only in small numbers.

The method of division in these forms is essentially similar
to that in the circulating blood, but the final division of the
protoplasmic body is very characteristic. Instead of the two
daughter individuals swinging out so as to be arranged kinetonucleus to kinetonucleus as in the majority of trypanosome
divisions, there is no longitudinal splitting of the parent organism, but the young specimen is pushed off at the posterior end
(Fig. 75, 17) and division is practically transverse.

After the 10th to the 15th day the slender forms that
constitute the proventricular type gradually develop from the
broader forms, and as their numbers increase move forward into
the proventriculus, where they are the dominant type. There
is only one important point in which they differ from their
predecessors. The body is long and slender, the cytoplasm
finely granular and much less dense than in the broader forms,
but the trophonucleus shews a distinct change. The karyosome has become much smaller and the membrane has become
much more marked and stains deeply. In the fully developed
slender types, division rarely seems to occur.

The infection·grows forward by sheer force of multiplication
until it fills the whole of the middle and hinder intestine and
the posterior part of the anterior intestine. The anterior
portion of the anterior intestine and the proventriculus shew

the typical long slender forms and are only invaded about the middle of the developmental cycle. There seems to be some difficulty in the trypanosomes reaching the proventriculus and once arrived there they cannot maintain themselves if the fly is exposed to too long a fast. If there is any considerable interval before another meal the trypanosomes gradually ebb backwards to the posterior part of the anterior intestine and only gradually recover their position again after the next feed. The intestinal infection is thus the focus from which the subsequent stages are derived.

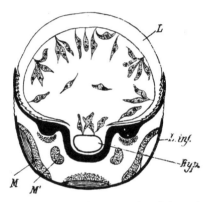

Fig. 76. Transverse section (semi-diagrammatic) of the proboscis of an infected *Glossina*. The section shews the arrangement and aspect of the trypanosomes attached to the walls of the labrum (*L*) and the hypopharynx (*Hyp*.). ( × about 700.) (After Roubaud.)
*L*, labrum ; *Hyp*. hypopharynx ; *M*, *M'*, muscles ; *L. inf*., under lip.

After becoming established in the proventriculus the slender forms pass up into the hypopharynx and then along the salivary ducts into the salivary glands. The period at which this happens depends upon the virulence of the trypanosomes, and early infectivity is generally a character found in a strain which produces many positive flies. The trypanosomes settle down in the salivary glands in the cellular part of the lumen immediately above the narrow tubular part of the duct. At first they are slender forms attached to the wall of the gland by their flagella, but later they gradually change into broad crithidial forms.

These crithidial flagellates multiply and finally fill up large portions of the gland with flagellates in all stages from typical crithidial forms, attached by the flagellum, to free-swimming trypanosomes closely resembling the blood type. The fly never becomes infective until the trypanosomes have invaded the salivary glands. The proventriculus and gut forms when injected into monkeys never produce an infection. The invasion of the glands usually occurs about the 20th day, but occasionally it may take place earlier, in one case a salivary gland being found infected on the 12th day. The *Glossina* seems to become infective two to five days after the trypanosomes have invaded the gland. During this period the parasites pass through the crithidial cycle, which seems to be a necessary feature in the development of the trypanosome in the invertebrate host before the latter can become infective.

The whole cycle from the ingestion of the trypanosomes to the appearance of young blood forms in the salivary glands generally occupies from 20 to 30 days, after which the *Glossina* becomes infective and probably remains so for the remainder of its life. When an infected fly bites an animal the young trypanosomes in the lumen of the salivary glands are passed down the duct together with the salivary secretion and thus injected into the wound caused by the mouth parts of the insect.

### *Prophylaxis of Sleeping Sickness.*

In spite of the experimental evidence to shew that *Glossina morsitans*, *G. fusca*, and *G. tachinoides*, and probably the other members of the genus, are all capable of transmitting sleeping sickness, the epidemiological evidence in support of the view that *G. palpalis* is the main carrier, is overwhelming. Accordingly, for the time being, in combating the spread of the disease, the other species of tsetse-flies may be ignored. The prophylactic measures fall into two main classes. In the first place we may prevent the access of trypanosome carriers to fly areas, and in the second, we may attempt the destruction of the fly.

With regard to the former of these two methods, the difficulties in the way of preventing the flies becoming infected have been enormously increased by the discovery that the wild game may serve as a reservoir for sleeping sickness. When it was discovered that the tsetse-flies along the shores of Lake Victoria were infected, the government of Uganda ordered the removal of all the population from the infested regions and by means of stringent regulations prevented any persons living on the lake shores or on any of the islands. Nevertheless three years later the tsetse-flies were still infected with sleeping sickness, although during this period they could not have had the opportunity of feeding on the blood of any human being suffering from the disease. It is evident, therefore, that the wild game serves as an efficient reservoir for sleeping sickness and as there is no possibility of exterminating all the mammals in the infected regions, the idea of eradicating the disease in this manner must be abandoned.

Nevertheless, it is very important to prevent any infected person entering a fly area in which sleeping sickness does not already exist. The danger of this has been well exemplified in the case of Uganda, where, owing to the entrance of a few infected natives from the Congo, the disease was introduced among the previously uninfected *Glossina palpalis*, along the shores of Lake Victoria. Dr Bagshawe in his excellent article on this subject, advises the removal of healthy persons from the vicinity of the fly, or their protection from fly bites. This may be effected in a variety of ways amongst which may be mentioned the following :

Whenever possible villages or markets should be removed to fly-free areas as has been done in Uganda. In many districts, however, the difficulties in the way of such a scheme are almost insuperable, and even in Uganda it has not been found practicable to deal in a similar way with the infected districts near the Albert Lake and White Nile. Needless to add, any camps, whether temporary or permanent, should not be pitched in the fly regions.

All occupations carried on in fly-areas should be discouraged or prohibited. The most important of these is fishing, as river and lake-side natives usually spend all their time in this occupation, unprotected by any clothes and constantly being bitten by the tsetse-flies. The rapid spread of sleeping sickness in Uganda was the result of the fishing habits of the natives. Fishermen should be recommended to cultivate the soil or raise stock, and regulations prohibiting fishing in fly infested regions should be enforced. Brumpt has suggested that the natives who live on fish might be persuaded to grow vegetables by importing dried sea fish in exchange for their vegetable produce. Rubber collecting in *palpalis* areas should also be abandoned and there is little doubt that the prevalence of sleeping sickness in the Congo is largely due to this occupation.

During the heat of the day all fly areas should be avoided as the insects are especially active during these hours. Any visits to the water that may be necessary should be made either in the early morning or late evening.

Whenever possible roads should be selected that do not traverse fly areas, and when travelling fly-infested ferries and fords should be avoided. If caravans are obliged to cross such rivers at hours when the fly is active, they should not be allowed to halt within a distance of at least 100 yards of the water. In the construction of railways, fly areas might also be avoided, for there is a great danger of these insects being carried very considerable distances in the carriages of trains. When trains have to travel through infested regions the carriages and trucks should be protected with wire gauze; similarly, steamers that ply on fly-infested lakes or rivers should have some portion of the upper deck protected. The protective effect of clothing is well known and the comparative immunity of Europeans and native chiefs is mainly due to their practice of wearing clothes. The peasants who go about for the most part naked are particularly liable to the bites of the flies, and therefore they should be instructed as to the protective effect of clothes. Europeans when travelling through infested regions should take great care to protect their legs and arms, and if the flies are numerous it is advisable to wear both veils and gloves. It is possible that some substance may be found which will be repellent to the fly and when rubbed on the skin will keep it away, but up to the present no satisfactory repellent has been discovered.

The instruction of the natives and also Europeans, as to the danger of being bitten by tsetse-flies, should be carried out systematically in all infected regions, for without the co-operation of all persons it will be impossible to prevent the occurrence of cases of sleeping sickness.

It is most important that no person harbouring trypanosomes in his blood should be allowed to travel from one district to another. All sick persons should be segregated in treatment camps, away from any species of tsetse-fly. The employment of these segregation camps in Uganda has greatly reduced the number of deaths from sleeping sickness, but unfortunately such methods can never entirely eradicate the disease.

It should be forbidden to recruit soldiers, carriers or labourers in infected districts and bring them into any other districts which contain fly areas. The importance of such preventive measures in the case of uninfected districts containing G. palpalis is obvious, but the passage of persons harbouring trypanosomes from one infected district to another should also be avoided. Dr Bagshawe has called attention to the importance of this measure, for the strains of T. gambiense vary in virulence. There is some evidence that in consequence of the introduction of a virulent strain into a region where a mild strain previously existed, a small endemic focus of sleeping sickness has been succeeded by a great epidemic. It is also possible that an epidemic which is gradually losing its virulence and tending to die out may be kept alive by the introduction of persons harbouring virulent trypanosomes in their blood.

The only effective way of suppressing sleeping sickness is by the extermination of the tsetse-fly, and, therefore, the most important of all prophylactic measures are those directed against the fly. In fact, the control of this disease is essentially a problem for the entomologists. There are no doubt enormous difficulties in the way of exterminating an insect ranging over some millions of square miles of Tropical Africa, but the manner in which Stegomyia and other mosquitoes are disappearing during campaigns against yellow fever and malaria should make one hesitate before considering such a task impossible. A complete knowledge of the bionomics of G. palpalis, including its natural enemies and diseases, would be of immense value, and yet up to the present comparatively little work has been done on this subject.

Bagshawe advises the use of the following measures against the fly :

(a) The clearing of fly-infested scrub.

(b) The filling up or draining of pools when it is practicable.

(c) The cultivation of plants noxious to the fly.

(d) The destruction of animals on which the fly feeds.

(e) The encouragement or introduction of animals or plants (Fungi) which attack the fly in its adult or pupal stages.

(f) The collection or destruction of pupæ or of the flies themselves.

The clearing of fly-infested scrub has been found to be of great value in Uganda, but it is rather difficult of application over wide areas. As the natural range of *palpalis* does not exceed 30 yards from the water, a clearance of this strip will cause the disappearance of the fly. According to Roubaud, in the Congo it is sufficient merely to thin out the vegetation on each side of the water, but in most localities it is necessary to remove thoroughly all brushwood and scrub which shelter the fly and its pupæ. The cleared areas must either be kept free from scrub-vegetation, or some crop planted which will not give the flies any shelter. Citronella is one of the most suitable, as the grass repays cultivation and its smell may be repugnant to the fly. No clearing should be attempted unless it is possible to make it efficient and keep the cleared spaces free from scrub, and before undertaking any such measure the locality should be carefully examined. The flies and pupæ may be restricted to certain parts of the shore, in which case it is only necessary to clear these areas. It is advisable to clear the following localities : boat and steamer landing-places on lakes or rivers ; dipping and washing places ; stations on railways that traverse *palpalis* areas ; ferries and fords ; and the sites of markets or camps.

The clearing should be performed during the dry season, because the flies are then less numerous.

In the Senegal, where clearing has been practised on a

large scale, whole tracts of country have been deforested, and in consequence, the streams have dried up and the tsetse-flies have disappeared.

The destruction of animals on which the flies feed is a proposal that needs very careful examination. Koch advocated the destruction of the crocodile, but as mentioned above (p. 264) it is very doubtful whether this scheme would be of much use, and the available evidence is decidedly against it. The destruction of the big game is not likely to affect the numbers of *G. palpalis*, for it rarely feeds on these animals, as they mostly come to the water at early morning or late evening, when the flies are not about. The main food supply of this insect has not yet been satisfactorily decided.

Minchin has suggested the introduction of jungle-fowl, which might scratch up the pupæ and devour them, but it is possible that the birds might find plenty of other food. In any case the experiment might be tried, for at present we know very few enemies of this redoubtable insect. A knowledge of the insectivorous birds that prey upon the tsetse-fly is much to be desired, for we are almost in complete ignorance of this subject.

With regard to the collection or destruction of the pupæ or of the flies themselves, there is little hope of any considerable reduction in numbers being effected by these means. Dr Balfour is of the opinion that fly-traps might be of some use and mentions an incident in support of this view. In the Sudan occurs a limited fly-belt, about twenty miles long and three or four miles in breadth. The fly is *G. morsitans* which in this locality haunts the neighbourhood of wells. " This limited and peculiar distribution is said by the natives to be due to the fact that the fly was intentionally brought here from the river for purposes of revenge ! This may or may not be true,...but certain it is that at the present time the natives trap the fly in gourds containing blood as a bait, and then liberate them in spots where the cattle or horses of their enemies are grazing or are collected together. The trap is a spherical gourd with a hole cut in the top. It is half-filled with blood, and carefully watched. As soon as a number of flies have entered it in quest of food the native rushes forward and claps his hand over the aperture. He then closes the hole in some more permanent fashion, and carries off the flies in triumph for the future discomfiture of those with whom he has a feud. This native custom would certainly seem to indicate that a blood trap is a feasible method of dealing with one of the greatest pests from which Africa, the land of pests, has ever had to suffer."

Mr Maldonado, manager of one of the estates in the Isle of Principe, caught large numbers of G. *palpalis*, by making his labourers wear a black cloth, coated with bird-lime, on their backs. This method of trapping tsetse-flies, however, has not given good results in other localities, for it has been shewn that a single fly-catcher can capture far more flies in a single day than twenty or thirty fly-papers.

## REFERENCES.

Bagshawe, A. G. (1908). *Sleeping Sickness Bulletin*, vol. I.

Balfour, A. (1908). *Third Report Wellcome Research Laboratories*. Khartoum.

Bruce and Nabarro (1903). Progress Report on Sleeping Sickness in Uganda. *Reports S. S. Comm. of Roy. Soc.* No. I.

Bruce, Hamerton and Bateman (1911). *Proc. Roy. Soc.* B, 564, pp. 311–327.

Bruce, Hamerton, Bateman, Mackie and Lady Bruce (1911). *Eleventh Report of S. S. Commission of the Royal Society.* H. M. Stationery Office, London.

Castellani (1903). *Rep. S. S. Comm. of Roy. Soc.* 1903.

Duke (1912). *Proc. Roy. Soc.* vol. LXXXV. pp. 156–69.

Dutton (1902). Trypanosoma in man. *B. M. J.* Jan. 4, p. 42.

—— and Todd (1903). First Report of the Trypanosomiasis expedition to Senegambia. *Liv. Sch. of Trop. Med.* Memoir XI.

Kleine (1909). *Deutsch. Med. Wochenschr.* May 27, pp. 924–25.

Laveran and Mesnil (1912). *Trypanosomes et Trypanosomiases.* Masson : Paris.

Martin, Lebœuf and Roubaud (1909). *Rapport de la Mission d'études de la maladie du sommeil au Congo Français, 1906–1908.* Masson : Paris.

Mense (1906). *Handbuch der Tropenkrankheiten.* vol. III.

Minchin (1908). *Quart. Journ. Micr. Sci.* vol. LII. pp. 159–260.

Robertson, M. (1912). *Proc. Roy. Soc.* B, 578, pp. 241–48.

—— (1913). *Trans. Roy. Soc.* B, vol. 23, pp. 161–84.

Ross and Thomson (1911). *Proc. Roy. Soc.* B, 563, pp. 187–205.

Sandwith (1912). *Sleeping Sickness.* Macmillan & Co. London.

Taute (1911). *Zeitschr. f. Hyg. u. Infektionskr.* vol. LXIX. pp. 553–558.

Trypanosoma rhodesiense Stephens and Fantham, 1910.

*General account.* Until 1909 it was generally supposed that human trypanosomiasis was restricted to regions in which *Glossina palpalis* occurs, for there were no records of any cases occurring outside such areas.

In that year Hearsey published an account of six cases of trypanosomiasis in persons who had not visited any *palpalis* region. The infections in every case must have been contracted either in Nyasaland or North-Eastern Rhodesia, or Portuguese East Africa. Subsequently a number of additional cases were recorded, especially along the shores of Lake Nyasa and in the Luangwa Valley.

In 1910, the first of these cases reached England and was studied at the Royal Southern Hospital, Liverpool. The history of this patient is of some interest as it was in his blood that this trypanosome was first observed, and it is the only strain of the virus which has yet reached Europe.

W.A., a male aged 26, first went to South Africa in July, 1904, living in Johannesburg till the end of 1906. He then went to Salisbury for two years. About the end of November, 1908, he left Salisbury for North-Eastern Rhodesia with a view to prospecting for minerals. On the journey northwards he passed through Fort Jameson, Landazi, and Chinsali to Kasama, arriving at the latter place about the beginning of June, 1909. During this journey the patient traversed an area infested with *Glossina morsitans*. He stayed two months at Kasama, a place apparently free from tsetse-flies. On the return journey he called at Mpika (where *Glossina morsitans* occurs), Serenje and Mzaza (*G. morsitans* present). On September 10, he left Mzaza and travelling along the Luangwa River reached Feira on September 28. During this part of the journey he would pass through an area infested with *Glossina fusca*, between Mzaza and Hargreaves.

The patient first became ill on September 20th, but after a rest of two days continued his journey. A short stay was made at Feira and then the return journey was continued through the Hartley District to Salisbury, where it was found that he was suffering from trypanosomiasis, parasites being found in his blood on November 17th, 1909.

The patient subsequently returned to England and in 1910 was admitted into the Royal Southern Hospital.

The same year Stephens whilst examining a stained specimen of the blood of a rat infected with this race of trypanosomes observed a marked peculiarity in its morphology, and in November, 1910, Stephens and Fantham gave a full description of this new species of human trypanosome under the name of *T. rhodesiense.*

The announcement of the discovery of a new species of human trypanosome has given rise to a great deal of discussion as to the nature of *T. rhodesiense* and its relation to pre-existing species of trypanosomes. Whereas some authors tend to regard it as merely a variety of *T. gambiense,* hardly distinct, others consider it to be a form of *T. brucei* that has acquired pathogenic properties for man. The latter view seems rather unlikely, for on two or three occasions man has been shewn to be immune against experimental infection with *T. brucei,* and, moreover, human serum has a curative action on nagana in experimental infections.

By means of cross-immunity reactions Laveran and Mesnil have shewn that *rhodesiense* is distinct from both *gambiense* and *brucei,* and therefore it must be regarded as a new species of human trypanosome.

There can be little doubt that *T. rhodesiense* has arisen within the last few years and that it is an interesting example of the origin of a new species at the present time. As the transmitting agent *G. morsitans* is widely distributed throughout Rhodesia and East Africa, there is no reason why this disease, had it previously existed, should not also have had a wide range of distribution, instead of being restricted to one or two valleys in Nyasaland and Rhodesia, and the symptoms are so characteristic that the disease could hardly have remained unnoticed.

Since the discovery of the trypanosome, however, its range of distribution has increased considerably and already cases have occurred south of the Zambesi. The sudden appearance of this disease in one small region, followed by such a rapid spread, can only be explained on the supposition that it is an entirely new form of sleeping sickness. Moreover, its extremely deadly effect on its vertebrate host, man, is further evidence in support of the same view.

*T. rhodesiense* is remarkably pathogenic to the majority of experimental animals, the duration of life of monkeys infected with this species being only about 8 to 14 days, as compared with 27 to 149 days in the case of *T. gambiense*. It is evident, therefore, that this new trypanosome is extraordinarily virulent, and it is also very resistant to treatment, atoxyl apparently having no effect on it.

In man the course of the disease is much more rapid than in the case of ordinary sleeping sickness (*T. gambiense*) and death usually takes place within three or four months of infection.

At present *T. rhodesiense* is restricted to Southern Nyasaland, North-Eastern Rhodesia, especially in the Luangwa Valley, and Portuguese East Africa, but it seems to be extending its range and unless effective preventive measures are discovered there is reason to fear that it may give rise throughout Africa to an epidemic, besides which the ravages of *gambiense* would appear almost mild in comparison.

*Morphology of the parasite.* *T. rhodesiense* in most respects resembles *T. gambiense*, but is characterised by the occurrence of stout or stumpy forms in which some have the trophonucleus at the posterior end. Stephens and Fantham give the following account of the parasite: " Rats inoculated with this Rhodesian strain usually shew a few long thin trypanosomes in the peripheral blood in about three days. The stumpy forms of trypanosomes with the trophonucleus posterior appear about the fifth or sixth day and from this time onwards somewhat increase in number up to the seventh or eleventh day. They then form about six per cent. of the trypanosomes present, but may decrease again, varying from day to day."

The dimensions of stumpy forms with a posterior trophonucleus vary from 17 to 21 microns in length by 2 to 3 microns in breadth. There is a well-marked kinetonucleus

and the flagellum terminates in a short free portion.  The cytoplasm is coarsely granular, especially at the anterior end.

In addition Stephens and Fantham mention the occurrence
of " snout " forms with an elongated posterior end.  These
forms are present especially during the first half of the infèction,
and although not absent from the ordinary strains of *T. gambiense* are much more numerous in the case of *rhodesiense*.

It is important to note that the posterior position of the
trophonucleus has never been observed in trypanosomes in the
blood of man, but only in experimental animals.  Wenyon and
Hanschell found that the percentage of posterior nuclear forms
varies very much, not only with the stage of infection but also
with the strain employed.  In three strains of *rhodesiense* in
rats the percentages of these forms were found to vary in one
strain from 0 to 0·9 per cent., in the second from 3 to 7 per cent.
and in the third strain from 13 to 40 per cent.

*T. rhodesiense*, like *gambiense*, is markedly dimorphic, for
there are long slender forms and short stumpy forms, together
with intermediate forms.  The numerical relations between
these various forms are extremely variable, depending on the
stage of infection. The dimensions of the parasites vary from
13 to 39 microns in length, but the majority of them fall between
17 and 30 microns.

*Mode of transmission.*  In 1912, Kinghorn and Yorke
demonstrated the transmission of *T. rhodesiense* by *Glossina
morsitans*, the experiments being carried out at Nawalia,
Northern Rhodesia, on the Nyamadzi River, a tributary of the
Luangwa.

About five per cent. of the flies were found to become infected
when fed on patients or animals containing trypanosomes.
The development in the fly is of the cyclical type, the insect
becoming infective after an incubation period of about fourteen
days.  Once infected a fly remains infective for the remainder
of its life and may infect fresh animals at each successive feed.

Temperature has a marked effect on the development of
*rhodesiense* in the intermediate host as shewn by the following
experiment.

" Two batches of wild *G. morsitans*, batch *A* 95 flies, batch

*B* 119, shewn to be non-infective by feeding upon clean monkeys, were fed for three days on a *rhodesiense*-infected guineapig. Each batch was then fed on a healthy monkey until the fortieth day, the mean temperature being 59° F. Neither monkey became infected. The 42 flies remaining of batch *A* were placed in the incubator at 85° F., and the 58 flies of batch *B* were left at laboratory temperature. Of the batch *A* flies, on the 43rd day only six were alive. From the 41st to the 47th day the flies of batch *A* were fed on a monkey (which died) ; from the 48th day on a rat. The rat became infected, shewing that batch *A* contained an infective fly on the 48th day, eight days after being placed in the incubator. The four flies still alive on the 53rd day were fed on four clean rats, three of which became infected.

On the 61st day the 38 flies of batch *B*, which had then failed to infect the monkey, were put in the incubator at 83° F., and from that day till the 75th were fed on a healthy monkey. The animal unfortunately died. All the flies were dissected as they died. One was found to harbour trypanosomes in the salivary glands and gut, and animals inoculated with the contents became infected. In the first part of the experiment the relative humidity in the incubator was 36 per cent., in the second, 72 per cent."

This experiment clearly shews that at a comparatively low temperature the early stages of the trypanosomes may persist in the alimentary canal of the fly for sixty days, but that for the completion of the cycle of development a higher temperature is required (75°—85° F.). The necessity of a certain degree of heat, before the fly can become infective, explains why Kleine was unable to transmit *T. gambiense* by *G. morsitans* on Lake Victoria, where the temperature is not high enough.

The life cycle of *T. rhodesiense* within the tsetse-fly has not been thoroughly worked out, but seems to present many points of resemblance to that of *T. gambiense* in *G. palpalis*. The trypanosomes first become established in the intestine and in every case the salivary glands are invaded before the fly becomes infective. The manner in which the glands become infected is uncertain, but it is apparently secondary to the intestinal infection, and it only occurs when the trypanosomes in the gut have reached a certain stage of development, and even then only when the conditions of temperature are suitable for the further development of the parasites. It was found that on every occasion on which the salivary glands were infective, the trypanosomes in the intestine were also virulent

As a large number of the wild game harbour *T. rhodesiense*, in nature the fly is frequently infected. In the Luangwa Valley, Kinghorn and Yorke found that about 0·18 per cent. of the *morsitans* were infected with *rhodesiense*.

Recently, however, Taute has published an important paper in which the validity of these results is questioned. This investigator carried out experiments at Lubimbinu, Portuguese Nyasaland, and found that a large proportion (16·2 per cent.) of the big game of that district was infected with a trypanosome closely agreeing with *T. rhodesiense* in its general characters. Nevertheless this parasite was shewn to be non-pathogenic for man, as Taute fed laboratory-bred *Glossina morsitans* on a monkey infected with the wild game strain, and subsequently on a number of animals and also himself. After the usual incubation period the flies became infective and all the experimental animals (goats, dogs, and monkeys) on which they were fed became infected and died of trypanosomiasis. On the other hand, although Taute fed these same tsetse-flies on himself for four days after they had been proved to be infective for animals, yet he remained well. This experiment was repeated, with the same results, and in addition the author injected himself with 2 c.c. of blood from a naturally infected dog, without ever developing any symptoms of trypanosomiasis.

These results suggest that game and domestic animals may not play the part in the spread of human trypanosomiasis that certain authors have supposed, and trypanosomes from such sources can only be regarded with certainty as factors in the spread of sleeping sickness when they have been shewn to be pathogenic for man.

## REFERENCES.

Hearsey (1909). *Nyasaland Sleeping Sickness Diary.* Part VIII.

Kinghorn and Yorke (1912). *Ann. Trop. Med. and Parasitology*, vol. VI. pp. 1–23, 301–15 and 317–24.

Laveran and Mesnil (1912). *Trypanosomes et Trypanosomiases*, 2nd edit. Masson : Paris.

Shircore, J. O. (1913). *Trans. Soc. Trop. Med. and Hyg.* vol. VI. pp. 131–42.

Stephens and Fantham (1910). *Proc. Roy. Soc.* B, 561, pp. 28–32.

Taute, M. (1913). *Arbeit a. d. Kais. Gesundheitsamte*, vol. LXV. pp. 102–112.

Wenyon and Hanschell (1912). *Jl. Lond. Sch. of Trop. Med.* vol. II. pp. 34–35

## Nagana (T. brucei Plimmer and Bradford, 1899).

*General account.* Nagana, or the " tsetse-fly disease," is the most widely distributed and best known of all the cattle trypanosomiases of Africa. For many years the common tsetse-fly, *Glossina morsitans*, was known to be the cause of the disease and the popular belief was that the fly injected into the bitten animal some poison that caused the well-known symptoms of the " fly disease."

In 1895, Bruce, together with his wife, investigated the disease as it occurred in Zululand and discovered that it was caused by the presence of a trypanosome in the blood. This parasite was found to be conveyed from diseased to healthy animals by the common tsetse-fly, and was present in the blood of all affected animals. Bruce gives the following account of the infection.

" Nagana, or the fly disease, is a specific malady appearing in horses, mules, donkeys, cattle, dogs, cats, and many other animals, and of which the duration varies from a few days to some weeks or even up to some months. It is invariably fatal in the horse, ass and dog ; but a small percentage of cattle recover. It is characterised by fever, by an infiltration of coagulated lymph into the subcutaneous tissue of the neck, abdomen or the extremities, giving rise to a swelling of these regions ; by a more or less rapid destruction of the red cells of the blood, an extreme emaciation, often blindness, and by the constant presence in the blood of an intusorian parasite—a trypanosome."

It is generally supposed that Bruce employed *Glossina morsitans* in these transmission experiments, but, according to Austen, from a consideration of the description and figures given in Bruce's Report on the tsetse-fly disease, or nagana, in Zululand, there can be little doubt that *G. pallidipes* was the species employed.

*T. brucei* is one of the best known of all the trypanosomes, as a dog infected with the parasite reached England in 1898, and subsequently was sent to most of the laboratories of Europe. As a result this parasite is the one most often employed in treatment experiments and other observations on the biology of trypanosomes under experimental conditions.

The disease is widely distributed in Africa, where, in addition to Zululand, it has been recorded from the basins of the Limpopo and Zambesi, Nyasaland, Northern Rhodesia, German and British East Africa, Uganda, Bahr el Ghazal, and in the region of the White Nile.

It is also possible that the disease may occur in Somaliland and Galla, for the trypanosome causing the camel disease known as *Aino* is indistinguishable morphologically from *T. brucei*.

Nagana is one of the most deadly of all trypanosomiases and the majority of animals succumb to the infection after a comparatively short illness.

With regard to the virus as it occurs in the laboratories of Europe, Laveran and Mesnil divide the mammals into three groups according to their susceptibility.

" (1)　Animals in which nagana produces an acute infection : mice, rats, marmots, hedgehogs, dogs and monkeys.

(2)　Animals in which nagana produces a sub-acute infection : rabbits, guinea-pigs, dormice, horses, donkeys, mules and pigs.

(3)　Animals in which nagana produces a chronic infection : cattle, goats and sheep."

In nature the disease affects horses, ruminants and dogs, and also the wild game, such as antelopes, waterbuck, etc., are frequently infected with the trypanosome. These wild animals, however, seem to have become immune against the disease, for they may harbour the parasite in the blood for long periods without suffering from any apparent ill-effects. The wild game, therefore, serves as a reservoir for the infection, as in the case of *T. gambiense*, and thus, in nature, generally a large proportion of *G. morsitans* and *pallidipes* are infected with *T. brucei*.

*The morphology of the parasite.* In the living state, *T. brucei* displays active movements, as its undulating membrane is well developed. Its translatory powers, however, are far inferior to those of *T. cazalboui* and it rarely moves out of the field of the microscope.

The dimensions of the parasite according to Bruce vary from 15 to 34 microns in length. Moreover the species is somewhat dimorphic, the short stumpy forms measuring from 2 to 5 microns in diameter and the elongated forms only about 1·5 microns in diameter. According to Laveran and Mesnil the average length of the parasite in horses is 28 to 33 microns and in dogs and the smaller rodents 26 to 27 microns.

In stained specimens the protoplasm usually contains numerous granules, especially in the anterior region of the body. The kinetonucleus is distinct, and is generally situated near the posterior extremity, especially in the shorter forms. The undulating membrane is much folded and the flagellum usually becomes free at its anterior extremity.

The trypanosome multiplies by simple longitudinal division.

*Mode of infection.* The experiments of Bruce in Zululand shewed that *Glossina pallidipes* and *morsitans* were able to transmit *T. brucei*, but the exact mode of infection remained unknown until Kleine's observations were published.

In 1909, Kleine shewed experimentally that *G. palpalis* is able to transmit this disease, and in addition that the trypanosome underwent a cyclical development in its invertebrate host. The account of the first experiment in which this important discovery was made is as follows :

Since nagana did not exist in the Kirugu region (in German East Africa) some sheep and a mule were brought from a place

seven days' march away; these animals had been naturally
infected with nagana by the bites of *G. morsitans*. Fifty *G.
palpalis* were fed on three of these infected animals for three
successive days and from the fourth day onwards daily on fresh
healthy animals. From the fourth to the seventeenth day
inclusive the flies fed on a new animal each day, but none of
them became infected. From the eighteenth to the twenty-
fourth day the flies fed on the same sheep, and from the twenty-
fifth to thirty-ninth day on the same ox. On the twelfth day
after the flies were put on this ox, numerous trypanosomes were
found in the blood and the sheep was also found to be infected.
All the other animals remained healthy. Continuing this experiment from the fortieth to the fiftieth day the flies, now reduced
in number to twenty-two, were fed on two goats, two calves
and two sheep. All these animals became infected after incubation periods varying from five to eight days.

This experiment clearly shews that *G. palpalis* remains non-
infective for many days after the ingestion of blood containing
*T. brucei*, but that after this negative incubation period the flies
become infective and may remain so for a considerable length
of time.

Later these experiments were repeated employing *Glossina
morsitans* instead of *palpalis*. It was found that the animals
bitten during the three days following the feed on an infected
animal, all became infected, the transmission being direct, as
in the case of the Zululand experiments. The animals bitten
from the fourth to the tenth day remained healthy, whilst all
those that were bitten by the flies from the eleventh to the
forty-fourth day became infected. Moreover, Taute has shewn
that *Glossina morsitans* may remain infective for at least
83 days.

The evolution of *T. brucei* within the intermediate host has
not been fully worked out, but the parasites seem to multiply
within the alimentary canal and subsequently invade the
proboscis in a manner similar to *T. gambiense*.

## REFERENCES.

Austen (1911). *Handbook of Tsetse Flies.*
Bruce (1895). *Preliminary Report on the Tsetse Fly disease or Nagana in Zululand.* Ubombo, Zululand. *Further Report,* 1896.
Bruce, Hamerton, Bateman and Mackie (1910). *Proc. Roy. Soc.* B, vol. LXXXIII.
Kleine (1909). *Deutsche Med. Woch.* Nos. 11, 21, 29 and 45.
Kleine and Taute (1911). *Arb. a. d. Kais. Gesundheitsamte,* vol. XXXI.
Laveran and Mesnil (1912). *Trypanosomes et Trypanosomiases.* Paris : Masson et Cie.

## Baleri (T. pecaudi Laveran, 1907).

*General account.* In 1904, Cazalbou observed a trypanosome in the blood of a horse from the Bani region of Northern Nigeria. This animal was suffering from a disease known by the natives as Baleri. In 1907, Laveran described the trypanosome under the name of *T. pecaudi,* and since this time Baleri has been recorded from many parts of Tropical Africa.

It is common in the Upper Senegal and Nigeria, especially in the basins of the Niger, Bani, and the Upper Volta. It has also been observed in the Lower Senegal, Ivory Coast, Dahomey, French Congo, and in the region of Chari. In Bahr el Ghazal, Balfour and Wenyon have observed in dromedaries and horses infections probably due to *T. pecaudi.*

Baleri is especially a disease of horses and donkeys, but cattle are also susceptible to infection. The disease is characterised by the occurrence of febrile attacks that are repeated every three, four or five days. The trypanosomes are generally numerous during the first attacks, becoming rare towards the end of the infection. In horses the disease is practically always fatal, after a duration of from three to four months. Donkeys are less susceptible and may remain infected for nearly two years before death supervenes.

A large number of animals may be experimentally infected with *T. pecaudi* and the symptoms vary according to the species. Cattle, goats, sheep and pigs are very resistant to the infection and generally recover. On the other hand, monkeys, dogs, cats, guinea-pigs, rats and mice are all susceptible and the infection is invariably fatal. In these animals the parasites are numerous in the late stages of the disease.

*Morphology of the parasite.* In the living state the movements of the trypanosome are very active. In stained preparations two types can be distinguished, namely, long thin forms and short broad forms.

The long thin forms measure about 25 to 35 microns in length by about 1·5 microns in breadth. The posterior extremity is drawn out to a point. The undulating membrane is very narrow and the flagellum anteriorly is free for about one-quarter of its length. The elongate trophonucleus is situated about the middle of the body and the kinetonucleus is some distance away from the posterior extremity. The cytoplasm is free from granules.

The short forms measure from 14 to 20 microns in length by 3 to 4 microns in breadth. They are stumpy in appearance and the undulating membrane is very well developed ; there is no free flagellum. The trophonucleus is large and round and the kinetonucleus is situated almost at the posterior extremity. The cytoplasm often contains numerous granules. In the Bahr el Ghazal strain, Wenyon found many forms in which the kinetonucleus was near to the trophonucleus and a few in which the latter was at the posterior end of the body.

Both the long and short forms multiply by ordinary longitudinal division.

*Mode of infection.* *T. pecaudi* is transmitted mainly if not entirely by tsetse-flies. The experiments of Bouet and Roubaud in Dahomey have shewn that, in this region, *G. longipalpis* is the most favourable intermediate host, but *tachinoides*, *palpalis* and *morsitans*, can also carry the disease.

These two authors found that the *longipalpis* caught on the banks of the Ouémé River, in the neighbourhood of Agouagon, were heavily infected with *T. pecaudi*. Thus batches of 45 flies and upwards, almost invariably produced infections of *pecaudi* when fed on susceptible animals. On the other hand, several hundred *palpalis* and *tachinoides* captured in the same area and similarly fed on susceptible animals never produced any infection, so it is evident from the epidemiological point of view that *longipalpis* is the species which in this region constitutes the reservoir fly of *T. pecaudi*, to the exclusion of the others.   The incubation period of the parasite in *G. longipalpis* is about 23 days.   In addition, 60 *G. tachinoides* were fed on a guinea-pig infected with *T. pecaudi* and then on a series of healthy guinea-pigs.   Two of these guinea-pigs became infected, giving an incubation period in the fly of 26 days, whereas the others remained normal.   In this region experiments with *G. palpalis* gave entirely negative results, but Bouffard previously succeeded in the transmission of *T. pecaudi* by means of this species, though only with difficulty.

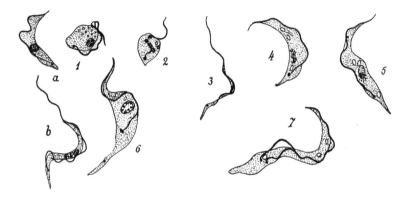

Fig. 77.   Culture of *T. pecaudi*, in the intestine of *G. palpalis* ( × 1200). *a, b*, normal forms from the circulating blood ; 1–5 forms 18 hours after ingestion ; 1, 2, involution forms ; 3, slender form ; 4, 5, large forms ; 6, 7, large forms 56 hours after ingestion. (After Roubaud.)

In the Nigerian Sudan, Bouet and Roubaud, during the dry season, found that the *morsitans* of that region were naturally infected with *T. pecaudi*.

It appears, therefore, that *longipalpis* and *morsitans* are the two most favourable hosts for this parasite, and that *tachinoides* and, exceptionally, *palpalis* may also be infected.

Every infected fly that was dissected contained flagellates along the whole of the digestive tract from the proboscis to the hinder intestine.   The trypanosomes multiply in the intestine up to 48 hours after ingestion in a modified form called by Roubaud the "intestinal trypanosome form." Under favourable conditions these multiply very rapidly and in seven to nine days invade the whole of the intestine as far as the pharynx. These flies are not infective until the parasites have invaded the proboscis and passed through the *Crithidia* and *Leptomonas* phase. These proboscis forms multiply and some reach the hypopharynx, where they assume the "salivary trypanosome form" and are then capable of infecting any susceptible animal.

REFERENCES.

Bouet and Roubaud (1910). *Bull. Soc. Path. Exot.* vol. III. p. 599.
—— (1911). *Ibid.* vol. IV. p. 539.
Bouffard (1908). *Ann. Inst. Pasteur*, vol. XXII. p. 15.
Cazalbou (1904). *Rec. de Méd. Vétér.* vol. LXXXI. p. 615.
Laveran (1907). *Compt. Rend. Acad. Sci.* vol. CXLIV. pp. 243–247.
Balfour and Wenyon (1908). *Rep. Wellcome Research Lab.* Khartoum.

## Souma (T. cazalboui Laveran).

*General account.* In 1904, Cazalbou described, from the Upper Niger Territories, a cattle trypanosomiasis known to the natives by the name of Souma. Two years later, Laveran described the trypanosome causing this disease under the name of *T. cazalboui*, and also gave an account of its biological properties.

The disease has subsequently been observed in most of the provinces of West Africa south of latitude 17° N., especially along the upper valleys of the Niger and Volta. It is common in Uganda and has also been recorded from the French Congo, Congo Free State and Rhodesia.

Souma is a very widespread disease affecting cattle, horses, mules, and donkeys; goats, sheep and antelope are also susceptible to the infection, but contrary to the general rule for the group of trypanosomes to which it belongs, dogs, cats, monkeys, pigs, rabbits, guinea-pigs, rats and mice are all refractory, and this constitutes one of the principal means of distinguishing *T. cazalboui* from allied forms.

*T. vivax* and *T. uniforme* are very closely related to this species and may subsequently prove to be identical, but at present it is impossible to unite them without increasing the confusion of the subject.

The incubation period is usually about seven days. The course of the disease is variable and may be either acute, subacute, or chronic. In the former case, cattle may succumb in as short a time as eight days after infection. The average duration of the malady is about two months, being terminated by the death of the infected animal, but in some cases the disease lingers on for more than a year, and recoveries are not unknown.

The parasites are usually rare in the peripheral circulation, but often increase in numbers previous to the death of the host.

*Morphology of T. cazalboui.* The movements of the living parasite are very active and it frequently darts across the field of the microscope.

It is a monomorphic species and its dimensions are very constant; in stained specimens about 24 microns in length, by 1·5 to 2 microns in breadth. The trophonucleus is oval and situated about the middle of the body, whilst the distinct and spherical kinetonucleus is situated very close to the rounded posterior extremity. The undulating membrane is not markedly folded, resembling that of *T. lewisi*; the flagellum is always free at the anterior extremity.

Division is of the usual longitudinal type.

*Mode of infection.* The principal agents for the transmission of Souma are tsetse-flies, four species of which, viz., *G. palpalis, tachinoides, longipalpis* and *morsitans*, have been proved capable of carrying the infection. In addition, Bouffard's experiments have shewn that *Stomoxys* may serve as a direct carrier (*vide* p. 362).

The distribution of Souma seems to shew that *Glossina palpalis* is the usual intermediate host, and Bouffard found that in Upper Guinea this species was commonly infected with *T. cazalboui*. Experimentally, both *G. palpalis* and *G. tachinoides* have been proved to be very liable to become infected when fed on an animal containing the trypanosomes in its blood, for

Bouffard found that out of 224 tsetse that ingested *T. cazalboui*, no less than 38·8 per cent. became infected. In Uganda, Bruce and his collaborators found that under similar circumstances about 20 per cent. of *palpalis* shewed a development of trypanosomes in the proboscis.

The effect of climate on the development of this trypanosome in the intermediate host is well shewn by the results of Bouet and Roubaud in Upper Dahomey and the Nigerian Sudan, during the dry season. In these regions only two species of *Glossina*, namely *tachinoides* and *morsitans*, were found during the summer, all *palpalis* having disappeared as a result of the dry weather. Experiments were undertaken to determine which of these species was most liable to infection with *T. cazalboui*. Although in Middle Dahomey *tachinoides* was as efficient a carrier as *palpalis*, in the dry regions of Upper Dahomey and the Nigerian Sudan the same species was only infected with great difficulty, the authors concluding that during the dry season, at any rate, *G. tachinoides* of the regions between 12° and 13° north latitude is unable, or only slightly able, to infect with the endemic viruses, or those which it is able to transmit outside these areas. On the other hand, about 50 per cent. of wild *morsitans* captured at random were found to be infected; the development of the trypanosome in this species, however, is somewhat slower than in *palpalis*, *tachinoides* and *longipalpis*, respectively. In the Katanga district the members of the Belgian Sleeping Sickness Expedition (1912) found an equally large percentage of *morsitans* infected with *cazalboui*.

The development of the trypanosome in the tsetse-fly is restricted to the proboscis, the flagellates never multiplying in any other part of the alimentary canal. *Palpalis*, *tachinoides*, and *longipalpis*, become infective about six to seven days after an infecting feed, whilst in the case of *morsitans* this developmental period is prolonged to eight to ten days.

In Uganda, the development of *T. cazalboui* is much slower than in the West African Provinces, for the members of the Sleeping Sickness Commission at Mpumu, found that the non-infective period varied from 11 to 35 days.

It is possible that this remarkable difference in the rate of development may be accounted for by the difference in climate, for Bamako, on the Niger, the locality where Bouffard performed his experiments, is less than 1000 feet above sea-level, whereas Mpumu is more than 4000. Moreover, the mean temperature of Uganda is far below that of Bamako and the influence of this factor is most important. .

After being ingested some of the trypanosomes remain in the proboscis of the fly and change into *Leptomonas* or Crithidial forms. These become attached to the walls of the labrum and undergo rapid multiplication, resulting in the production of large clusters of flagellates, which may almost obstruct the cavity of the proboscis. Under the influence of the salivary secretion some of these fixed flagellates develop into small actively motile trypanosomes closely resembling the blood forms. These free trypanosomes are found in the hypopharynx and escape together with the salivary secretion when an infected fly feeds on any host.

Once a fly becomes infected it may remain infective for at least two and a half months and probably for the remainder of its life. If the air is very dry, however, the flagellates may disappear from the proboscis and the fly cease to be infective. Thus Bouet and Roubaud found that in Upper Dahomey during the dry season about 50 per cent. of freshly caught *morsitans* shewed infection of the proboscis, but when these flies were kept and examined 20 to 31 days later the proportion of infected flies was only two in thirteen.

Roubaud has performed some very interesting experiments on the effects of various conditions on the development of *T. cazalboui* in *G. palpalis*, which supplement the observations of Bouet and Roubaud in Upper Dahomey. Twelve *G. palpalis*, caught in nature, were placed in a dehydrated atmosphere. Twelve hours later and twice in the three succeeding days they were allowed to feed on a goat infected with *T. cazalboui*. Four days later they were fed on a healthy kid for two days. On the ninth day the flies were dissected and found to be uninfected and also the kid remained healthy. In another experiment eight flies were fed for two days on the infected goat and then placed in a partially dehydrated atmosphere. They were fed every day on a healthy kid until the ninth day when they were dissected and four were found to be infected. In another similar experiment three out of fifteen flies became infected and the kid succumbed to trypanosomiasis caused by their bites In two control experiments, during which the flies were kept in the ordinary atmosphere, eight out of twelve and eight out of nine flies shewed flagellates and also infected a succession of healthy kids on which they were fed.

In another experiment, six flies hatched from pupæ that had been kept in dry air from their formation, were fed on July 7, 8, and 9 on an infected goat and then returned to dry air. On the 18th and 19th they were allowed to bite a healthy kid and on the 27th and 28th yet another normal kid. The next day the flies were dissected and two out of six were found to be infected, moreover both kids suffered from a very severe attack of trypanosomiasis. Roubaud accordingly is of the opinion that if the modifying influence, such as dry air, acts for a long time before the infecting feed is given, the saliva regains its suitability as a medium for the development of the trypanosomes.

The action of saturated air was similarly tested and respectively, one fly in eight and one in fifteen became infected, without, however, infecting a kitten on which they were fed. These results tend to explain the author's observation that, in nature, during the dry season more flies were found to be infected than during the wet.

REFERENCES.

Bouet and Roubaud (1911). *Bull. Soc. Path. Exot.* vol. IV. p. 539.
Bouffard, G. (1909). *Bull. Soc. Path. Exot.* vol. II. p. 599.
——— (1910). *Ann. Inst. Pasteur,* vol. XXIV. p. 276.
Cazalbou, L. (1905). *Compt. Rend. Soc. Biol.* vol. LVIII. pp. 564–565.
Laveran, A. (1906). *Compt. Rend. Acad. Sci.* vol. CXLIII. pp. 94–97.
——— (1910). *Bull. Soc. Path. Exot.* vol. III. p. 80.
Rodhain, Pons, van den Branden and Bequaert (1912). *Bull. Soc. Path. Exot.* vol. V. pp. 45–50 and 281–84.
Roubaud, E. (1909). *Thèse de doctorat ès sci. nat.* Paris, June, 1909.
——— (1910). *Compt. Rend. Acad. Sci.* 1910, pp. 729–32.

### Trypanosoma vivax Ziemann, 1905.

In 1905, Ziemann described under the name of *T. vivax* a trypanosome occurring in the blood of cattle, sheep, and goats in the Cameroons. The symptoms of the disease it produces are almost identical with those of Souma, and moreover, in its morphology, *T. vivax* closely resembles *cazalboui*. But Ziemann definitely states that rats are susceptible to *T. vivax*, eight of them dying from the infection after eight, nine and eleven days. Also a dog and a pig both shewed a temporary infection. On the other hand, rats are absolutely refractory to *T. cazalboui* and this constitutes a method of distinguishing the two.

Bagshawe has called attention to the resemblance between the two forms, and inclines to consider them as constituting a single species. This view has been opposed by Laveran, and certainly as long as " species " of trypanosomes are distinguished mainly on the basis of cross-immunity reactions and the susceptibility of laboratory animals, it is impossible to unite two forms differing so markedly in the latter feature.

Bruce and his colleagues on the basis of a microscopic examination of Ziemann's slides came to the conclusion that *T. cazalboui* Laveran was synonymous with *T. vivax* Ziemann. Accordingly throughout their reports they have employed the latter name for a trypanosome which is undoubtedly identical with the *T. cazalboui* of the French and Belgian authors. A careful comparison of Ziemann's original description with the accounts of *cazalboui*, shew that although very closely related the two forms may be easily distinguished by their respective animal reactions. Thus, all small laboratory animals and the pig are refractory to *cazalboui*, whereas rats are very susceptible to *vivax* and die within eleven days ; also a dog and a pig shewed a temporary infection.

As rats as well as the other small experimental animals are not susceptible to the Uganda virus, it is evident that the species of that region, which has been referred to as *T. vivax*, should be known correctly as *cazalboui*.

Undoubtedly the two forms are closely related, but as long as the reaction of experimental animals constitutes one of the means of distinguishing varieties of trypanosomes, it is only increasing the confusion of the subject to unite *vivax* and *cazalboui* on purely morphological grounds.

REFERENCES.

Bruce, Hamerton, Bateman and Mackie (1910). *Proc. Roy. Soc.* B, vol. 556, p. 368 and vol. 561, p. 1.
Bruce, Hamerton, Bateman and Lady Bruce (1911). *Eleventh Report Sleeping Sickness Comm. of Roy. Soc.*
Yorke and Blacklock (1911). *Ann. Trop. Med. and Parasit.* vol. v. p. 413.
Ziemann, H. (1905). *Centralbl. f. Bakter.* I. Orig. vol. xxxviii. p. 9.

## Trypanosoma uniforme Bruce, Hamerton, Bateman and Mackie, 1911.

This parasite was first noticed in the blood of oxen in Uganda. It closely resembles *T. cazalboui*, but may be distinguished by its smaller size.

*T. uniforme* causes a very fatal disease, for two naturally infected cattle died after 5 and 79 days respectively. Goats inoculated with the parasite lived on an average 29 days, but out of three sheep inoculated only one became infected. Fraser and Duke found that two out of 30 bushbuck and sitatunga (*Tragelaphus spekei*), obtained within two miles of the shore of Lake Victoria, were naturally infected with *T. uniforme*. Monkeys, pigs, dogs, cats, guinea-pigs and white rats are all refractory to this parasite, another characteristic in which this species resembles *cazalboui*.

According to Laveran and Mesnil, *uniforme* is probably the same as *cazalboui*, but its small size seems to be a sufficient means of distinction.

*Morphology.* *T. uniforme* is a small and active trypanosome with marked translatory movement, though inferior to that of *cazalboui*. The parasites are remarkably uniform in size and appearance, the average dimensions being 16 microns in length by 1·5 to 2·5 microns in breadth. The extreme range of variation in the length is only from a minimum of 12 to a maximum of 19 microns. The free part of the flagellum is from 1 to 5 microns in length. In all other characters *T. uniforme* is the same as *cazalboui*, with the exception that there is no marked narrowing opposite the trophonucleus as in the case of the latter species.

*Mode of infection.* Fraser and Duke have shewn that the *Glossina palpalis* in the neighbourhood of Lake Victoria are naturally infected with this trypanosome, for after 1020 flies from the lake-shore had been fed on a goat it became infected with *T. uniforme*. Also it was shewn experimentally that laboratory-bred *palpalis* were capable of transmitting this species of trypanosome from infected to healthy animals. Of six experiments four were successful. The flies became infective in from 27 to 37 days, and the infection in the fly was always limited to the proboscis as in the case of *cazalboui*.

REFERENCES.

Bruce, Hamerton, Bateman and Mackie (1911). *Proc. Roy. Soc.* B, 563, p. 176.
Fraser and Duke (1912). *Ibid.* B, vol. LXXXV. p. 1.

### Trypanosoma dimorphon Laveran and Mesnil, 1904.

*Synonyms.* *T. confusum* Montgomery and Kinghorn, 1909. *T. frobeninsi* Weissenborn, 1911.

*General account.* In 1902, Dutton and Todd in the course of their expedition to the Gambia observed trypanosomes in the blood of some of the horses in that region.

Under the title of " Horse trypanosome " they described and figured the parasites occurring in one of these horses. The remarkable feature about the infection was the occurrence of small tadpole-shaped trypanosomes without any free flagellum, side by side with long and slender forms with a long free flagellum. Dutton and Todd did not name their horse trypanosome, a fortunate omission, since there is practically no doubt that several distinct species were in their hands. One of these infected horses was sent over to Liverpool and from here the strain was sent across to Laveran and Mesnil in Paris, where they studied the morphology of the trypanosome, and, in 1904, published a description of it under the name of *T. dimorphon*.

The name *T. dimorphon*, therefore, is only applicable to the trypanosome which reached Europe and was described by Laveran and Mesnil. This parasite, as pointed out by the authors, differs considerably from Dutton and Todd's description of the " Horse trypanosome," especially in the absence of any forms provided with a free flagellum. *T. dimorphon* Laveran and Mesnil, is the ordinary *dimorphon* of the laboratories of Europe, and it is important that the use of this name should be absolutely restricted to trypanosomes agreeing with Laveran and Mesnil's original description (1904). Montgomery and Kinghorn wish to reserve the name *T. dimorphon* for the forms described by Dutton and Todd and apply the term *T. confusum* to the parasite described by Laveran and Mesnil. Such a course, however, is illegitimate, for the name *dimorphon* was only applied to the latter, and never to Dutton and Todd's original description.

The occurrence of mixed infections in many animals is a source of great difficulty in identifying the species of trypanosomes, for Yorke and Blacklock have shewn that *dimorphon* and *cazalboui* may occur side by side in horses from the Gambia.

*T. dimorphon* is widely distributed throughout West Africa and has been recorded from the following localities : Gambia, Senegal, Casamance, Upper Gambia, French Guinea, Sierra Leone, Ivory Coast, Togoland, Dahomey, French Sudan and French Congo. In the Congo Free State, Rhodesia, Zululand, Portuguese East Africa, Zanzibar, Bahr el Ghazal, and Somaliland, trypanosomes of the *dimorphon* type have been observed, but it is difficult to say whether they should all be referred to *T. dimorphon* Laveran and Mesnil.

Horses, mules, cattle, goats, sheep, pigs, dogs, cats, monkeys, and all the smaller laboratory animals are susceptible to infection with *T. dimorphon*. As a rule, in the larger animals, the course of the disease is slow, and death only occurs after trypanosomes have been present in the blood for several months. In some cases the animals recover and trypanosomes may be present in the peripheral circulation for some years, without apparently producing any pathogenic symptoms.

*Morphology of the parasite.* In the fresh state,the dimorphic nature of this species is easily recognisable. The most common forms are only 12 to 14 microns in length and 1 micron in breadth, with a rounded posterior extremity and a body which gradually tapers towards the anterior extremity. These short forms present a somewhat characteristic movement ; after progressing forward for some little distance, wriggling after the manner of a tadpole, they stop abruptly, and then move on again in the same fashion. The undulating membrane is very slightly developed.

The long forms of *dimorphon* are less common than the preceding and may occasionally be absent. They range from 20 to 25 microns in length, by 1·5 microns in breadth. The undulating membrane is only slightly developed and the parasites, although more active than the short forms, do not present as lively motions as *T. brucei.*

These two forms are connected by intermediate stages, and therefore the short trypanosomes might be regarded as a young form of the large, were it not for the fact that they both reproduce by longitudinal fission.

In Giemsa-stained specimens, a remarkable feature of *dimorphon* is the extremely dense blue colour of the protoplasm. The kinetonucleus is situated close to the rounded posterior extremity. The undulating membrane is never very marked and in every case the protoplasm is continued along to the extremity of the flagellum. This latter feature, together with the dimorphism, is very characteristic. Division is of the usual longitudinal type.

*Mode of infection.* Bouet, in 1907, succeeded in transmitting *T. dimorphon* by the bites of *Glossina palpalis* that had fed on an infected animal 24 hours previously. In this experiment the transmission was merely mechanical.

In Dahomey, Bouet and Roubaud have demonstrated the part played by *G. palpalis, tachinoides* and *longipalpis* in the transmission of this parasite. *Palpalis* captured in nature, were fed on two dogs, a sheep, and a kid, and these animals became infected with *dimorphon* after incubation periods varying from 14 to 20 days. The same flies were fed on guinea-pigs but produced no infection, thus shewing that these animals are only slightly susceptible to this trypanosome.

*G. morsitans* is also capable of transmitting *T. dimorphon*, and thus four species of tsetse-flies in West Africa are all efficient intermediate hosts for the parasite. The experiments with regard to the infection of the fly are somewhat inconclusive, but from an examination of " wild " tsetse it appears that *longipalpis* is the most often infected, then *tachinoides*, whilst the proportion of *palpalis* containing *dimorphon* is very much less, being only about one per cent.

In Dahomey, the negative period of incubation in the fly is said to be more than 18 days, but as Bouet and Roubaud worked entirely with wild flies the exact period could not be decided.

The infection in each species of fly is what is known as " total." The trypanosomes become established in the hind intestine and gradually extend forwards until they reach the proboscis, when they become fixed and assume the *Leptomonas* or Crithidial form. These proboscis forms of *dimorphon* may be distinguished from those of *congolense* by the frequent occurrence of giant forms like those of *cazalboui*, but differing in the flattened appearance of the posterior prolongation. The inoculation of intestinal forms produced no infection, whereas when the proboscis was inoculated a positive result was obtained.

It is evident, therefore, that the evolution of *T. dimorphon* in *Glossina longipalpis, tachinoides, palpalis*, and *morsitans*, respectively, is of the usual type, first a multiplication of trypanosomes in the intestine, during which period the fly is non-infective, followed by an invasion of the proboscis where the *Leptomonas* or Crithidial stage is gone through, after which the fly becomes infective.

REFERENCES.

Bouet (1907).   *Ann. Inst. Pasteur*, vol. XXI. p. 474.
——— and Roubaud (1910).   *Bull. Soc. Path. Exot.* vol. III. p. 722.
Dutton and Todd (1903).   *Liverpool Sch. of Trop. Med.* Memoir XI.
Laveran and Mesnil (1904).   *Compt. Rend. Acad. Sci.* vol. CXXXVIII. p. 732.
Montgomery and Kinghorn (1909).   *Lancet*, Sept. 25, 1909.
Yorke and Blacklock (1911).   *Ann. Trop. Med. and Parasit.* vol. V. p. 413 and vol. VI. p. 107.

## Trypanosoma pecorum Bruce, Hamerton, Bateman and Mackie, 1910.

*General account.* In 1910, Bruce and his collaborators observed a trypanosome in the horses and cattle of Uganda. This parasite was supposed to be identical with *T. dimorphon* and *T. congolense*, and, therefore, all three were united under the name *T. pecorum*. Laveran, however, has shewn by means of cross-immunity reactions that *T. pecorum* is a distinct species, but is closely related to *dimorphon, congolense* and *nanum*.

Recently Kinghorn and Yorke have found *T. pecorum* present in the wild game of the Luangwa Valley, North-Eastern Rhodesia.

The incubation period in cattle inoculated with *T. pecorum* is on an average about six to seven days. The duration of the disease may vary from 26 up to as long as 287 days. It is invariably fatal, the symptoms being weakness and emaciation, accompanied by anaemia. Cattle, goats, sheep, monkeys, dogs, rabbits, guinea-pigs, rats and mice are all susceptible to infection with *T. pecorum*, and this constitutes a means of distinguishing it from *nanum*. Duke's experiments have shewn that the bushbuck is also susceptible and may remain infective for at least 323 days, therefore the wild game may serve as a reservoir for this trypanosome.

*Morphology of the parasite.* In the living state *T. pecorum* is remarkable for its habit of exhibiting alternate periods of quiescence and activity. When quiescent it usually buries itself under clumps of red cells and is thus difficult to detect. The movements are active but, as in the case of *T. congolense*, not translatory ; therefore, the parasites do not travel across the field of the microscope.

In stained specimens the trypanosome is practically indistinguishable from *T. nanum* and *T. congolense*.

It is a monomorphic species ; the extreme variations in length are 8 to 18 microns, but the average dimensions, comprising the majority of individuals, are 14 microns in length by about 3 microns in breadth, including the undulating membrane. The posterior extremity is rounded ; the anterior is more or less tapering. The undulating membrane is well developed, being larger than that of *T. nanum*, and there is no free flagellum. The oval trophonucleus is situated about the middle of the body and the small spherical kinetonucleus is at the posterior extremity. The cytoplasm is generally homogeneous and not very granular.

*Mode of infection.* The results of Kinghorn and Yorke in the Luangwa Valley have shewn that *Glossina morsitans* is probably the most important agent for the spread of this infection. By collecting large numbers of these tsetse-flies and feeding them on healthy monkeys, out of 3202 flies at least two were found to be infected with *T. pecorum*.

Under experimental conditions, *Glossina palpalis* can also serve as the intermediate host for this species and animals may be infected by the bites of *palpalis* that have previously ingested blood containing *T. pecorum*. The mode of transmission is indirect, that is to say the trypanosome undergoes a cyclical development within the alimentary canal of the fly, but this development is so extremely slow that it is evident that *G. palpalis* is not the usual intermediate host of this parasite. It is also significant that wild *palpalis* has never been found naturally infected with *pecorum*. The stages in the development of *T. pecorum* in the alimentary canal of *G. palpalis* have been observed by Fraser and Duke, and also by Miss Robertson.

Although these two species of *Glossina* have thus been proved capable of transmitting this infection, there is considerable evidence to shew that the disease can exist in the absence of tsetse. Thus Bruce and other members of the Sleeping Sickness Commission saw an outbreak of *T. pecorum* infection under the following circumstances. The cattle belonging to this Commission grazed at the foot of Mpumu Hill, half to the east and half to the west. *Tabanus* and *Hæmatopota* were occasionally seen but always in very small numbers. In September, 1909, swarms of *Tabanus secedens* Walk. suddenly appeared to the west of the hill and a month later to the east. Soon afterwards the cattle, which had been healthy for a year, shewed signs of *T. pecorum* infection, first those which grazed to the west, then those which grazed to the east. It should be noted that there were a few pre-existing cases of infection in the herd. Afterwards a few *Glossina palpalis* were found at the foot of the hill. Nevertheless, although this circumstantial evidence is so strong, all attempts to transmit the disease experimentally by the bites of either Tabanids or *Stomoxys* have given uniformly negative results.

*Development within the intermediate host.* The development of *T. pecorum* within the alimentary canal of *Glossina palpalis* in all essential features resembles that of *T. nanum*, but is excessively slow, so that it seems probable that this species of tsetse only exceptionally serves as its intermediate host.

The parasites develop in the hinder intestine and give rise to a large number of trypanosomes of very varying size. Eventually, the slender forms are produced and these are extraordinarily attenuated; in addition the nuclear changes occurring at this stage in the cycle of *T. gambiense*, also take place in *T. pecorum*. The invasion of the proventriculus usually occurs about the 45th day and no proboscis infection was found before the 76th day. The Crithidial phase is passed through in the proboscis, as in the case of *T. nanum*, and the salivary glands are never invaded.

LITERATURE.

Bruce, Hamerton, Bateman and Mackie (1910). *Proc. Roy. Soc.* B, vol. LXXXII. p. 468.
Duke, H. L. (1912). *Proc. Roy. Soc.* B, vol. LXXXV. p. 554.
Kinghorn, A. and Yorke, W. (1912). *Ann. Trop. Med. and Parasit.* vol. VI. pp. 301 and 317.
Laveran, A. (1910). *Bull. Soc. Path. Exot.* vol. III. p. 718.
Robertson, M. (1913). *Trans. Roy. Soc.* B, vol. CCIII. pp. 161–184.

### Trypanosoma nanum Laveran, 1905.

*General account.* This parasite was first discovered by A. Balfour in 1904, in the blood of cattle from the Anglo-Egyptian Sudan. It has since been recorded from various other localities of this region and also in Uganda, where Bruce and his collaborators found it in the blood of cattle.

Kleine and Fischer, in the region of Lake Tanganyika, have found both sheep and antelopes naturally infected with a trypanosome that seems to agree with *nanum* in its characters.

In cattle, *T. nanum* produces a disease which develops slowly; the main symptom is the well-marked anaemia, which is accompanied by a gradual emaciation and usually ends in the death of the infected animal.

The parasites are usually present in the peripheral circulation, sometimes in considerable numbers, and can be easily recognised.

*T. nanum* can readily be inoculated into cattle and goats, but all the smaller laboratory animals are refractory to infection, for monkeys, dogs, rats and mice have been inoculated without becoming infected.

*Morphology of the parasite.* Laveran has given the following diagnosis of *Trypanosoma nanum* :

" The trypanosomes measure 10 to 14 $\mu$ in length, by 1·5 to 2 $\mu$ in breadth. Their structure is that of flagellates belonging to the genus *Trypanosoma* ; yet, contrary to the rule, the protoplasm is prolonged at the anterior end, in such a manner that there is no free flagellum, or the free part of the flagellum is extremely short. The undulating membrane is very narrow and in consequence only slightly evident. The posterior extremity is conical, not drawn out, otherwise a little variable in form."

" The oval nucleus is situated about the middle of the body of the parasite. The centrosome (= kinetonucleus), rounded and rather large, is found almost at the posterior extremity.

" The protoplasm is homogeneous, without granulations.

" Some of the forms, a little larger than the others, shew two centrosomes and a flagellum divided for a greater or lesser extent from the origin in the centrosome ; these are evidently multiplication forms."

In Uganda the length of the parasite may extend up to 16 microns as shewn by Bruce, Hamerton, Bateman and Mackie, and also by Duke.

*Mode of transmission.* The experiments of Duke in Uganda have shewn that *Glossina palpalis* may serve as the intermediate host for *T. nanum*. Laboratory bred flies were fed on an infected sheep and subsequently on a calf, which developed a typical infection with this trypanosome. About five per cent. of the flies fed on this sheep were found to be infected.

Kleine and Fischer are of the opinion that *Glossina morsitans* is the intermediate host of *T. nanum* in the region of Lake Tanganyika.

*Development of the parasite.* In the blood the trypanosome multiplies in the usual manner by means of longitudinal division.

When taken into the gut of *G. palpalis* the resulting changes are exactly comparable with those that take place in the case of *T. gambiense*, described above. The trypanosomes begin to develop in the hinder intestine and by the 10th day numerous parasites may be found in the hinder and middle intestine. The slender forms begin to be produced from the 10th to the 14th day onwards, and the proventriculus is usually invaded about the 20th day. The proventricular forms are not quite so uniformly slender as in the case of *T. gambiense*. Moreover, there are no marked changes in the appearance of the nuclei of *T. nanum*. About the 25th day the trypanosomes invade the proboscis, where they may be found attached to the labrum, often lying in clusters. They then pass through the Crithidial phase, many of them being extremely long and slender. Subsequently trypanosome forms are produced which may be found free, sometimes in the hypopharynx and at other times in the labrum.

The salivary glands never become infected in the case of *T. nanum*, the proboscis infection apparently playing the same part as the gland infection in the cycle of *T. gambiense*.

LITERATURE.

Laveran, A. (1905). *Compt. Rend. Soc. Biol.* vol. LVII. p. 292.
Balfour, A. (1904). *B. M. J.* Nov. 26, 1904.
Bruce, Hamerton, Bateman and Mackie (1910). *Proc. Roy. Soc.* 1910, B, vol. LXXXIII. p. 180.
Duke, H. L. (1912). *Proc. Roy. Soc.* B, vol. LXXXV. p. 4.
Kleine and Fischer (1911). *Zeitschr. f. Hyg. u. Infectionskr.* vol. LXX. p. 18.
Robertson, M. (1913). *Phil. Trans. Roy. Soc.* B, vol. CCIII. p. 161.

### Trypanosoma congolense Broden, 1904.

This parasite, which very closely resembles *T. pecorum* and *T. dimorphon*, was first described by Broden, who found it occurring in the blood of a donkey and sheep in the Congo Free State. Subsequently the parasite was also observed in the blood of cattle and dromedaries in the same locality and also in cattle, sheep, goats and dogs in the French Çongo, where, according to Martin, Lebœuf and Roubaud, it is widely distributed. In North-East Rhodesia, Montgomery and Kinghorn have observed *T. congolense* in the blood of cattle. It is doubtful whether the trypanosomes occurring in dogs on the shores of Tanganyika should be referred to this species or to *T. pecorum*.

*T. congolense* is only distinguishable from *T. pecorum* by cross-immunity reactions, for Laveran and Mesnil shewed that a goat immune against *T. congolense* was susceptible to infection with *pecorum*. Otherwise the two forms are practically identical and it is questionable whether they should be regarded as distinct species.

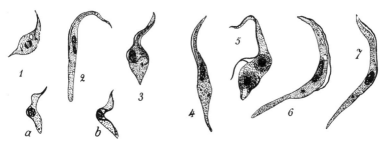

Fig. 78. Culture of *T. congolense* in the intestine of *G. palpalis*. ( × about 1600). *a, b*, normal forms from the circulating blood ; 1, 2, forms 24 hours after ingestion ; 3, 5, forms after 48 hours ; 6, 7, forms after 56 hours. (After Roubaud.)

In addition to cattle, sheep, goats and dogs, all the usual experimental animals may be infected with *congolense*, but the course of the disease is usually very slow, resembling that of *dimorphon*. The constant susceptibility of guinea-pigs is, however, in marked contrast with that of other laboratory animals, for Laveran and Mesnil found that the average duration of the disease in this species was only two weeks and invariably resulted in the death of the animal.

*Morphology of the parasite.* The living parasite exhibits active wriggling movements without, however, progressing across the field of the microscope. The trypanosomes are often attached to the leucocytes by their anterior extremities.

The dimensions of the majority of the individuals vary between 10 to 13 microns in length, by 1 to 2 microns in breadth, and the largest forms are never more than 17 microns in length, a means of distinguishing this species from *dimorphon*. In stained specimens the posterior extremity is rounded and anteriorly the body of the parasite gradually tapers, the protoplasm being prolonged to the extremity of the flagellum.

The trophonucleus is situated about the middle of the length of the parasite ; the kinetonucleus is very distinct and is usually close to the posterior extremity. The protoplasm is somewhat clear and rarely contains chromatophilous granules.

*Mode of infection.* There is some little doubt as to whether *G. palpalis* is capable of transmitting *congolense,* for the only positive experiments with this species of tsetse-fly that have been recorded up to the present are those of Roubaud, and this author states that the observations were made with " *T. congolense* (vel *dimorphon*)."

In the alimentary canal of *G. palpalis* Roubaud observed the commencement of a development of this trypanosome somewhat resembling that of *T. gambiense,* but the parasites all disappeared by the end of the third day.

Rodhain, van den Branden, Pons and Bequaert, found that the *G. morsitans* in the Katanga region were naturally infected with *congolense.* In addition an experiment was made with 23 flies born in the laboratory. These were fed on an infected goat and subsequently on healthy animals. After an incubation period of 23 days one of the flies became infective. This individual on dissection was found to present an " infection totale " of the alimentary canal. The parasites in the intestine were nearly all of the trypanosome type and some were of the blood form. In the proboscis the hypopharyngeal tube was filled with small trypanosomes of the *congolense* type without any free flagellum, whilst the parasites that swarmed in the labrum were of the *Leptomonas* type.

REFERENCES.

Broden, A. (1904). *Bull. Soc. d'Études Coloniales*, Bruxelles, February, 1904.
Laveran and Mesnil (1912). *Trypanosomes et Trypanosomiases.*
Montgomery and Kinghorn (1909). *Ann. Trop. Med. and Parasit.* vol. III. p. 349.
Rodhain, van den Branden, Pons and Bequaert (1912). *Bull. Soc. Path. Exot.* vol. V. p. 281.
Roubaud (1909). *Thèse de doct. ès sci. nat.* Paris, pp. 153 and 161.

## Trypanosoma simiæ Bruce, Harvey, Hamerton, Davey and Lady Bruce, 1912.

*Synonym. T. ignotum* Kinghorn and Yorke, 1912.

*General account.* This species of trypanosome has been recorded from Nyasaland, Central Angoniland, and North-Eastern Rhodesia, where a large percentage of *Glossina morsitans* are naturally infected with the parasite. Its pathogenic properties are very remarkable, since it only affects such widely different animals as monkeys and goats. Oxen, baboons, dogs, guinea-pigs, and white rats, seem to be immune.

In goats *T. simiæ* sets up a chronic disease, but in monkeys the infection is rapidly fatal, for in a series of 19 the average duration of life after the trypanosomes were first seen in the blood was only 2·9 days.

*Morphology.* When living the parasite shews active progressive movements, some individuals passing completely across the field of the microscope. The dimensions of the trypanosomes as found in the monkey and the goat, are found to vary from 14 to 24 microns in length, by 1 to 2·75 microns in breadth, the mean being 18 microns in length by 1·75 in breadth. The parasites are monomorphic and, as a rule, fairly uniform in shape. The authors give the following summary of its characters :

" Elongated, narrow, undulating body ; posterior extremity bluntly pointed or rounded ; anterior extremity pointed ;

nucleus oval ; micronucleus small, round, situated about 1·5 microns from posterior extremity, placed laterally, protuberant ; undulating membrane marked, thrown into bold folds ; flagellum frequently not projecting beyond undulating membrane, sometimes 1 to 2 microns of the extremity apparently free."

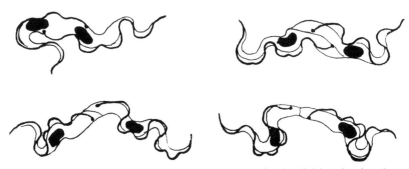

Fig. 79. *Trypanosoma simiæ.* Successive stages in the division shewing the peculiar manner in which the two daughter trypanosomes seem to " slip " past each other, until they are only joined by their non-flagellate ends. (After Bruce, Harvey, Hamerton, Davey and Lady Bruce.)

In the blood of the monkey these trypanosomes swarm in enormous numbers and numerous division forms can be seen, often four or five in a field. When dividing the trypanosomes appear to slip past one another until they are only joined by their posterior extremities, as shewn in Fig. 79. Multiplication often takes place so rapidly that the individual trypanosomes have not time to disengage themselves and thus large multi-

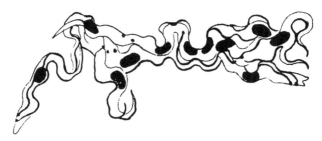

Fig. 80. *Trypanosoma simiæ.* Large multinucleate form. (After Bruce, Harvey, Hamerton, Davey and Lady Bruce.)

nucleate masses are·produced, sometimes filling the whole field of the microscope (Fig. 80).

The life history of this parasite in its intermediate host, *Glossina morsitans*, has not yet been worked out. Its extreme pathogenicity in monkeys is very remarkable and suggests that *T. simiæ* is a species that has only recently become adapted to its present mode of life.

### LITERATURE.

Bruce, Harvey, Hamerton, Davey and Lady Bruce (1912). *Proc. Roy. Soc.* B, vol. LXXXV. p. 477.

Kinghorn and Yorke (1912). *Ann. Trop. Med. and Parasit.* vol. VI. pp. 301–315 and 317–324.

# CHAPTER XIX

## STOMOXYS

*General description.* The members of the genus *Stomoxys* may be distinguished from other blood-sucking Muscidæ by the following characters :

The proboscis protrudes horizontally in front of the head and is pointed towards its anterior extremity. The maxillary palps are cylindrical and slender, less than half the length of the proboscis. The first longitudinal vein opens into the wing about mid-way along its length, almost opposite the small transverse vein. The first posterior marginal cell opens widely at the tip of the wing. Between the posterior transverse vein and the margin of the wing the fourth longitudinal vein is arched like a bow with the concavity facing the third longitudinal vein (Fig. 81).

The flies belonging to this genus are all moderate sized (5 to 7 mm.) dull-coloured insects that generally feed on the blood of cattle. They closely resemble the house-fly (*Musca domestica*) in general appearance, but may be readily distinguished by the presence of the proboscis, and also *Stomoxys* rests with its wings widely divergent whilst in *Musca* they are held closer together.   The most abundant species is *Stomoxys calcitrans*, the common stable-fly of this country, but in addition to this insect, *S. nigra* is also supposed to be concerned in the spread of disease.

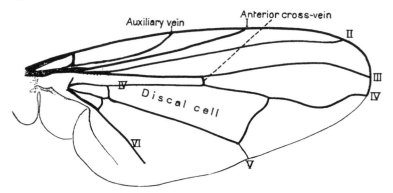

Fig. 81.   Wing venation of *Stomoxys calcitrans*.

## *Stomoxys calcitrans* Linn.

*General description.*   This insect closely resembles the common house-fly in colouration and general appearance, but as mentioned above, may be easily recognised by the presence of the biting proboscis and the attitude of the wings. In addition *S. calcitrans* is distinguished by the following characters :

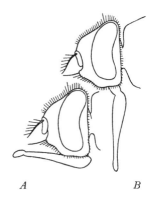

Fig. 82.   Side view of head of Stable-fly ;   *A*, proboscis in resting position ;   *B*, proboscis extended.   (After Graham-Smith.)

The lower part of the face is white, frequently with a yellowish tint, which is especially visible upon the sides of the forehead. The latter is marked with black or reddish-brown stripes ; the antennæ are brown, at times lighter dorsally. The maxillary palps are short, scarcely protruding, and yellow in colour. The dorsal surface of the thorax is marked with four dark longitudinal stripes, two on each side, extending from the shoulders to the scutellum, but interrupted in the middle of their length by the transverse suture. The abdomen has a yellowish-brown tint and is marked with three indistinct dark spots on the second segment and some on the following segments. The legs are blackish-brown with reddish-yellow knees. According to Austen, the African examples of this species are smaller than British specimens and the abdominal spots shew considerable variation in size and shape. The insect varies from about 5·5 to 7 mm. in length.

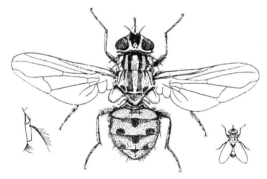

Fig. 83. Stable-fly, *Stomoxys calcitrans* (× 5). On the left, magnified view of antenna. On the right, view of the fly in its resting position. (Nat. size.) (After Graham-Smith.)

*Distribution.* S. *calcitrans* has been recorded from almost every part of the world, occurring throughout both temperate and tropical countries and even extending as far north as Lapland. It is especially abundant, however, in warmer countries, or during the summer months of more temperate regions.

*Habits.* The common name of this insect, the stable-fly,

gives a true indication of its usual habitat, and during the summer large numbers of *Stomoxys* may generally be found around the cow-sheds and stables of any farmyard ; in warm weather, however, it may be found wherever cattle are grazing ; and during late summer and autumn they are frequently found in houses, where they are known as "Biting House-flies." When resting on a wall, *Stomoxys* generally points the head upwards, and thus may be distinguished from the house-fly which usually takes the opposite position.

The fly may feed on the juices from any decaying organic matter, and also on the blood of vertebrates. It is possible that its blood-sucking habits have been somewhat over-estimated, for Newstead kept a careful watch on both horses and cattle in a farmyard where *Stomoxys* were plentiful without seeing even one settle on an animal. During hot weather, however, the flies become very troublesome to animals and may even attack human beings. The voracious habits of *Stomoxys* are well shewn when a number are kept together in captivity. Under these circumstances if an individual suffers any injury, the others at once try to feed on it and, if successful in piercing the integument, suck all the contents out of their unfortunate companion.

Unlike many blood-sucking flies, the female *Stomoxys* will lay fertile eggs without ever having fed on blood.

*Life history.* Newstead has recently given a complete description of the metamorphosis of this insect from which the following account is taken. The female generally lays its eggs a few inches below the surface in stable manure, decomposing vegetable matter, or similar materials. Although the flight of this insect is usually noiseless, when the female is preparing to oviposit the noise of its wings is distinctly audible, resembling the hum made by most other members of the Muscidæ. The eggs are generally laid in an irregular heap and their number is usually about 50 to 70. The egg is 1 mm. in length, very elongate, shaped somewhat like a banana, being curved on one side and deeply grooved on the other. This groove widens towards the anterior end. The colour of the egg is white when first laid, but subsequently becomes creamy-white.

The larva escapes by splitting the egg membrane at the broad end of the groove.   During August, with an average temperature of 72° F. in the day and 65° at night, the incubation period varies from two to three days.

The young larva is round, smooth, and almost transparent, and of the usual acephalous muscid type (Fig. 6, p. 20).   It may be distinguished by the appearance of the two posterior stigmata, which are small, circular and situated rather far apart. Its length when full grown is about 11 mm.   The duration of

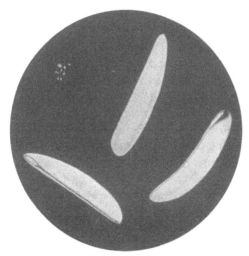

Fig. 84.  *Stomoxys calcitrans*.  Eggs.   The small group in the top left hand corner represents their natural size.  (After Newstead.)

the larval stage under favourable conditions, is from two to three weeks, but the absence of plentiful moisture or exposure to light retards the development very considerably, to at least a period of 78 days.   Such larvæ produce abnormally small pupæ and correspondingly small adults.

The process of pupation is completed within two hours. The larva first burrows to some little depth and then shortens itself by contraction of the front segments, thus becoming barrel-shaped (Fig. 9, p. 22).   The colour of the pupæ is at first terra-cotta, but it subsequently darkens to a chestnut-brown. The length varies from 5 to 5·5 mm. The duration of the pupal stage varies from nine to thirteen days under favourable conditions, but may be considerably prolonged by cold.

A few days before the emergence of the insect the pupal case darkens and splits anteriorly along the lateral and median lines and also across the fourth segment. The front region then falls away and the fly escapes after undergoing a final moult within the puparium. On emergence the fly at first tries to make its way to the surface of any rubbish with which it may be covered. This is chiefly accomplished by means of the frontal sac, which is alternately inflated and deflated, and at the same time the insect pushes itself forward by means of its legs. After it has become free the hairs of the arista are carefully combed out, and also the frontal sac and rudimentary wings are cleaned by means of the front pair of legs. Subsequently the frontal sac contracts and the head assumes a more normal appearance, and then the insect stretches itself to the full extent and pumps air into its body. This air is forced along the nervures of the wings and these finally unfold, being aided by the use of the hind-legs. The fly then remains quiescent for some time and when the integument and wings are sufficiently hardened it takes flight.

The duration of the whole life-cycle from egg to imago varies from 25 to 37 days, under favourable conditions of temperature and moisture.

*Methods of destruction.* The methods which have been used for the destruction of the common house-fly are also applicable to *Stomo ys*, with this difference, that whereas in the case of the former, middens and ashpits are notorious breeding places, the stable-fly rarely selects these localities, but chiefly breeds in stable manure and heaps of decomposing vegetation. The numbers of the insect would be considerably reduced in any particular locality, if all stable manure, etc. were carefully removed at least every seven days, during May to October inclusive. By this means the fly would be prevented from breeding, as the immature stages would be removed together with the manure. In the case of farmyards and country districts, where the removal of manure is impracticable, the manure heaps should be sprayed periodically with some insecticide, in order to destroy any eggs, or larvæ, that may be present.

REFERENCES.

Austen (1909). *African Blood-sucking Flies.* London : Brit. Mus
Bouffard, G. (1907). *Compt. Rend. Soc. Biol.* vol. LXII. p. 71.
Newstead, R. (1907). *Ann. Trop. Med. and Parasit.* vol. I. p. 76.
Tulloch (1906). *Proc. Roy. Soc.* vol. LXXVII. B. p. 523.

# CHAPTER XX

## INFECTIONS TRANSMITTED BY STOMOXYS

### 1. Trypanosomiases.

There is no doubt that under experimental conditions the direct transmission of various trypanosomiases from infected to healthy animals, is comparatively easily effected by means of the bites of *Stomoxys*, but with regard to the importance of this insect in the spread of disease, opinion is still very divided. Surra (*T. evansi*) is generally stated to be transmitted by *Stomoxys* as well as *Tabanus*, and yet Mitzmain in the Philippines made a most exhaustive series of experiments on the transmission of this disease by *Stomoxys calcitrans* and obtained uniformly negative results. In Africa, Bruce, Grieg and Gray, Bevan, and others have also been unsuccessful in attempts to transmit various trypanosomiases by this insect. Nevertheless a number of observers are of the opinion that *Stomoxys* plays an important part in the transmission of certain infections. Thus in Java, according to Schat, Surra is mainly spread by the agency of *Stomoxys calcitrans* Linn. and *Lyperosia exigua* de Meijere, but experimental proof is lacking. Similarly, Musgrave and Clegg stated that in the Philippines it has been " conclusively shewn that *Stomoxys calcitrans* and other biting flies transmit the disease," but this statement is somewhat exaggerated.

Bouffard at Bamako on the Upper Niger experimented on the transmission of Souma, a trypanosomiasis of cattle caused by *T. cazalboui* (*vide* p. 335). A calf was inoculated with this parasite and shewed numerous trypanosomes in its blood on the eighth day. A healthy calf was then segregated with the other calf in a fly-proof stable, the animals being separated by a distance of one and a half metres. Forty wild *Stomoxys* were then put in the stable and were observed to feed on two afternoons, after which they died. Twelve days later trypanosomes appeared in the blood of the healthy calf so that it seems evident that *Stomoxys* is able to carry *T. cazalboui*. Whether the flies were naturally infected or not when caught, was not decided.

In French West Africa, Bouet and Roubaud succeeded with difficulty in the direct transmission of *T. cazalboui* and *T. pecaudi* by means of *Stomoxys*, but failed to transmit *T. dimorphon*. On the other hand, the trypanosomes of the Sahara were easily transmitted by means of this insect as shewn by their results. Employing *T. soudanense*, out of five experiments performed under laboratory conditions, with no intervals between the bites of the flies, four gave positive results. In another experiment at least 24 hours were allowed to elapse between the feed on the infected and on the healthy animal, in this case a dog. This animal became infected a month later shewing that the flies were still infective after 24 hours. In addition one experiment was made under natural conditions. A healthy puppy from which all ectoparasites had been carefully removed was kept on a chain during the day beside an infected dog in a place infested with *Stomoxys* ( ? *calcitrans* and *nigra*) ; at night it was removed and placed in a fly-proof cage to prevent any nocturnal flies feeding on it. The experiment lasted from the 11th to the 19th of August and both animals were frequently bitten by *Stomoxys*. On August 24th the puppy became infected.

The results were similar on employing a strain of *T. evansi* (Surra) obtained from some camels at St Louis. In three experiments the *Stomoxys* were transferred from an infected to a healthy rat and a minute later to another healthy rat. In two cases the first animal became infected whilst the second did not ; but in the third experiment, in which only a single *Stomoxys* was used, both animals became infected after one bite. In addition positive results were obtained in the transmission of this virus after intervals varying up to at least three days. As Dr Bagshawe remarks, these experiments demonstrate that the trypanosomes of the Surra type in French West Africa may be transmitted by *Stomoxys* and that the flies may retain the infection for at least three days. But it is so obvious that some of the flies may have been infected when caught, that definite conclusions as to the period during which *Stomoxys* retains infection, may be as misleading as were those drawn from similar experiments with *G. palpalis*.

Nevertheless, the fact that a single *Stomoxys* was capable of transmitting the infection shews that under certain conditions this insect might be an important agent for the spread of the disease. By means of interrupted feeding, that is, the fly beginning its meal on an infected animal and at once finishing it on another, various authors have succeeded in the experimental transmission of *T. brucei*, *T. gambiense*, *T. equiperdum*, in addition to *T. evansi*, *T. cazalboui* and *T. soudanense*.

In India, Leese is of the opinion that Surra (*T. evansi*) may be naturally spread by the bites of *Stomoxys*, but the results of experiments shew that *Tabanus* is a much more efficient carrier as far as direct transmission is concerned (*vide* p. 237). In Mauritius, where *Stomoxys nigra* Macq. is very abundant, this species is believed to be concerned in the spread of the same disease, but experimental evidence is lacking. Finally it should be noted that in practically all experiments with *Stomoxys* in Africa, no distinction has been made between *S. calcitrans* and *S. nigra* both species being used indiscriminately.

## REFERENCES.

Austen, E. (1909). *African Blood-sucking Flies*.
Bagshawe, A. G. (1912). *S. S. Bulletin*, vol. IV. p. 273.
Bevan, Ll. (1910). *Ibid.* vol. II. p. 252.
Bouet and Roubaud (1912). *Bull. Soc. Path. Exot.* vol. V. p. 544.
Bouffard (1907). *Compt. Rend. Soc. Biol.* vol. LXII. p. 71.

Bruce, Hamerton, Bateman and Mackie (1910).  *Proc. Roy. Soc.* B, 558, p. 468.

Greig and Gray (1905).  *Rep. S. S. Comm. Roy. Soc.* No. 6.

Leese, A. S. (1912).  *Journ. Trop. Vet. Sci.* vol. II. p. 19.

Manders, N. (1905).  *Journ. R.A.M.C.* vol. v. p. 623.

Martin, Lebœuf and Roubaud (1908).  *Bull. Soc. Path. Exot.* vol. I. p. 356.

Minchin, Gray and Tulloch (1907).  *Reports S. S. Comm. Roy. Soc.* No. 8, p. 124.

## 2.  Filaria labiato-papillosa Alessandrini, 1838.

*Synonyms.* *Filaria cervina* Dujardin, 1845. *F. terebra* Diesing. *Stomoxeos* von Linstow, 1875.

*Habitat.* The adult worm inhabits the peritoneal cavity and occasionally the eyes of cattle and various species of deer. The embryos are constantly present in small numbers in the peripheral circulation.

*Description.* The adult filaria is white and filiform with the integument shewing fine transverse striations. The body tapers towards both extremities, the anterior being blunter than the posterior. The mouth is surrounded by a chitinous ring and immediately behind it are four small depressions, from each of which arises a tactile papilla. The male measures 4 to 6 cms. in length. Its tail is especially twisted and on each side are three pre-anal, one ad-anal and five post-anal papillæ, behind which is situated a well-developed conical process. The female measures 6 to 12 cms. in length Its tail is also twisted but not so much as in the male. The caudal extremity bears a large number of fine processes, in front of which are situated two strong conical processes.

*Life history.* This filaria is viviparous and the embryos when born measure 140 to 250 microns in length. Noè has investigated the further evolution of these embryos and finds that it takes place in the body of *Stomoxys calcitrans*. When this fly ingests blood containing the embryonic filariæ, the latter bore through the gut wall and make their way into the thoracic muscles. Here they accomplish their larval development and when it is complete, the young filariæ travel into the labium of their intermediate host. When an infected *Stomoxys* bites another animal the filariæ escape from the labium and probably bore through the skin of the host in the same way as *F. bancrofti*, but this part of the life-cycle has not yet been observed. Noè found that in Italy, where his experiments were performed, only three to four per cent. of the *Stomoxys* became infected, the remaining 96 to 97 per cent. being apparently immune to infection.

Although there is little doubt that *S. calcitrans* is capable of transmitting this filaria, it is important to add that up to the present no one has been successful in actually infecting cattle by the bites of infected flies.

REFERENCES.

Alessandrini. *Rendiconti Accad. d. Lincei*, vol. XII. pp. 387–393.
Neumann-Macqueen (1905). *Parasites and Parasitic Diseases of Domesticated Animals.* London : Baillière, Tindall & Cox.
Noè, G. (1903). Studî sul ciclo evolutivo della Filaria labiato-papillosa. *Rend. Accad. d. Lincei*, vol. XII. pp. 387–393.

### Poliomyelitis.

*Synonyms.* Epidemic Poliomyelitis ; Infantile Paralysis ; Epidemische Kinderlehrnung.

*History.* Poliomyelitis has been endemic in Northern Europe for many years, especially in Scandinavia, but it was only in 1907 that the disease suddenly began to extend its range of distribution. During the past two or three years many countries in different parts of the world have been visited by epidemics, the origin of which has remained quite unexplained. In America there is no previous history of a general epidemic until 1907, although local outbreaks had occasionally been noticed. Since this date, however, the disease has been prevalent during the summer and autumn in many parts of the United States and Canada. It is possible that the infection may have been introduced from Scandinavia, for the two great centres of the recent epidemic were the Atlantic coast towns and the state of Minnesota, both of which received large numbers of Scandinavian emigrants. But there is no apparent reason why the disease should not have broken out previously to 1907, for large numbers of emigrants had been arriving for many years before that date, and also why the infection should have suddenly appeared in many other parts of the world. Since this date, however, the disease has taken on fresh activities in its original home, and in 1911, Sweden was visited by a very severe epidemic.

*Distribution.* Poliomyelitis is especially prevalent in Scandinavia and Northern Europe but, in addition, epidemics have occurred in England, France, Germany, Italy, Austria, and Spain ; in America large numbers of cases have been recorded from New York and Boston in the east, to San Francisco in the west, and a large outbreak occurred in Cuba in 1909. The disease has also been recorded from various parts of Australia.

*Causal agent.* Although the most varied methods of staining and cultivation have been employed, no parasite has ever been detected in patients infected with poliomyelitis, but the scarcity of polymorphonuclear leucocytes in the altered cerebro-spinal fluid and spinal cord and the large increase in the number of mononuclears suggest that the parasite is protozoal in nature. The filterable nature of the virus has since been demonstrated, for if the spinal cord of a recently paralysed monkey is made into an emulsion with either distilled water, or normal saline, and passed through a Berkefeld filter, the resulting filtrate is still infective. Moreover, its activity is very considerable, for one thousandth of a cubic centimetre of a filtered 2·5 per cent. suspension of the spinal cord of an infected monkey is sufficient to produce infection and paralysis when injected into another monkey. The resistance of the virus is extraordinary, for in dust, especially within protein matter, it remains virulent for months. In diffuse daylight it survives indefinitely and resists the action of pure glycerine and 0·5 per cent. phenol for many months.

The virus may be preserved by passage through monkeys, as these animals are easily infected by the intra-cerebral injection of an emulsion of the brain or spinal cord of an animal suffering from poliomyelitis. The susceptibility of monkeys has enabled Flexner, in conjunction respectively with Lewis and Clark, and also Landsteiner and Levaditi, to make some observations on the development of the virus within the body of an infected subject.

The disease is essentially one of the central nervous system as evidenced by both the clinical and pathological features of the infection. If the virus is injected into the sciatic nerve of a monkey, it has been shewn that it multiplies in the nerve, first at the site of the injection and then progresses along the nerve until it reaches the spinal cord, when it causes paralysis of the hind-quarters. When the virus is placed on the uninjured nasal mucous membrane, the infective agent travels up the olfactory nerves and subsequently causes general paralysis. It is evident, therefore, that nervous tissue is the one in which the organism chiefly multiplies. From the brain and spinal cord it passes into the cerebro-spinal fluid and thence into the blood circulation and lymphatic system, but in these positions it does not seem to persist for any length of time, except in the lymphatic nodes. The presence of the virus in the lymphatics explains why the nasal secretion becomes infected, for it has been shewn that poliomyelitis escapes with the secretions of the nose and throat and the discharges from the intestine of an infected person.

*Method of infection.* Considering the infectivity of the various secretions of a patient suffering from poliomyelitis, it is only reasonable to suppose that the disease may be directly transmitted from one person to another without the aid of any intermediate host. Flexner supports the view that the nasal mucous membrane is the chief site of infection, for the virus is able to survive in the form of dust and thus might be inhaled, and, in fact, the sweepings of a room occupied by a poliomyelitis patient have been shewn to be infected.

On the other hand, as a result of very thorough epidemiological studies conducted by the Massachusetts State Board of Health, evidence has been collected which supports the theory that the disease is spread by insects. Rosenau has recently (1912) been able to transmit poliomyelitis from infected to healthy monkeys by the bites of *Stomoxys calcitrans*. Several monkeys infected with the disease by intracerebral inoculation were daily exposed to the bites of several hundred *Stomoxys*, at the same time exposing twelve healthy monkeys to the bites of these flies. Of these twelve monkeys, six developed symptoms characteristic of poliomyelitis, namely, illness, followed by more or less extensive paralysis. Two monkeys died, and in the spinal cord of one of them was found the characteristic lesions of this disease, *i.e.*, perivascular infiltration and destruction of the motor cells of the anterior cornu.

Anderson and Frost have confirmed these experiments of Rosenau and their results will be given in detail. On October 3rd, a rhesus was inoculated intracerebrally with an emulsion of the spinal cord of a monkey that had died of poliomyelitis. Two hours after inoculation it was exposed to the bites of about 300 *Stomoxys* collected in Washington. Each day until the death of the monkey on October 8th, it was exposed for about two hours to the bites of these flies, together with additional ones that were added as they were caught. This monkey developed the characteristic complete paralysis on October 7th and died on October 8th. Another monkey similarly inoculated on October 5th was then daily exposed to the bites of the same lot of flies from October 7th until October 9th, when the second monkey died. Thus from October 4th to the 9th inclusive, the *Stomoxys* had been able to feed on two monkeys infected with poliomyelitis.

Beginning on October 4th, two fresh monkeys (Java and rhesus) were exposed daily for about two hours to the bites of these same flies; and on October 5th yet a third monkey (rhesus) was similarly exposed. On October 12th the Java monkey was found completely paralysed and died the same day. The second rhesus monkey also developed paralysis during the day and was anæsthetised. The first rhesus monkey died on October 13th after presenting the typical symptoms of poliomyelitis.

Thus three monkeys exposed daily to the bites of several hundred *Stomoxys*, which at the same time were allowed to feed on two infected monkeys, developed typical symptoms of poliomyelitis seven, eight and nine days, respectively, from the date of their first exposure to the bites of the flies.

These results are of great interest and shew that the

disease may be transmitted by the bites of *Stomoxys*.   It should be added, however, that the transmission has only been effected under experimental conditions and it remains to be seen whether this is the usual method of infection in nature, for cases of poliomyelitis have occurred in the absence of any *Stomoxys*.

### REFERENCES.

Anderson and Frost (1912).   Transmission of poliomyelitis by means of the stable-fly (*Stomoxys calcitrans*). *Public Health Reports, Washington*, vol. xxvii. No. 43.

Brues and Sheppard (1912).   The possible etiological relation of certain biting insects to the spread of infantile paralysis. *Journ. Econ. Entom.* vol. v. No. 4.

Kling, Wernstedt and Pettersson (1912).   Recherches sur le mode de propagation de la paralysie infantile épidémique. *Zeitschr. f. Immunitätsforschung*, vol. xii. pp. 316–323 and 657–670.

Kling and Levaditi (1913).   Études sur la poliomyélite. *Publ. de l'Inst. Pasteur.* 126 pp. Paris : Maretheux.

Rosenau (1913).   *Public Health Reports, Washington*, vol. xxvii.

# CHAPTER XXI

## LYPEROSIA

*General description.*   The genus *Lyperosia* is closely related to *Stomoxys*, from which it may be distinguished by the shape of the maxillary palps, which are more or less spatulate, and as long, or almost as long, as the proboscis.   When the insect is resting the palps ensheath the proboscis, as in the case of *Glossina*, and as a result the combined structures appear as a stout rod-like process in front of the head.   The proboscis is long and tapering, chitinous throughout, and the labella are small.   The arista is feathered only on the dorsal surface. The third longitudinal vein is without bristles and the fourth longitudinal is gently curved distally so as to leave the first posterior cell wide open.

All the known species of *Lyperosia* are small, dull, inconspicuous insects, not exceeding about 4 mm. in length.

They are very common on domestic animals and generally cluster on any small sores. They also take advantage of the wounds caused by the bites of Tabanids, etc. In the Philippines, Mitzmain has observed these insects to wait for a *Tabanus* to finish feeding and then immediately suck up the drop of blood that oozed from the open wound caused by the larger insect. They are also capable of obtaining blood for themselves, and the only European species, *L. irritans* Linn., has the habit of clustering in a dense mass about the base of the horns of cattle. *Lyperosia* rarely attacks man, but regarding a Uganda species, *L. punctigera*, Austen records the following observation by the collector (the late Dr W. A. Denshaw) : " These flies were noticed in great numbers in one camp only near the Nile, and were very troublesome to my boys early one sunny morning ; they clustered thickly on any small sore, and quickly filled themselves ; though preferring to feed in this way, they seemed also to insert the proboscis into sound skin."

*Life-cycle.* The life-history of *Lyperosia irritans* Linn. has been investigated in America by Riley and Howard. The eggs are laid singly on the surface of freshly dropped cow-dung. They are light reddish-brown in colour and vary from 1·25 to 1·37 mm. in length, by 0·34 to 0·41 mm. in breadth. As soon as they hatch the larvæ penetrate into the dung and in this situation complete their development. The fully-grown larva is dirty white in colour and about 7 mm. in length. The posterior stigmatic plates, situated on the terminal segment, are large, very dark brown, and almost circular, but with their inner adjacent margins almost straight, and each has a circular central opening. On the ventral surface of the anal segment is a dark yellow chitinous plate bearing six irregular paired tubercles, and the whole plate is surrounded by an area of coarsely granulated skin.

The pupæ are found in the ground beneath the dung, at a depth of about 2 cms. The puparium resembles that of the house-fly, being dark brown in colour and barrel-shaped. Its dimensions vary from 4 to 4·5 mm. in length, by 2 to 2·5 mm. in breadth.

## LYPEROSIA *and Disease*

There is no direct experimental evidence in support of the view that *Lyperosia* carries any infection, but certain authors have suggested that this fly may occasionally be responsible for the spread of various trypanosomiases of animals. Schat is of the opinion that *Lyperosia exigua* de Meijere, takes a part in the spread of Surra in Java. Montgomery and Kinghorn, in Rhodesia, record an outbreak of trypanosomiasis occurring under the following circumstances. A herd of cattle in Northern Rhodesia which had been in good health for a year was kept on a farm two-and-a-half miles from the nearest tsetse area. In April six bullocks were sent on a journey and as they passed through a fly belt were probably bitten by tsetse. These bullocks returned to the farm a few days later. In June, three of these animals and also one which had not been away shewed trypanosomes. In July, fifteen animals were infected so all the healthy cattle were isolated in a place that seemed free from biting-flies. Five more of these animals shewed trypanosomes in August and were removed, but the balance continued to remain uninfected. The average duration of the disease was about 30 days, and the parasite is described as *T. dimorphon.* The authors write :

" From an examination of all conditions, we think it probable that one or more of the six cattle that went to Mwomboshi in April contracted the disease on the road and brought it to the farm, where, in the presence of *Stomoxys* and *Lyperosia* in the kraals, the animals, including cows and bulls, which did not leave the place, became infected, and that the segregation from these flies checked its spread to the fourteen cattle which remained healthy." Montgomery and Kinghorn believe that in this case, *Lyperosia* was partly responsible for the transmission, the trypanosomes being directly carried from infected to healthy animals.

In India, Leese has given an interesting account of an outbreak of Surra in the Bikanir State in the desert of Rajputana. During this outbreak the Imperial Service Camel Corps, out of 500 camels, had only 205 survivors and of these 130 were suffering from chronic Surra. Only 40 camels had been outside the State and the great majority of them had been in the Corps so long that they could not have been infected when purchased, therefore the infection must have chiefly spread within the State itself. Bikanir is about 200 miles square, and there is only one small locality in which *Tabanus* is known to occur. Leese proved that the outbreak occurred and spread when the camels were grazing in the desert portion of the State at least 100 miles from any fly zone. In this region the only biting fly present was *Lyperosia minuta* Bezzi, which swarmed on the animals and caused great irritation so that the camels rubbed against each other in order to dislodge them. It seems probable, therefore, that Surra can spread in the presence of *Lyperosia* alone, and Leese believes that the transmission is probably mechanical.

REFERENCES.

Austen, E. (1909). *African Blood-sucking Flies*, p. 160.
Leese, A. S. (1912). *Journ. Trop. Vet. Sci.* vol. VII. p. 19.
Montgomery and Kinghorn (1908). *Ann. Trop. Med. and Parasit.* vol. II. p. 130.
Riley, C. V. and Howard, L. O. (1889). *Insect Life*, vol. II. p. 93.
Schat, P. (1903). *Mededal. Proefstation Oost-Java*, 3rd ser. No. 44.

## CHAPTER XXII

### *Family* HIPPOBOSCIDAE (Tick-Flies).

*Description.* The members of this family may be regarded as Muscidæ that have become adapted to an entirely parasitic mode of life on birds and mammals. As a result certain marked changes in structure and reproduction have taken place and the flies form such a distinct group that they are frequently placed in a separate sub-order, the Pupipara, characterized by their viviparous mode of reproduction. The Hippoboscidæ may be distinguished by the following characters :

The head is generally flattened and usually fits into an emargination of the thorax. The antennæ are apparently one-jointed and are inserted in pits or depressions, situated near the border of the mouth. The maxillary palps ensheath the proboscis, which closely resembles that of *Glossina*, but never projects in front of the head. The eyes are round or oval, and are widely separated in both sexes ; ocelli may be present or absent. The thorax is flattened, strongly chitinised, and leathery in appearance ; the scutellum is broad and short. The abdomen is unsegmented. The legs are rather short and very strong, broadly separated by the abdomen and end in powerful claws. The wings may be well-developed, rudimentary, or entirely absent ; when present the veins are always concentrated towards the anterior margin. The halteres are small or rudimentary.

The length of the adult insect may vary from about 3 mm. up to 11·5 mm.

*Bionomics.* The Hippoboscidæ live amongst the fur or feathers of either mammals or birds, and by means of their strong legs and claws are enabled to cling to their hosts. As a result of the adoption of this parasitic mode of life, the wings have gradually become rudimentary and in *Melophagus ovinus*, the common "sheep-ked," they are entirely wanting. They run about on the surface of their hosts, and even when possessing well-developed wings make little use of them. They feed entirely by sucking the blood of birds and mammals, and except for some special reason, such as the death of the host, rarely leave its body. The bites of Hippoboscidæ are not very painful to man, but the sensation produced by their sharp claws hanging to the skin is most unpleasant. However, none of the species, except fortuitously, ever attack man.

*Reproduction.* As in the case of *Glossina*, the female Hippoboscid at certain intervals gives birth to a fully grown larva which at once proceeds to pupate. The body of the larva exhibits practically no trace of segmentation and thus differs from those of the true Muscidæ. The female may deposit its larva either amongst the hair of its host (*e.g. Melophagus*) or on the ground (*e.g. Lynchia*), but precise information on this subject is lacking. After a variable incubation period the pupa, which is of the usual Cyclorrhaphous type, splits off a cap at the anterior end and the perfect insect emerges from the circular aperture thus formed.

*Hippoboscidæ and disease.* Up to the present no truly pathogenic organisms have been shewn to be carried by Hippoboscidæ, but two species of *Hippobosca* are said to transmit *Trypanosoma theileri* occurring in cattle in the Transvaal, and three species of *Lynchia* have been shewn to carry the pigeon halteridium, *Hæmoproteus columbæ*. The insects, therefore, are of little importance from the point of view of disease-carriers, but some of them are of economic interest because of the harm they do to domestic animals, through mere irritation.

*Classification.* The Hippoboscidæ may be divided into thirteen genera as follows :

*Synopsis of the genera of Hippoboscidæ after Speiser*[1].

A. *Wings well developed and functional.*

1 {Claws with the usual two points (heel and tip) ; parasitic on mammals = 2
{Claws with three teeth ; parasitic on birds .. .. .. .. = 3

2 {┌Head of normal form, not broadly impinging on thorax, freely movable ;
{│   ocelli absent ; wings always present .. .. = *Hippobosca.*
{│Head flat, broadly impinging on thorax ; ocelli present ; wings sometimes
{└   becoming detached (in female) leaving only a shred = *Dipoptena.*

3 {Ocelli present .. .. .. .. .. .. .. = 4
{Ocelli wanting (no anal cell) .. .. .. .. .. .. = 5

4 {Anal cell present .. .. .. .. .. .. .. = 6
{Anal cell absent .. .. .. .. .. .. = *Ornithophila.*

5 {┌Wings of a peculiarly pointed form (*vide* Fig. 85), the tip rounded = *Lynchia.*
{┤Wings of the ordinary form but less expanded than in *Ornithomyia*, with
{└   broadly rounded tip .. .. .. .. .. = *Olfersia.*

6 {┌Third longitudinal vein not elbowed at the anterior transverse vein
{│                                                          = *Ornithomyia.*
{┤Third longitudinal vein abruptly bent forwards at the level of the anterior
{└   transverse vein                                       = *Ornithœca.*

B. *Wings rudimentary or wanting.*

1 {Wings present, but rudimentary and functionless ; halteres present = 2
{Wings and halteres absent .. .. .. .. = *Melophagus.*

[1] Modified from Alcock's *Entomology for Medical Officers*, p. 187.

2   { Claws with the usual two points (heel and tip)    ..    ..    .. =3
     { Claws with three teeth   ..    ..    ..    ..    ..    ..    .. =4

3   { Ocelli present.   Wings always well developed, but always in the female
         and generally in the male becoming detached, so that only shreds
         remain resembling rudimentary wings    ..    ..       =*Lipoptena*.
      { Ocelli wanting.   Wings rudimentary.   Legs much enlarged or elongated
                                               =*Allobosca*.

4   { Ocelli present.   Wings narrow, nearly ten times as long as broad, and
         longer than the abdomen   ..    ..    ..    ..    =*Stenopteryx*.
      { Ocelli absent.   Wings not more than three times as long as broad   .. =5

5   { Wings as long as, or longer than, the abdomen    ..    =*Oxypterum*.
     { Wing rudiments much shorter than the abdomen    ..    ..    .. =6

6   { Veins of the wings distinct.   Asiatic species   ..    ..   =*Myiophthiria*.
     { Veins of the wings indistinct.   North American species =*Brachypteromyia*.

## *Genus* LYNCHIA *Weyenbergh.*

Speiser[1] gives the following diagnosis of the genus : " Head without frontal eyes, antennal prolongations frequently bearing characteristic brushes. Scutellum squarely cut off from the thorax, almost four times as broad as long, often with conspicuous hairs. Legs normal, claws with accessory teeth and rather large basal protuberances. Wings narrowly tapering, consequently the venation is striking and characteristic. The posterior basal cell is quite open, the posterior transverse vein absent. The veins appear somewhat more compressed towards the anterior border than in *Olfersia* Leach. Spec. typica : *L. penelopes* Weyenbergh."

Certain members of this genus have been shewn to transmit *Hæmoproteus columbæ* and are probably responsible for the spread of other kinds of Halteridia.

*L. lividicolor*, Bigot (1885)[2] has been shewn to transmit *H. columbæ* in Brazil. It is easily distinguished from the other members of its genus by the brownish colour of the wings instead of the usual milky-white.

[1] Speiser (1902). Studien über Diptera pupipara. *Zeitschr. f. syst. Hymenopterologie u. Dipterologie*, vol. II. p. 155.
[2] Bigot (1885). *Ann. Soc. Ent. France*, p. 238.

## *Lynchia maura* (Bigot), 1885.

## *Olfersia maura* Bigot, 1885.

*Description.* Bigot gives the following diagnosis of this species :

" Antennæ chestnut-coloured with yellowish setæ ; epistome and vertex testaceous ; frons brown, shining on either side. Thorax brownish-black, scarcely shining, with the shoulders and scutellum dirty fulvous. Abdomen obscurely infuscate ; apex of the second segment with a fulvous margin. Legs testaceous ; upper surfaces of femora slightly infuscated and with scanty black setæ ; posterior femora marked on the outside with a slender brownish line. Wings nearly hyaline ; costal and first four longitudinal veins tinctured with black along the whole length, and the fifth vein as far as the first black transverse vein."

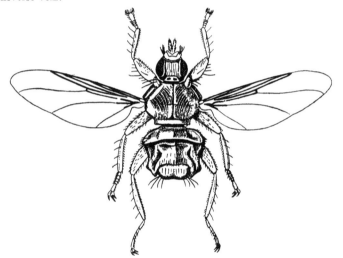

Fig. 85. *Lynchia maura* ♀. ( ×6.) Drawn from Bigot's type specimen.

*Bionomics.* L. *maura* generally occurs on young pigeons about 15 to 20 days old, in which the feathers have commenced to grow. As many as 50 or 60 may be found on a nestling pigeon, whereas it is uncommon to find any on the adult birds.

The insects usually remain hidden amongst the plumage and their smooth flat body enables them to glide under the feathers. If the bird is taken in the hand, or shakes itself very thoroughly, the *Lynchia* take flight. They change hosts readily and their flight is very rapid.

The insect seems to be unable to live on any other bird than the pigeon, and in captivity usually dies within 48 hours after being removed from its host.

The copulation takes place either during repose or whilst the insects are flying and lasts a very long time ; during the act the female raises its wings in order to permit the access of the male.

*Life-cycle.* The larva is laid amongst the dry dust in the pigeon-house, never in the moist excrement. When freshly laid the larva appears as a white ovoid body with a black spot in the form of a six-rayed star at the posterior pole. Pupation is usually complete within an hour of the larva being born, and is accompanied by darkening of the integument, which becomes black. The pupa measures about 3 mm. in length by 2·5 mm. in breadth, and closely resembles a small grain of seed. The surface of the pupa is marked by a network of fine lines giving it the appearance of crushed morocco.

The pupa hatches after an incubation period of 23 to 28 days, when it is kept at a temperature of 24 to 30° C. When pupæ are kept at the body temperature of the pigeon (42° C.) they invariably die without hatching, therefore it is very unlikely that they occur amongst the feathers on the body of the host.

*Lynchia and disease.* Three species belonging to this genus, viz. L. *maura, brunea* and *lividicolor,* have been shewn capable of transmitting *Hæmoproteus columbæ.* It is also probable that certain other protozoal infections of pigeons, such as trypanosomes and *Leucocytozoa* may also be carried by these insects, but up to the present there is no experimental proof in support of this supposition.

LITERATURE.

Bigot (1885). *Ann. Soc. Entomol. de France,* 6th series, vol. v. p. 237.
Sergent, Ed. and Et. (1907). *Ann. Inst. Pasteur,* vol. XXI. p. 251.

*Hippobosca rufipes* v. Olfers, 1816.

This species is about 1 cm. in length and is characterised by the markings on the thorax and scutellum. The thorax is a rich chestnut-brown colour and is bordered by a ring of yellowish-white spots ; in addition there is a white spot in the middle of the dorsal surface. The scutellum is marked by a median red spot, on each side of which is a yellowish-white spot.

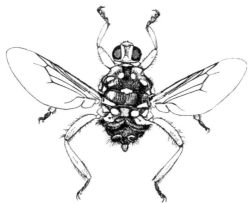

Fig. 86.    *Hippobosca rufipes.*    ( × 3.)

*Bionomics.*  *H. rufipes* is the common parasite of cattle and horses in South Africa.  According to von Olfers, the type of this species was taken on an ostrich, but he suggests that the fly may have come from a quagga, as these animals used to mingle with the flocks of ostriches.

According to Theiler it is often found on cattle, on which it usually settles between the hind-legs, but may occur running over any part of the body.

This species may occasionally stray on to other hosts, for Mr Distant states that in the Transvaal this fly often attached itself to his neck.

A pupa of *H. rufipes* has been described by Austen.  It is 5·6 mm. in length by 4·8 mm. in breadth and is roundly ovate in shape.  The colour is a dark seal-brown with the exception of the posterior end which bears a black cap, separated off from the rest of the surface by a distinct groove. The anterior end is surrounded by a darker line, marking the line of dehiscence of the cephalic cap. There is a longitudinal row of six punctures on each side, above and below, near the lateral margin.

*Hippobosca and disease.* In addition to being the carrier of *Trypanosoma theileri* (*vide infra*), Mr Hutcheon states that a local form of anthrax, which is very common in horses in parts of Griqualand West, is most probably due to infection caused by *Hippobosca rufipes*. There is no experimental evidence in support of this statement.

*Hippobosca maculata*, Leach, also occurs parasitic on horses and cattle in many parts of the world, including South Africa, where, however, it is comparatively uncommon. It is probable that this species as well as *rufipes* is capable of transmitting *T. theileri*, and in his experiments Theiler used a mixture of the two. As, however, *rufipes* is the more common species in South Africa, where *T. theileri* is especially prevalent, it is only reasonable to assume that it is the usual carrier of the infection.

# CHAPTER XXIII

## INFECTIONS TRANSMITTED BY HIPPOBOSCIDAE

### 1. Hæmoproteus columbæ Celli and San Felice, 1891.

*General account.* *Hæmoproteus columbæ*, the halteridium of the pigeon, is very common in many parts of the world, having been recorded from Italy, France, North Africa, India and Brazil. It is apparently non-pathogenic, for pigeons may shew large numbers of the parasites in the blood circulation for years, without any obvious harmful effects being produced. Et. and Ed. Sergent, in 1906, shewed that in Algeria the parasite is transmitted by *Lynchia maura* Bigot, one of the Hippoboscidæ. In 1908, Aragão worked out the life-cycle of the parasite both in the blood of the pigeon and in the invertebrate hosts of this infection in Brazil, viz., *Lynchia brunea* and *L. lividicolor* (Oliv.). Aragão's account is somewhat incomplete but such as it is does not support Schaudinn's observations on the life-cycle of a closely related parasite, *Hæmoproteus noctuæ*, occurring in the little stone owl, *Athene noctua*.

*Life-cycle*. Owing to the presence of infected flies in the nests of the pigeons, the young birds frequently become infected, the parasites appearing in the blood after an incubation period of from 20 to 30 days.

The first stages of development take place in the white blood corpuscles and if smears are made of the lungs of a pigeon 13 or 14 days after it has been bitten by an infected insect, the young forms of the *Hæmoproteus* can generally be found within the leucocytes. At this stage the parasite appears as a small mass of protoplasm about 3 to 4 microns in diameter, containing one or two nuclei. This form lives within the cytoplasm of a leucocyte and by repeated division gives rise to a number of parasites, each of which contains a single nucleus and is provided with a more or less distinct membrane. This stage may be found in the pigeon from 15 to 17 days after the bite of the insect. Each of these bodies then commences to grow very rapidly and produces a large mass of cytoplasm 8 to 12 microns in diameter, containing several small particles of chromatin, and surrounded by a more or less definite cyst-wall. The leucocytes containing the parasites undergo hypertrophy and become very large, up to 60 microns in diameter. This phase of development is present about the eighteenth or nineteenth day. According to Aragão, at this stage it is possible to distinguish two kinds of cysts by their staining reactions, one of which will give rise to the female and the other to the male-producing merozoites.

From the twentieth to the twenty-fourth day of development the cysts increase enormously in size, up to as much as 50 microns in diameter. The membrane is now very distinct and the numerous nuclei are uniformly scattered throughout the cytoplasm. The cysts cease to grow and their protoplasm breaks up into a number of polygonal masses with the nuclei arranged along their edges (Fig. 87, *18*), thus closely resembling the young malaria sporoblasts. This change takes place on the twenty-fifth day and is immediately succeeded by the division

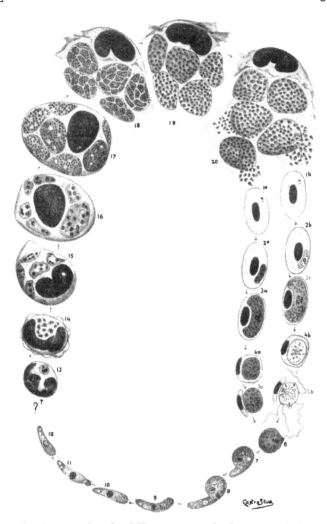

Fig. 87.  Developmental cycle of *Hæmoproteus columbæ*.  1*a* and 1*b*, young
halteridia in the blood corpuscles;  1*a* to 4*a* and 1*b* to 4*b*, stages in the
growth of the female and male gametocytes, respectively;  5*a*, female
gamete;  5*b*, formation of male gametes;  6, fertilization;  7, zygote;
8 to 12, stages in the extrusion of granules from the oökinete;  13, youngest
stage in a leucocyte from the lung of a pigeon;  14 to 20, stages in its
multiplication, accompanied by hypertrophy of the leucocyte;  20, the
liberation of large numbers of uninucleate forms which enter the red cells
and there become the young halteridia.  (After Aragão.)

into merozoites.  Each nucleus, together with a small mass of cytoplasm, becomes separated off, and thus, in the inside of the cyst, hundreds of merozoites are formed (Fig. 87, *19*).  The cysts, together with the leucocyte that contains them, then rupture, and the merozoites are set free in the blood stream of the pigeon about 26 days after the bite of an infected insect (Fig. 87, *20*).

The merozoites then invade the red blood corpuscles and develop into the typical halteridium forms that are found in the circulating blood (Fig. 87, *1–3*), and these are incapable of any further development within the body of the pigeon.  Accordingly there is no cycle of schizogony such as occurs in the case of the malarial parasites, but after the completion of development within the leucocytes in the internal organs, the merozoites, as soon as they have entered the red blood corpuscles, develop into the sexual forms, male and female.

The appearance of the male and female gametocytes of *Hæmoproteus* is practically the same as that of the corresponding stages of *Plasmodium*.  The macro-gametocytes stain intensely and contain a large amount of reserve food material in the form of granules, whilst the micro-gametocytes are much lighter and almost free from granules.

When taken into the stomach of the invertebrate host the gametocytes escape from the red cells and give rise to the gametes.  The macro-gamete is a large rounded body containing a single nucleus near the middle of the cytoplasm (Fig. 87, *5a*). The nucleus of the micro-gametocyte (Fig. 87, *4b*) breaks up into a number of small particles arranged in pairs, and each pair, together with a small quantity of cytoplasm, becomes separated off in the form of an elongate vermiform micro-gamete. These swim about until they come in contact with a ripe macro-gamete when fertilization takes place, the result of the fusion being an oökinete.  The liberation of the micro-gametes and the process of fertilization may be observed by placing a small quantity of infected blood on a glass slide and watching it under the microscope.  Probably as a result of the diminution in temperature, the ripening of the gametes and fertilization take place in the same way as if the blood had been ingested into the stomach of its invertebrate host.

The oökinetes may be observed in the gut of *Lynchia* within three hours after a meal of infected blood. Each oökinete is an elongate, somewhat gregarine-like body, that moves about by means of undulations of its body. The pigment granules, that originally are scattered throughout the whole of its cytoplasm, become concentrated in a clump at the posterior extremity (Fig. 87, *9–11*), which eventually is separated from the rest of the body. In this manner the oökinete gets rid of the waste granules in its cytoplasm. The subsequent history of this form is not certain, but in all probability it does not undergo any further development in the invertebrate host. When an infected *Lynchia* bites a pigeon, the oökinetes present in the front part of the insect's alimentary canal, are introduced into the blood of the bird and undergo further development in the leucocytes. The cycle within the vertebrate host is then repeated, the parasite multiplying in the leucocytes of the pigeon in the manner described above.

It will be noticed that *Hæmoproteus columbæ* possesses only one method of multiplication, there being no distinct schizogonic and sporogonic cycles as in the case of *Plasmodium*. The parasite is apparently unable to multiply within the body of its invertebrate host, *Lynchia*, all multiplication taking place in the vertebrate host.

*H. columbæ* is not hereditarily transmitted to the offspring of infected *Lynchia*, for large numbers of freshly-hatched insects may be fed on a healthy pigeon without producing any infection.

The number of halteridia appearing in the blood circulation of a pigeon is directly proportional to the number of infected *Lynchia* that feed on the bird. The bite of only one insect produces a very mild infection, whereas when 50 are fed on a pigeon, almost every corpuscle becomes infected.

### REFERENCES.

Aragão (1908). Der Entwicklungsgang und die Übertragung von *Hæmoproteus columbæ*. *Arch. f. Protistenkunde*, vol. XII. p. 154.
Mayer, M. (1910). Die Entwicklung von *Halteridium*. *Arch. f. Schiffs. u. Tropenhyg.* vol. XIV. p. 197.
—— (1911). Ein Halteridium und Leucocytozoon des Waldkauzes. *Arch. f. Protistenkunde*, vol. XXI. p. 232.
Sergent, Ed. and Et. (1907). Les Hématozoaires d'Oiseaux. *Ann. Inst. Pasteur*, vol. XXI. p. 251.

## 2. Trypanosoma theileri Laveran, 1902.

*Synonym.* *T. transvaaliense* Laveran.

*General account.* This trypanosome was discovered by Theiler in 1902, occurring in the blood of cattle in the Transvaal. It was named and described by Laveran, in 1902, who at the same time distinguished two species of trypanosomes occurring in the blood of cattle in the Transvaal, viz. *T. theileri* and *T. transvaaliense.* Theiler has shewn that the latter is merely a young stage in the development of *T. theileri*, for when blood containing *transvaaliense* was injected into cattle the latter developed infections of typical *theileri*.

The pathogenic effects of this trypanosome are so slight, that no difference can be detected between normal and infected cattle.

Since the discovery of *T. theileri*, non-pathogenic trypanosomes have been found in the blood of catt e from all parts of the world. In the majority of cases the parasites are present in such scanty numbers that their presence can only be detected by means of culturing the blood of the infected animals, but in others the trypanosomes are in sufficient quantity to be evident on ordinary microscopic examination. Considering the fact that cattle infected with *T. theileri* in Africa frequently shew very many parasites in the circulating blood, whereas in the case of infections with *T. americanum, franki, rutherfordi*, etc., the trypanosomes are always excessively rare, the specific identity of these forms seems a little doubtful. However, there is a possibility that the numerous non-pathogenic trypanosomes, described under different names[1] from practically every part of the world, only constitute one species, and therefore the observations in this chapter only refer to *T. theileri* as observed in the Transvaal.

*Morphology of the parasite.* *T. theileri* is remarkable because of its relatively enormous size. The large forms measure as much as 60 to 70 microns in length by 4 to 5 microns in breadth. The *transvaaliense* forms, which are probably stages

---

[1] Among these may be mentioned *T. himalayanum, indicum* and *muktesari* Lingard, 1904; *T. franki* Frosch, 1909; *T. wrublewskii, T. americanum,* Crawley, 1909; *T. rutherfordi* Hadwen, 1912.

in the development of these large trypanosomes vary considerably in their dimensions. The smaller parasites measure about 18 microns in length by 2 microns in breadth, and all stages in their increase in size may be observed. In the small forms the kinetonucleus is frequently situated alongside the tropho-

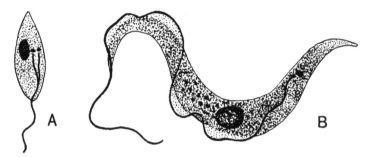

Fig. 88. *Trypanosoma theileri.* × about 1500. A. Small crithidial form; B. Large individual from the blood of a cow. (After Theiler.)

nucleus in the middle of the body of the trypanosome, and the undulating membrane is only slightly developed. In the larger parasites of the *theileri* type, the kinetonucleus is situated towards the posterior extremity and the trophonucleus about the middle of the body. The undulating membrane is very large and thrown into bold folds ; anteriorly the flagellum is free for a distance equal to about one-quarter the length of the body of the parasite. The protoplasm contains large numbers of granules and stains very deeply.

The only mode of multiplication that has been observed is simple longitudinal division, which is of the normal type.

*Mode of transmission.* Theiler has shewn that this trypanosome may be carried from one animal to another by means of *Hippobosca.* " For this purpose some flies were kept overnight in order to make them hungry, and were then placed on the groins of an infected calf. To give the experiment every chance of success, the spot where the flies were put to feed was first shaved, as was also the spot on a clean animal where they were placed for infection. Feeding by turns on a sick and on a clean animal was thus repeated several times, in order to secure an infection. Out of four experiments made in this way, two were successful. It must be stated here that the experimental animals were kept together with control animals in a stable, to exclude spontaneous infection, and that none of the control animals shewed a spontaneous infection. The incubation periods coincided typically with the period which is observed after artificial infection with small quantities of virus " (Theiler).

Two specimens of the *Hippobosca* used in these experiments were identified by Speiser as *Hippobosca rufipes* v. Olfers, and *H. maculata* Leach, respectively. As the latter is excessively rare in South Africa, it is probable that *H. rufipes* is the usual carrier of *T. theileri*.

The parasite may also be experimentally transmitted to cattle by the injection of small quantities of infected blood. Under these circumstances the incubation period depends, to a large extent, on the number of trypanosomes introduced ; it averages between four and six days, but in one case a period of 18 days was noticed.

The trypanosomes are only present in the peripheral circulation for a comparatively short time and then disappear, leaving the animal immune against any further infection. The longest period in which the presence of the parasite was observed in the blood was 13 days, the average nine days, and the shortest period, one day. While present the numbers of the parasites may rise to 30 trypanosomes in each microscopic field, but the average is about five per field. The disappearance of the parasites is only apparent, however, for the blood of a cow has been shewn to be still infective 11 months after the animal was inoculated.

REFERENCES.

Laveran, A. (1902).   *Compt. Rend. Acad. Sci.* vol. cxxxiv. p. 512.
Theiler, A. (1903).   *Journ. Com. Path. and Therap.* vol. xvi. p. 193.

# INDEX

*Where more than one reference is given the most important is printed in black figures*

Acalyptratæ  24, 239, **240**
Acanthocera  231
Acanthomeridæ  225
Acartomyia  109
Acroceridæ  225
Aëdes  63, 71, 72, 109
  calopus  See *Stegomyia fasciata*
Aedimorphus  109
Aëdinæ  76
Aëdomyia  109, 110, 114
Aestivo-autumnal malaria  See *Plasmodium falciparum*
African trypanosomiasis  *See* Sleeping Sickness
Agchylostoma duodenale  214
Ague  *See* Malaria
Aïno  31, 287, 329
Aldrovanda vesiculosa  72
Allobosca  375
Ambassis ranga  152
Anabas  151
Andersonia  109
Anisócheleomyia  111
Anopheles  62, 63, 76, 78, 79, 95, 123, 134, 136, 144, 145, 148, 149, 154
  Enemies of  144
Anopheles aconita  87, 88, 96
  — var. *cohæsa*  87, 96, 99
  aitkeni  26, 80, 96, 105, 107, 140
  albimana  94, 96, 97, 99, 107, 142
  albipes  27, 94, 96, 215
  albirostris  26, 87, 88, 96, 97, 99, 142
  albitarsis  94, 96
  alboannulatus  85, 96
  albofimbriata  94, 96
  albotæniatus  84, 85, 96, 97
  algeriensis  26, 81, 96, 142
  annularis  85, 96
  annulimanus  81, 96
  annulipalpis  95, 96
  annulipes  Walker  95, 96, 103, 142
  annulipes  Arrib.  95, 96
  antennatus  95, 96
  ardensis  91, 93, 96

Anopheles argyrotarsis  27, 90, 94, 96, 97, 99, 142, 215
  arabiensis  26, 89, 96, 142
  arnoldi  96
  asiatica  83, 96, 138
  atratipes  83, 96
  atropos  81, 96
  aureosquamiger  91, 96
  aurirostris  96
  austenii  89, 96
  azriki  96
  bancroftii  84, 96
  barberi  81, 96
  barbirostris  27, 84, 96, 140, 215
  barianensis  81, 96
  bellator  96
  bifurcatus  Linn.  26, 80, 81, 96, 99, 107, 141, 143, 222
  bifurcatus  Meigen  96, 101
  bigotii  94, 96, 105
  bisignata  96
  boliviensis  95, 96
  bozasi  94, 96
  brachypus  85, 96
  braziliensis  94, 98
  brunnipes  95, 98
  cardamatisi  89, 98
  ceylonica  95, 98
  chaudoyei  Theobald  27, 89, 98, 99, 142
  chaudoyei  Billet  89, 98
  christophersi  87, 98, 141, 162
  christophersi  var. *alboapicalis*  87, 98
  christyi  95, 98
  cincta  94, 98
  cinereus  89, 98, 101
  claviger  81, 98, 221
  cleopatræ  89
  cohæsus  95, 98
  corethroides  80, 98
  costalis  27, 88, 91, 92, 93, 98, 101, 142, 215
  costalis  var. *melas*  91, 98, 135
  coustani  85, 98

Anopheles crucians 81, 82, 98, 99
  cruzii 87, 98
  cubensis 94, 98
  culicifacies 26, 87, 88, 98, 101,
    103, 137, 140, 142
  culiciformis 80, 98
  deceptor 95, 98
  distinctus 89, 98
  distinctus var. melanocosta 89, 98
  d'thali 27, 87, 98
  dudgeoni 92, 98
  eiseni 81, 82, 98
  elegans 95, 98
  error 95, 98
  fajardoi 95, 98
  farauti 95, 98
  ferruginosus 81, 98
  flava 92, 98
  flavicosta 87, 98
  fluviatilis 87, 98
  formosaënsis I 26, 87, 98, 142
  formosaënsis II 26, 95, 97, 98
  formosus 83, 98
  fowleri 91, 92, 98
  fragilis 80, 100
  franciscanus 83, 100
  freeræ 91, 92, 100
  fuliginosus 27, 91, 92, 100, 101,
    142
  funesta 26, 86, 87, 88, 100, 101,
    142
  funesta var. subumbrosa 87, 100
  funesta var. umbrosa 87, 88, 100
  funesta var. neiriti 100
  gambiæ 92, 100
  gigas 82, 83, 100
  gilesi 93, 100
  gorgasi 94, 100
  grabhamii 84, 100
  gracilis Theobald 95, 100
  gracilis Dönitz 92, 100
  grisescens 81, 100
  halli 92, 100
  hebes 87, 100
  hispaniola 27, 87, 88, 100, 105,
    142
  hyemalis 83, 100
  immaculatus 81, 100
  implexa 95, 100
  impunctus 87, 100
  indefinata 90, 100, 105
  indica 87, 92, 100
  indiensis 92, 100
  intermedia 92, 100
  intermedium 86, 100
  jacobi 94, 100
  jamesii Theobald 91, 100
  jamesii Liston 92, 100
  jehafi 87, 100
  jesoënsis 85, 100
  jeyporensis 89, 100

Anopheles karwari 91, 92, 100, 103
  kochii 91, 92, 100, 101
  kumassii 87, 100
  leptomeres 87, 100
  leucopsus 92, 100
  leucosphyrus 95, 102
  lindesayi 83, 102
  lindesayi var. maculata 83, 102
  lineata 92, 95, 102
  listoni 26, 86, 87, 88, 95, 99, 102,
    137, 142
  longipalpis 87, 102
  ludlowi 27, 90, 102, 103, 138, 142
  lutzi Cruz 93, 95, 102
  lutzi Theobald 27, 87, 93, 95, 99,
    102, 138, 142
  maculatus 27, 87, 91, 92, 102, 105,
    107
  maculicosta 95, 102
  maculipalpis Giles 91, 102, 142
  maculipalpis James and Liston 92,
    102
  maculipalpis var. indiensis 27, 92,
    101, 102, 103
  maculipennis 26, 51, 62, 65, 70,
    71, 80, 81, 97, 99, 101, 102,
    105, 141, 142, 156, 219, 222 ;
    Pupa 22
  maculipes 85, 86, 102
  malefactor 86, 102
  mangyana 90, 102
  marshallii 91, 93, 102
  martini 95, 102
  masteri 95, 102
  mauritianus 27, 84, 85, 99, 102,
    105, 107
  mediopunctatus 28, 86, 102
  merus 91, 93, 102
  metaboles 92, 102
  minimus 89, 102
  minutus 27, 85, 102
  multicolor 95, 102
  muscivus 95, 102
  myzomyfacies 27, 89, 102, 142
  natalensis 95, 102
  neavei 88
  neiriti 95, 101
  nigerrimus Giles 27, 85, 102
  nigerrimus James and Liston 85,
    102
  nigra 93, 102
  nigrans 92, 102
  nigrifasciatus 89, 102, 105
  nigripes 81, 102
  nigritarsis 93, 102
  nili 87, 88, 102
  nimba 79, 80, 104
  nivipes 91, 92, 104
  nursei 89, 104
  ocellatus 95, 104
  occidentalis 104

*Anopheles palestinensis* 89, 104
*pallida* 80, 104
*pallidopalpi* 83, 104
*paludis* 84, 85, 103, 104
*paludis* var. *similis* 84, 85, 104
*parva* 93, 104
*peditæniatus* 27, 85, 104, 215
*perplexans* 83, 104
*pharoënsis* 93, 94, 97, 104, 142
*pharoënsis* var. *alba* 94, 104
*philippinensis* 91, 92, 104
*pictus* Ficalbi 85, 104
*pictus* Lœw 85, 104
*pictus* Macdonald. 87, 104
*pitchfordi* 89, 104
*plumbeus* 81, 103, 104
*plumiger* 85, 104
*pretoriensis* 91, 92, 104
*pseudobarbirostris* 84, 104
*pseudocostalis* 91, 93, 104
*pseudomaculipes* 28, 86, 104
*pseudopictus* 27, 84, 85, 104, 105, 222
*pseudopunctipennis* 26, 83, 104
*pseudosquamosa* 95, 104
*pseudowillmori* 92, 104
*pulcherrima* 93, 94, 104
*punctatus* 95
*punctipennis* Bigot MSS. 94, 104
*punctipennis* Say 28, 83, 101, 104, 141
*punctulata* 95, 104, 105
*pursati* 26, 95, 104
*pyretophoroides* 87, 104
*quadrimaculatus* 81, 104
*rhodesiensis* 87, 88, 104
*rossii* 26, 86, 90, 104, 107, 137, 138, 140, 215
*rossii* var. *indefinata* 90, 104
*separatus* 85, 104
*sergentii* 89, 104
*simlensis* 83, 104
*sinensis* 27, 83, 84, 85, 97, 101, 103, 105, 106, 107, 141, 215
*sinensis* var. *indiensis* 84, 85, 101
*smithii* 81, 106
*squamosus* 94, 106
*squamosus* var. *arnoldi* 94, 97, 106
*stephensi* 91, 92, 93, 101, 103, 106, 138, 140, 142
*stigmaticus* 95, 106
*strachani* 84, 106
*subpictus* 95, 106
*superpictus* 27, 89, 106, 142, 222
*tarsimaculatus* 27, 94, 106
*tenebrosus* 85, 106
*tessellatum* 95, 99, 106, 107
*theobaldi* 27, 91, 92, 106
*thorntonii* 95, 106
*tibani* 92, 106
*tibiomaculata* 93, 106

*Anopheles transvaalensis* 89, 106
*treacheri* 80, 106
*trifurcatus* 81, 106
*turkhudi* 27, 87, 88, 106
*umbrosa* 87, 106
*umbrosus* 27, 84, 106
*unicolor* 106
*vagus* 90, 106
*vanus* 85, 106
*villosus* 81, 106
*vincenti* 95, 106
*walkeri* 81, 106
*waponi* 92
*watsonii* Edwards 106
*watsonii* Leicester 95, 106
*wellcomei* 95, 106
*wellingtonianus* 83, 106
*willmori* James 27, 91, 92, 99, 101, 106, 137, 142
*willmori* Leicester 92, 106
*willmori* var. *maculosa* 106
*ziemani* 85, 106
Anophelinæ 26, 76, 215
Dichotomous table showing natural grouping of species of 79
Table showing detailed tabulation of species of 79
Introduction of natural enemies of 151
Measures directed against adult mosquitoes 151
Obliteration of breeding-places 149
Anopheline-transmitted diseases 119
Anthomyidæ 241
Anthrax 3, 31, 379
Antimosquito campaigns 149
Apioceridæ 225
*Apocampta* 231
*Aporoculex* 110
*Apotolestes* 231
Arista 14
*Arribalzagia* 77, 78, 79, 85 See *Anopheles*
*maculipes* 77, 85
Asilidæ 224, 225
*Athene noctua* Blood parasites of 200

*Babesia canis* 155
*Bacillus icteroides* 181
*Bacillus X* 181
Baleri. General account 332 ; References to literature on 335 ; see also *Trypanosoma pecaudi*
*Banksinella* 109, 111
*Bathosomyia* 109
*Bdellolarynx* 31, 243
*Bembex* 270
*Bibio* 34
Bibionidæ 33
Bilious remittent fever *See* Yellow Fever

Bird Malaria 196
  General account 196
  References to literature 199
  See also *Plasmodium præcox*
*Bironella* 77, 95 ; see *Anopheles*
  *gracilis* 77
Biting-Flies as Carriers of Disease 25
Blepharoceridæ 33
Blood-sucking Muscidæ 241
*Bolbodimyia* 230
Bombyliidæ 225
*Brachypteromyia* 375
Breeze-Flies See Tabanidæ
*Boycia* 110

*Cacomyia* 109
*Cadicera* 231
*Calvertina* 77, 92, 95
  *lineata* 77, 92
Calyptratæ 24, 239, **240**
  Synopsis of families of 240
*Cecidomyia* 34
Cecidomyidæ 33
*Cellia* 77, 78, 79, 90, 93, 95 ; see
  *Anopheles*
  *argyrotarsis* 90
Celli's formula 124
*Ceratopogon* 26
*Chagasia* 77, 95 ; see *Anopheles*
  *fajardoi* 77
Chalcididæ 270
Chaoborinæ 76
Chironomidæ 26, 33
*Chironomus* 34
*Chætura pelagica* 74
*Christophersia* 77, 91 ; see *Ano-
  pheles*
  *kochii* 77, 91
*Christya* 77, 95 ; see *Anopheles*
  *implexa* 77
*Chrysops* 28, **231**, 238
*Cinchona* 120
*Cincindela* 270
*Citronella* 319
Classification of Diptera 23
Cleggs See Tabanidæ
*Cœlodiazesis barberi* 81
Commensalism between fungus and
  mosquito 68
*Conopomyia* 110
*Corethra* 76
*Corizoneura* 231
Crescents 161, 162
*Crithidia* 7
*Culex* 2, 62, 63, 109, 110, 115, 175,
  176, 191, 198
  *concolor* 115
  *fatigans* 1, 28, 115, 122, 195, 196
    198, 215
  *fatigans* Distribution of 193
  (*Leucomyia*) *gelidus* 28, 215

*Culex jepsoni* 214
  *malaria* 222
  (*Culicada*) *nemorosus* 28, 198, 199
  *penicillaris* 222
  *pipiens* 28, 62, 66, 70, 71, 115,
    198, 200, 203, 209, 215, 222
  (*Leucomyia*) *sitiens* 28, 215
*Culicada* 109, 114
*Culicelsa* 109
*Culicidæ* 13, 17, 26, 28, 33, 50
  Affect of colours 68
  Biology of adult 67
  Circulatory system 62
  Classification 75
  Definition 50
  Digestive organs 56
  Egg 62
  Enemies of 72
  External Anatomy 50
  Flight 72
  Food-habits 67
  Habitats 70
  Hibernation 71
  Influence of sound on 70
  Internal Anatomy 56
  Larva 63
  Life-cycle 62
  Longevity 71
  Mating habits 71
  Method of feeding 67
  Modes of dissemination 70
  Nervous system 62
  Publications of importance in con-
    nection with nomenclature and
    systematic work on 115
  Pupa 66
  References 75
  Reproductive organs 61
  Respiratory system 61
  Resting position 70
  Salivary apparatus 59
Culicinæ **165**, 215
  Diseases transmitted by 177
  References 177
*Culiciomyia* 110, 115
*Curupira* 33
Cyclical evolution of parasites 9
Cyclical transmission 4
*Cycloleppteron* 76, 78, 84, 85 ; see
  *Anopheles*
  *grabhamii* 84
Cyclops 11
Cyclorrhapha 23
Cyclorrhapha Aschiza 24
Cyclorrhapha Schizophora 24, 30,
  224, **239**
  General description 239
Cypriondontidæ 151

*Danielsia* 109
*Dasybasis* 230

*Dasymyia* 111
Definitive host 4
Dendromyinæ 76
Dengue 28, **190**
  Causal agent of 192
  Distribution and Epidemiology 190
  History 190
  Mode of Infection 194
  References to literature on 196
  Synonyms 190
*Dermococcus* 218
*Desvoidya* 109, 114
Deuteroanopheles 86
Development of parasite in the invertebrate host 9
Dexiidæ 241
*Diachlorus* 230
*Diatomineura* 231
*Dichelacera* 231
Dichoptic 13
*Dicrania* 231
*Dipoptena* 374
  Diptera
  Abdomen 15
  Alimentary canal of 19
  Antennæ 14
  Classification of 23
  Definition of 12
  Eggs 20
  General description of 12
  General morphology 13
  Head 14
  Heart 19
  Internal Anatomy of 19
  Larvæ 21
  Legs 15
  Mouth-parts 14
  Nervous system 19
  Pupa 21
  Reproduction 20
  Reproductive organs 19
  Respiratory system 19
  Surface of body 19
  Thorax 15
  Wings 15
Direct transmission 2
Dixidæ 33
Dixinæ 76
Dolichopodidæ 74, 226
*Dolomedes* 270
*Dorcalæmus* 231
Double Quartan Fever 160
Dourine 236
Drainage 153
*Duttonia* 109
Dytiscidæ 73
*Dytiscus* 73

*Ecculex* 109
El Debab 2, 233, 235
Elephantiasis **217**

Empididæ 74, 226
Empodium 15
Entomophtoraceæ 58
Epidemic poliomyelitis See Poliomyelitis
Epipharynx 14
*Erephrosis* 231
*Esenbeckia* 232
*Eumelanomyia* 111
Eumyiid Flies 24

*Feltinella* 77, 83 ; see *Anopheles pallidopalpi* 77, 83
*Filaria* 10, 11
*Filaria bancrofti* 1, 5, 26, 27, 176, **202**, 365
  Conditions affecting development in mosquito 214
  Description 204
  Distribution 203
  Effect on mosquito 216
  History 203
  Life-cycle in mosquito 209
  Life-cycle in vertebrate host 206
  Pathological effects 217
  Periodicity 207
  Possibility of another indirect mode of transmission by mosquito 216
  References to literature on 219
  Synonyms 202
*Filaria canis cordis* See *F. immitis*
  *diurna* 209
*Filaria immitis* 26, **219**
  Description 220
  Distribution 220
  General account 219
  Life-cycle 221
  Pathogenic effects 223
  References to literature on 223
  Synonyms of 219
*Filaria labiato-papillosa* 31, **364**
  Description 364
  Habitat 364
  Life-history 364
  References to literature on 365
  Synonyms 364
*Filaria loa* 29, 238
  *medinensis* 11
  *nocturna* See *F. bancrofti*
  *perstans* 304
  *philippinensis* See *F. bancrofti*
  *recondita* 223
  *sanguinis hominum nocturna* See *F. bancrofti*
Filariasis **202**
*Finlaya* 109
Fish as mosquito destroyers 150, 151, 152

Gad-Flies *See* Tabanidæ

*Gastrophilus* 240
*Gastroxides* 232
*Gilesia* 109
*Glossina* 20, 233, 242, **243,** 297, 373
  and disease 250, **293, 300**
  Determination of the species of 247
  Diagnosis 243
  Distribution 247
  General description 243
  References to literature on 252
  Synopsis of species of 248
  *austeni* 248
  *brevipalpis* 31,243,248,249,287,**288**
    Bionomics 288
    Description 288
    Distribution 288
    References to literature on 293
    Reproduction 291
    Synonyms 288
    and disease 292
  *Glossina caliginea* 248
  *Glossina fusca* 248, 249, 288, 315, 322
  *fusca* (Austen 1903) See *Glossina
    brevipalpis*
  *fuscipleuris* 249
  *Glossina longipalpis* 30, 249, 251,
    **274,** 283, 333, 334, 336, 337,
    344, 345
    Bionomics 274
    Description 274
    Distribution 274
    References to literature on 276
    Reproduction 275
    and disease 275
  *Glossina longipennis* 31, 243, 249,
    **286,** 288
    Bionomics 287
    Description 286
    Distribution 287
    References to literature on 287
    and disease 287
  *medicorum* 249
  *Glossina morsitans* 8, 30, 246, 247, 248,
    249, 250, 251, 272, 273, 306,
    310, 315, 320, 322, 325, 326,
    327, 328, 329, 330, 331, 333,
    334, 336, 337, 338, 345, 347,
    350, 352, 353, 355
    Bionomics 278
    Description 276
    Distribution 277
    Primary Fly Centres 280
    References to literature on 286
    Reproduction 283
    Synonyms 276
    and disease 285
    var. *pallida* 249, **277**
    var. *paradoxa* 248, 249, **277**
  *Glossina pallicera* 248
  *pallidipes* 30, 249, **271,** 305, 329, 330
    Bionomics 271

*Glossina pallidipes*
  Description 271
  Distribution 271
  References to literature on 274
  and disease 273
*Glossina palpalis* 30, 233, 244, 245,
  246, 248, 250, 251, 252, **256,**
  300, 305, 306, 308, 315, 318,
  319, 320, 330, 331, 333, 334,
  336, 337, 338, 342, 344, 345,
  347, 348, 349, 350, 352, 363
  Bionomics 260
  Breeding localities 268
  Description 256
  Distribution 258
  Internal Anatomy 258
  Longevity 266
  Natural enemies 269
  References to literature on 271
  Reproduction 266
  Synonyms 256
  var. *wellmani* 257
  and Disease 270
  *tabaniformis* 248, 249
*Glossina tachinoides* 30, 243, 248,
  251, **253,** 315, 333, 334, 336,
  337, 344, 345
  Bionomics 253
  Description 253
  Distribution 253
  Prophylaxis against 255
  References to literature on 255
  Reproduction 255
  Synonyms 253
*Goniops* 231
*Grabhamia* 114
*Gualteria* 109
*Gyrinidæ* 73

*Hæmamœba* See *Plasmodium*
*Hæmatobia* 31, 243
*Hæmatobosca* 31, 243
*Hæmatopota* 28, 227, **230,** 233, 234,
  236, 237, 243, 347
*Hæmogregarines* 10
*Hæmoproteus* 122, 200
  *columbæ* 10, 31, 201, 374, 475,
    **379**
    General account 379
    Life-cycle 380
    References to literature on 383
  *noctuæ* 28, 380
*Hæmosporidium* See *Plasmodium*
*Hæmazoin* 127
*Halteridium* See *Hæmoproteus*
*Haplochilus panchax* 152
*Harpagomyia* 111
*Heptaphlebomyia* 110
*Hereditary transmission* 6
*Hexatoma* 230
*Hibernation of Anophelines* 144

*Hippobosca* 374, 385
  and disease 379
  *maculata* 31, 379, 386
  *rufipes* 31, 378, 386
  Bionomics 378
Hippoboscidæ 23, 31, 372
  Bionomics 373
  Classification 374
  General description 372
  References to literature on 377
  Reproduction 373
  Synopsis of genera of 374
  and disease 374
*Hispidimyia* 110
*Hodgesia* 111
Holoptic 13
Horse-Flies See Tabanidæ
*Howardina* 110, 114
Humidity 144
Hydrophilidæ 73
Hypopharynx 14
Hypopygium 15

Incubation period 9
Indirect transmission 4
Infantile paralysis See Poliomyelitis
*Ingramia* 111
*Inimetoculex* 109
Intermediate host 5
Intermittent-fever See Malaria

*Janthinosoma* 109

*Kelloggina* 34
*Kerteszia* 77, 95
  See *Anopheles*
  *boliviensis* 77
*Kingia* 109, 111

Labium 15
Labrum 14
*Lælaps* 12
Larvæ 21
Larvicides 151
*Lasioconops* 110
*Laverania* 90
  See *Plasmodium*
*Lebias dispar* 150
*Leicesteria* 109, 114
*Lepidoplatys* 109
*Lepidoselasa* 230
*Lepidotomyia* 109
Leptidæ 29, 224, 225
*Leptomonas* 7, 144
*Leslieomyia* 109
*Leucocytozoon* 12, 200, 202, 377
  *ziemanni* 28
*Leucomyia* 110
Lice 11
*Lipoptena* 375
*Lispa sinensis* 74

*Lonchopteridæ* 226
*Lophomyia* 83
*Lophoscelomyia* 77, 83
  See *Anopheles*
  *asiatica* 77, 83
*Ludlowia* 110
Lunula 13
*Lutzia* 66, 74, 110
*Lynchia* 10, 373, 374, 375, 383
  and disease 377
  *brunea* 377, 379
  *brunnipes* 31
  *lividicolor* 31, 375, 377, 379
*Lynchia maura* 31, 376, 379
  Bionomics 376
  Description 376
  Life-cycle 377
  References to literature on 377
  *penelopes* 375
*Lyperosia* 31, 243, 369
  General description 369
  Life-cycle 370
  References to literature on 372
  and disease 371
  *exigua* 31, 361, 371
  *irritans* 370
  *minuta* 31, 372
  *punctigera* 370

*Maillotia* 110
Mal de la Zousfana 29, 236
Malaria 26, 27, 28, 119
  Bionomics of mosquitoes in relation
    to 136
  Definition 119
  Historical 119
  Immunity against 146
  Influences affecting through trans-
    mitting host 143
  Life-cycle of parasite 125
  Literature on 162
  New Aetiological Standpoint 124
  Prevention of 148
  Racial tolerance to 147
  Reservoirs of 154
  Segregation 125, 154
  Susceptibility to 146
  Synonyms 119
  Tropica See *Plasmodium falci-
    parum*
Malaria and Nonimmune immigration
    146
  in relation to man 145
Malarial parasite See *Plasmodium*
  Affect of temperature on Develop-
    ment of 143
  Asexual cycle 126
  Development of sexual forms
    in blood 129
  Intravenous inoculation of 121
  Life-cycle of 125

## 394 INDEX

Malarial parasite
  Schizogony **126**
  Sexual cycle **132**
  Sporogony **132**
*Malaya* 111
Malignant tertian See *Plasmodium falciparum*
Malignant tertian malaria 121
Mandibles 15
*Manguinhosia* 77, 95
*Manguinhosia lutzi* 77
*Mansonia* 115
  *annulipes* 29, 215
  *uniformis* 29
  *uniformis* (? *africana*) 215
*Mansonioides* 110, 114
Matlazahuatl 178
Maxillæ 15
Maxillary palps 15
Mbori 236
Mechanical transmission 2
Mediterranean Fever 28
Megarhininæ 75
*Megarhinus* 15, 74
*Melanoconion* 110
Melaxeny 122
*Melophagus* 373, 374
  *ovinus* 244, 373
Metanotopsilæ 76
Metanototrichæ 76
Miasm theory 120
*Micraëdes* 111
*Microculex* 110
*Mimomyia* 110, 111
Mites 74
Modes of infection 11
*Molpemyia* 109
Mosquitoes See Culicidæ
*Mucidus* 109, 111
*Musca domestica* 355
Muscidæ 13, 30, **241**, 373
  (Blood-sucking) 241
  (Blood-sucking) Synopsis of families of 242
Mycetophilidæ 33
*Mycetophilus* 34
Mydaidæ 225
*Myiophthiria* 375
Myodaria 239
*Myxosquamus* 109
*Myzomyia* 76, 78, 79, 86, 90, 93, 95
  See *Anopheles*
*Myzorhynchella* 77, 79, 86, 93
  See *Anopheles*
  *nigra* 93
*Myzorhynchus* 76, 78, 79, 83, 84, 85
  See *Anopheles*

Nagana 236
  General account 328
  References to literature on 332

Nagana
  .See also *Trypanosoma brucei*
Nemestrinidæ 225
Neoanopheles 94
*Neocellia* 77, 78, 91, 95
  See *Anopheles*
*Neomelanoconion* 110
*Neomyzomyia* 77, 78, 79, 95
  See *Anopheles*
  *elegans* 77, 95
*Neopecomyia* 109
Nonimmune immigration 146
*Notonotricha* 86
  See *Anopheles*
  *intermedium* 86
*Nosema* 144
*Numomyia* 114
*Nuria danrica* 150
*Nyssorhynchus* 77, 78, 79, 90, 91, 95
  See *Anopheles*

*Ochlerotatus* 109, 114
*Oculeomyia* 110
Oesophageal diverticula 58
  Function of 67
Oestridæ 240
*Olfersia* 374, 375
  *maura* See *Lynchia maura*
*Ophiocephalus* 151
*Ornithodorus moubata* 6
*Ornithoëca* 374
*Ornithomyia* 374
*Ornithophila* 374
*Orphnephila* 34
Orphnephilidæ 33
Orthorrhapha 23
  Brachycera 23, 29, **224**
  Synopsis of Families of 225
Orthorrhapha Nematocera 23
  Classification 32
  Definition 32
  Synopsis of Families 33
*Oscillaria* See *Plasmodium*
*Oxypterum* 375

Paludism See Malaria
*Pangonia* 28, **231**, 234, 235
Pangoniinæ **231**
Pappataci Fever 26, **44**
  Causal agent 47
  Distribution 45
  History 44
  Mode of infection 46
  Prophylactic measures 47
  References 48
  Symptomatology 45
  Synonyms 44
Pappataci Flies See *Phlebotomus*
*Paraplasma flavigenum* 186
*Patagiamyia* 76, 77, 78, 79, 82
  See *Anopheles*

*Pecomyia* 109
*Pectinopalpus* 110
*Pheidole megacephala* 270
*Pelecorhynchus* 231
Pellagra 26
*Phagomyia* 109
*Philæmatomyia* 31, 242
*Phlebotomus* Breeding localities 41, 42
  Definition of genus 36
  Eggs 40
  General account 35
  Larva 40, 41
  Life-cycle of 39
  Pupa 41
  References 48
  Synopsis of species 42, 43, 44
  and disease 42
  and reptiles 39
Phlebotomus Fever   *See* Pappataci
  Fever
*Phlebotomus antennatus* 43
  *argentipes* 43
  *cruciatus* 44
  *duboscquii* 43
  *himalayensis* 43
  *intermedius* 44
  *longipalpis* 44
  *major* 43
  *malabaricus* 43
  *mascittii* 43
  *minutus* 43, 46
  *nigerrimus* 42
*Phlebotomus papatasii* 20, 26, 43
  Bionomics of 37
  Wing venation 36
  *perniciosus* 43, 46
  *perturbans* 44
  *rostrans* 44
  *squamipleuris* 43
  *squamiventris* 44
  *vexator* 44
Phoridæ 226
*Piroplasma* See *Babesia*
Piroplasmidæ 10
*Pityocera* 231
*Plasmodium* 10, 181, 196
*Plasmodium falciparum* 129, 130, 141, 143, 156, **160**
  Description of 160
  Synonyms of 160
*Plasmodium malariæ* 129, 141, 143, 156, **158**
  Description of 158
  Synonyms 158
  *præcox* 28, 176, **197**, 200
  Development in the mosquito 198
  *relicta* See *P. præcox*
*Plasmodium vivax* 129, 141, 143, **155**, 162, 197
  Description of 155

*Plasmodium vivax*
  Distribution 158
  Synonyms of 155
Poliomyelitis 31, **365**
  Causal agent 366
  Distribution 366
  History 365
  Method of infection 367
  References to Literature on 369
  Synonyms 365
*Polyleptiomyia* 109
*Polymitus* 133
Primary Fly centres 280
*Pristorhynchomyia* 242
*Pronopes* 232
*Proteosoma* 1, 122
  See *Plasmodium præcox*
Protoanopheles 78
*Protoculex* 109
*Protomacleaya* 109
*Protomelanoconion* 110
*Pseudoculex* 109
*Pseudoficalbia* 111
*Pseudograbhamia* 109
*Pseudohowardina* 109
*Pseudomyzomyia* 77, 79, 86, 90
  See *Anopheles*
  *rossii* 77, 86, 90
*Pseudoskusea* 109
*Pseudouranotænia* 111
Pseudovacuolæ 197
*Psorophora* 63, 66, 74, 109
Psychodidæ 26, **33**
  Definition 35
Ptilinum 13
*Pulex irritans* 223
  *serraticeps* 223
Pulvillus 15
Pupa 21
Pupipares 13, 20, 25
*Pyretophorus* 77, 78, 79, 88
  See *Anopheles*
  *costalis* 88

Quartan Fever See *Plasmodium malariæ*
  malaria 120
Quinine prophylaxis 153
Quinine treatment of the sick 153
Quotidian malaria See *Plasmodium falciparum*

*Radioculex* 110
Rainfall 144
*Reedomyia* 109
Relations between parasite and host 7
Reservoirs of infection 7
*Rhinomyza* 232
*Rhipicephalus siculus* 223
Rhyphidæ 33
*Ryphus* 34

Sabethinæ 76, 115
Salticus 74
Sand-Flies See Phlebotomus
Sarcophagidæ 241
Sayomyia 76
Scenopinidæ 226
Schiner's nomenclature 18
Schüffner's dots 155
Scione 231
Scutellum 15
Scutomyia 109, 114
  albolineata 29, 215
Segregation 154
Selasoma 230'
Sepsis 240
Seroot-Flies See Tabanidæ
Silvius 232
Simuliidæ 26, 33
Simulium 26, 74
Sleeping Sickness 300
  Definition 300
  Distribution 306
  History 300
  Prophylaxis 315
  References to literature on 321
  Synonyms 300
  See also Trypanosoma gam-
    biense and T. rhodesiense
Souma 236, 251
  General account 335
  References to literature on 339
  See also Trypanosoma cazalboui
Spiders 74
Spirochæta 200
  duttoni 6, 11
  recurrentis 11
Stable-fly See Stomoxys
Stegoconops 109
Stegomyia 2, 62, 71, 109, 111, 198
  216
  and dengue 196
  africana 113
  albocephala 113
  albolateralis 113
  albomarginata 114
  amesii 114
  annulirostris 112
  apicoargentia 113
  argenteomaculata 112
  argenteopunctata 114
  assamensis 113
  auriostriata 113
  crassipes 114
  desmotes 112
  dissimilis 113
  dubia 113
Stegomyia fasciata 8, 28, 67, 112,
  165, 166, 177, 181, 198, 214,
  215, 219, 222
  Description 166
  Egg 172

Stegomyia fasciata
  Feeding habits of 170
  Fertilization and egg-laying 171
  Habitat of 168
  Larva 174
  Length of life 171
  Life-cycle 172
  Pupa 176
  Synonyms 166
  and disease 176
  fusca 114
  gebeleinensis 112
  gracilis 29, 215
  grantii 113
  hatiensis 114
  imitator 113
  lilii 112
  mediopunctata 113
  minuta 114
  minutissima 113
  nigeria 112
  nigritia 113
  periskeleta 112
  perplexa 29, 215
  pollinctor 113
  poweri 113
  pseudonigeria 112
  pseudonivea 113
  pseudoscutellaris 29, 112, 175, 209,
    213, 214, 215, 216
  punctolateralis 114
  quasinigritia 113
  scutellaris 29, 112, 215
  simpsoni 112
  tasmaniensis 114
  terrens 113
  thomsoni 112
  tripunctata 114
  W-alba 112
  wellmanii 112
Stenopteryx 375
Stenoscutis 109
Stethomyia 76, 78, 79
  See Anopheles
  nimba 79
Stomoxys 233, 234, 236, 237, 242,
  243, 336, 348, 355, 365
  General description 355
  and disease 361
Stomoxys calcitrans 20, 31, 238, 244,
  356, 362, 363, 364, 365, 367,
  368, 369
  Distribution 357
  General description 356
  Habits 357
  Life-history 358
  Methods of destruction 360
  Pupa 22
  References to literature on 361
  and S. nigra 31
Stomoxys nigra 234, 362, 363

Stratiomyidæ 225
Streptococcus 218
Stridulating organ 55
Stygeromyia 31, 243
Surra 232, **236**, 237, 238

Tabanidæ 29, 224, 225, **226**
  Classification 230
  Description 226
  Habitat 227
  Life-cycle 228
  References to literature 239
  Synopsis of genera 230
    and disease 232
Tabaninæ **230**
Tabanus 231, ,235, 236, 237, 347,
    361, 363, 370, 372
  Wing venation of 17
  atratus 29, 238
  biguttatus 28, 229, 236
  ditæniatus 29
  fumifer 29, 236
  kingi 227, 228, 229
  minimus 29, 237
  nemoralis 29, 235
  par 228, 230
  partitus 29, 236
  secedens 29, 233, 347
  striatus 29, 232, 238
  tæniatus 236
  tomentosus 29, 235
  vagus 29, 236
Tachinidæ 241
Tæniorhynchus 109, 110, 115
  domesticus 29, 215
Tarsus 15
Tertian malaria 120, **155**
Thapsia 235
Theobaldia 109, 110, 115
  annulata 71
Therevidæ 225
Thermotropism in mosquitoes 67
Three-Day Fever 26
  See Pappataci Fever
Tick-Flies See Hippoboscidæ
Tipula 34
Tipulidæ 33
Transmission, General conditions
  affecting 6
Trichogaster fasciatus 152
Trichopronomyia 110
Trichoprosoponinæ 76
Trichorhynchus 110
Triple Quartan Fever 160
Trypanosomata 200
  Biological characters 296
  Classification 297
  Cross immunity reactions 297
  Diagnosis of genus 293
  General description 294
  Key to African pathogenic 298

Trypanosomata
  Mode of division 295
  References 299
  Sero-diagnostic methods 297
Trypanosoma americanum 384
  boylei 8
Trypanosoma brucei 1, 9, 29, 30, 31,
    235, 270, 273, 286, 287, 292,
    294, 298, 323, **328**, 344, 363
  Mode of Infection 330
  Morphology 330
  See also Nagana
Trypanosoma cazalboui 9, 29, 30,
    236, 250, 251, 252, 255, 270,
    275, 286, 294, 298, 330, **335**,
    340, 341, 343, 362, 363
  Mode of infection 336
  Morphology 336
  confusum See T. dimorphon
Trypanosoma congolense 286, 299,
    344, 345, 346, **351**
  General account 351
  Mode of infection 352
  Morphology 352
  References to literature on 353
Trypanosoma dimorphon 30, 31, 233,
    234, 250, 251, 255, 270, 273,
    275, 286, 287, 299, **342**, 346,
    351, 362, 371
  General account 342
  Mode of infection 344
  Morphology 344
  References to literature on 345
  Synonyms 342
Trypanosoma equiperdum 29, 298,
    363
  evansi 29, 31, 236, 238, 295, 298,
    361, 362, 363, 372
  var. mbori 29, 298
  franki 384
Trypanosoma gambiense 8, 9, 28, 30,
    176, 250, 251, 252, 255, 270,
    286, 292, 299, 300, 304, **306**,
    323, 350, 363
  Life-history in vertebrate host—
    Endogenous cycle 306
  Life-history within the inverte-
    brate host—Exogenous cycle
    310
Trypanosoma himalayanum 384
  ignotum See T. simiæ
  indicum 384
  lewisi 11, 12, 294, 296
  muktesari 384
Trypanosoma nanum 30, 270, 299,
    346, 347, **348**
  Development 350
  General account 348
  Mode of transmission 349
  Morphology 349
  References to literature on 350

*Trypanosoma pecaudi* 30, 31, 234, 235, 270, 275, 286, 299, **332**, 362
  Mode of infection 333
  Morphology 333
*Trypanosoma pecorum* 29, 30, 233, 270, 286, 299, **346**, 351
  Development within the invertebrate host 348
  General account 346
  Mode of infection 347
  Morphology 346
  References to literature on 348
*Trypanosoma rhodesiense* 30, 251, 285, 294, 299, **322**
  General account 322
  Mode of transmission 325
  Morphology of 324
  References to literature on 328
  *rutherfordi* 384
*Trypanosoma simiæ* 30, 286, 296, 299, **353**
  General account 353
  Morphology 353
  References to literature on 355
  Synonyms 353
  *soudanense* 29, 31, 233, 235, 298, 362, 363
*Trypanosoma theileri* 31, 374, 379, **384**
  General account 384
  Mode of transmission 385
  Morphology 384
  *togolense* 298
  *transvaaliense* See *T. theileri*
  *ugandense* 305
*Trypanosoma uniforme* 335, **341**
  Mode of infection 342
  Morphology 341
  References to literature on 342

*Trypanosoma vivax* 335, **340**
  References to literature on 34
*Trypanosoma vivax* Bruce See *T. cazalboui*
  *wrublewskii* 384
Trypanosomes **293**
Trypanosomiasis 361
Trypanosomiases, Conditions affecting transmission by tsetse-flies 250
Tsetse-Flies 243
Tsetse-Fly Disease See Nagana
Typhus icteroides See Yellow Fever

*Udenocera* 230
*Uranotænia* 109, 111
Uranotæninæ 76
*Utricularia* 72

Venation 15
Verruga Peruviana 26, **42**

*Wyeomyia smithii* 66

Yellow Fever 8, 28, 176, **177**
  Causal Agent of 186
  Development of virus within mosquito 187
  Distribution 179, **182**
  Endemic centres of 182
  General account and history 177
  Immune serum 189
  Mode of infection 184
  References to literature 189
  St Nazaire epidemic 183
  Synonyms 177
  Vaccination 188
  Virus of 10
Yellow Jack See Yellow Fever

9 780521 235648